ELEMENTS OF BIOMETRICAL GENETICS

About the Author

Arvind R. Dabholkar (*b.* 1937) obtained his Masters degree in Agricultural Botany from Vikram University, Ujjain in 1963. He was awarded gold medal for securing First position in 1963 examinations of Agriculture Faculty. He got his Ph.D. from University of Indore in 1979. He graduated in agricultural sciences from Agra University in 1956.

Since 1963 he is engaged actively in breeding of sorghum, in various capacities. Presently he is Associate Professor/Scientist in Jawaharlal Nehru Krishi Vishwa Vidyalaya, Campus Indore. He is officer-in-charge of Sorghum Project and also Head, Plant Breeding and Genetics Department, College of Agriculture, Indore. He has guided several students for their M.Sc. (Ag.) thesis work. He has taught Advanced Gentics and Biometrical Genetics for more than 20 years to the post graduate students.

He has more than 40 research papers at his credit in journals of repute.

ELEMENTS
OF
BIOMETRICAL GENETICS

(Revised and Enlarged Edition)

DR. A.R. DABHOLKAR
College of Agriculture,
Indore - 452001 (M.P.)

CONCEPT PUBLISHING COMPANY NEW DELHI - 110059

ISBN 81-7022-667–8 (H.B.)
ISBN 81-7022-668–6 (P.B.)

First Published 1992

Revised and Enlarged Edition 1999

Published and Printed by
Ashok Kumar Mittal
Concept Publishing Company
A/15-16, Commercial Block, Mohan Garden
New Delhi-110059 (India)

Phone : 5648039, 5649024
Fax : 091-(11)-5648053

PREFACE TO THE SECOND EDITION

I had made an humble attempt in the first edition of this book to present elementary topics of this subject in such a way that the beginner can easily comprehend. I am happy and also encouraged by the response extended to me for this work, not only by the post graduate students of several Agricultural Universities but also by a few senior members of Agriculture Faculty.

A few requests were communicated to incorporate some additional topics in the book. However, I wish to very honestly add that this work of mine was only an elementary introduction to a difficult but interesting and valuable subject of biometrical genetics. This was especially aimed just to help the beginner to understand the subject. Some new topics have, nevertheless, been added in the book.

Mr. R.C. Jain "Badnasib" did an excellent job in the preparation of typescript of the first edition of book as well as some additions to the second edition for which I am thankful.

I would utterly fail in my duties if I do not acknowledge the encouragement and inspiration offered to me by my wife, daughter and son during the preparation of manuscript and proof-reading. I acknowledge the help extended by Dr. (Mrs) Usha Sexena for the proof-reading.

Although I have taken all the care to bring the book to its perfection, I humbly admit that there is no reason why there could not be a few errors, deficiencies which have unknowingly crept into the text. I solely owe the responsibility of whatever errors, deficiencies and inferences that may not be widely acceptable. Kindly make the work even more better by suggesting such drawbacks.

Indore
30 July, 1998

A.R. DABHOLKAR

PREFACE TO THE FIRST EDITION

I have been teaching a course in biometrical genetics to the post–graduate students. Students felt need for a book on this aspect of genetics which could be understood with relative ease. Several authoritative works on the subject are available. However, a single book does not cover the entire course. Several experimental techniques developed to study the genetic properties of the population or specific genotypes, and being popularly empolyed, have not been presented in a single text-book. The English language of the foreign writers is relatively hard for an average Indian student of the Agricultural Universities. An humble endeavour was therefore made by me to present the subject-matter in a relatively simple language. Most of the widely used experimental designs and procedures have been explained through worked examples. Theoretical background has also been provided for these procedures in addition to the interpretation of information derived from various analyses. There may be some disagreement on the discussion and interpretations. Interpretations differ from person to person. Constructive criticism on various aspects described in this work is most welcome.

Chapters of this book have been sequenced in a logical fashion rather than chronological. Most of the discussion in various chapters centres around population in Hardy-Weinberg equilibrium. Symbols of Falconer (1960) have been adopted for such populations. On the other hand, while describing properties of the populations developed by selfing the successive generations derived from F_1, back-crossing or sib-mating, symbols proposed by Fisher *et al.* (1932) have been used.

There is no hesitation to confess that I have taken full liberty to lean on excellent expositions on the subject by Mather (1949), Kempthorne (1957), Falconer (1960), Mather and Jinks (1971, 1977 and 1982) and several others, to present the contents of the book before the students of biometrical genetics.

I accept all the responsibility of any omission, deficiency and lacunae that may have crept inspite of the best efforts and intentions.

Generous helping hand has been extended to me by a number of colleagues either directly or indirectly while bringing out this book. It may not be possible to name them all. I shall be failing in my duty if I do not thank Dr. L.S. Somani and S.B.S. Tikka who inspired me to write this book. Dr. V.N. Shroff, Dean, College of Agriculture, Indore, also encouraged me in this effort. Help accorded by Mr. S.W. Telang and Rajesh Julka has also to be acknowledged. My wife and children provided me moral support without which I would not have succeeded to complete this work.

A.R. DABHOLKAR

CONTENTS

LIST OF TABLES

LIST OF FIGURES

1

INTRODUCTION

1.1 Multiple Factor Hypothesis

Mendel was the first to offer a simple and reasonable explanation for the process of heredity. His success was due in part to his use of sweet pea varieties that differed in clear-cut visible traits, categories of which did not overlap. The flower colour, for example, in his pea varieties was either red or white.This permitted Mendel to make accurate counts of individuals showing one or the other of the alternative traits. Mendel's successors continued to deal in main with such clear-cut qualitative differences and they succeeded in unravelling many complex cases of gene interaction.

If we observe segregation in F_2 generation of hybrid between tall and short strains of sweet pea,–one of the trait differences investigated by Mendel,–we would be struck by two aspects of variation in height among the plants. Firstly, there is such a gap between the tall and short segregates that the difference could be regarded as qualitative one. Hence, accurate classification into tall and short categories could be made by quick visual estimation of plant stature. The analysis can proceed along familiar genetic lines and difference is found to be governed by a single gene pair with tall being dominant to short. The second and perhaps less obvious aspect of variability is the variation within the short and tall groups. Examination of a number of short individuals would reveal that there exist all intermediate degrees between shortest "shorts" and tallest "shorts", middle expression being most common with frequency falling off towards either extreme. A similar graduated series for tallness is observed among the tall individuals.

In fact most of the quantitative characters follow a 'normal' distribution curve ranging from low to high values without sharp separation in values between the many classes within this range.

Many characters of economic importance with which plant breeders must work vary in such a way that they show continuous variation of phenotypes and easily distinguishable alternatives do not exist. For example, if a large collection of varieties of wheat is observed with respect to agronomic characters such as kernel yield, plant height, days required for 50 percent flowering, all degrees of intermediacy between one extreme and the other will be observed. The plants in F_2 generation between two diverse parents, will show continuous distribution. Variation of this sort without natural discontinuity is called continuous variation. The characters which exhibit it are called "quantitative characters" or "metrical characters" because these characters can be specified accurately only in terms of metrics such as length, time, weight etc.

Mendel himself and the rediscoverers of Mendelism, deliberately avoided the study of continuous variation in their material because they recognised that it would only confuse their analyses. Francis Galton, a cousin of Charles Darwin was, however, interested in the variation of this kind. In respect of physical and mental characteristics of human beings Galton observed that such measurable or "metrical" characters were at least partly inherited. The taller individuals, for example, produced taller children on the average. To measure the degree to which such characters were inherited, new biometrical techniques such as correlation and regression were developed by Galton and his students. Thus, although segregation and assortment of individual hereditary factors could not be determined, the "biometricians" were able to demonstrate statistically that there was resemblance between relatives with respect to numerous quantitative attributes. They concluded that individuals were mixtures of parental characteristics, who were in turn a mixture derived from their grand parents etc. In the absence of detailed knowledge about genes, it appeared to them that many of these quantitative attributes were determined by mixing or "blending" process.

After the discovery of Mendel's work (independently by De Vries in Holland, Correns in Germany and Tschermak in Austria) the different views formed the basis for the two main groups among geneticists, namely "Mendelians" who proposed that all the evolutionarily important heritable characters were qualitative and discontinuous in distribution and "Biometricians" who believed that the heritable variation was basically quantitative and continuous in distribution. The latter group denied that genes existed as separate units. It seemed very much difficult to reconcile these views at first because there was no evidence that genes which are presumably particulate and discontinuous in nature could account for the inheritance of phenotypes that are continuous in distribution.

One clue to resolve the conflict between "Mendelians" and "Biometricians" was provided by the detailed breeding analyses of a quantitative character in beans by Johannsen. Johannsen (1903), a Danish geneticist, showed that heritable and non-heritable agencies were jointly responsible for variation in seed weight of beans and that their effects were of the same order of magnitude. Johannsen measured weight of Princess bean (*Phaseolus vulgaris*) in a commercial seed lot and observed variation in size ranging from "light" (15 centigrammes) to "heavy" (90 centigrammes). Johannsen established 19 pure lines derived from 19 seeds of original seed lot by self-fertilising successive generations of plants that were derived initially from single seeds. As regards seed weight, these lines revealed two main features. Firstly, it was observed that each seed lot had a characteristic mean seed weight. For example, line 1 was heaviest with an average seed weight of 64 centigrammes and line 19 was lightest (mean seed weight 35 centigrammes). All intergrades were observed between 64 and 35 centigrammes. Secondly, it was noticed that within each line seeds of various sizes occurred. However, variability within each progeny was much less than that observed in original seed lot. Johannsen provided evidence to show that this variability was not genetic in origin but was due to slight differences in various environmental factors which affected individual plants to different degrees.

Johannsen's experiment thus helped to explain that continuous variation observed for quantitative characters resulted from joint action of genotype and environmental agencies. Although basically genetic in origin, distinction between Johannsen's pure lines could not be ascribed to particular genes because none could be genetically isolated. The genetic basis of quantitative variation thus remained disputed and unresolved.

In 1906 Yule proposed that continuous quantitative variation could result from a large number of genes, each having a small effect on the character measured. Nilsson-Ehle, a Swedish plant breeder, provided a naturally occurring model for the type of inheritance suggested by Yule. He found that in wheat and oats there were hereditary factors whose action was very similar, if not exactly alike. There were three individual gene pairs involved in the determination of kernel colour of wheat, i.e. *Aa, Bb* and *Cc*, with genes for red kernel colour (*ABC*) being dominant over genes for white (*abc*). Each of these gene pairs segregated in a Mendelian fashion such that selfing the heterozygote *Aa* produced offspring in a ratio 3 red (*A*-): 1 white (*aa*). When two gene pair differences were involved in simultaneous segregation, i.e., *AaBb* × *AaBb*, the result followed Mendelian principles, giving a ratio 15 red (*A-B-, A-bb, aaB-*) :1 white (*aabb*). Likewise a cross between heterozygotes for three gene pairs produced a close fit to a predicted ratio 63 red:1 white. It made little difference which of the red genes was segregating, *A, B* or *C*, because all three appeared to act similarly. Thus a variety of red genotypes occurred, some red phenotypes containing more genes for red kernel colour and others less. The action of each gene was to add a degree of redness to the kernel. Hence the phenotypic distribution of this attribute tended to approximate the normal distribution expected for quantitative characters. The reason for this "normalcy" arises from the random fashion in which genes segregate and assort.

The factors studied by Nilsson-Ehle had effects sufficiently large which made Mendelian analysis possible. It was realised by Nilsson-Ehle and also by East, that factors similar to those for kernel colour of wheat could account for the inheritance of quantitative characters, provided a large number of genes influencing same character were involved in action. Each factor would be inherited in Mendelian fashion and its change would be discontinuous or qualitative. With large number of genes with similar and additive action, many different dosages could be possible of which intermediate phenotypes would be most frequent. With phenotypic expression proportional to the factor dosage, phenotypic variation would be continuous and follow Galton's frequency curve. Continuity would be completed by the blurring effect of non-heritable agencies, which would of course make phenotypic ranges of various genotypes overlap. Because there are usually many genes of this type for any one quantitative character, they were appropriately named "multiple factors". During the next 10 years this multiple factor hypothesis, as it was called, was applied to data from a variety of organisms, notably by East and his collaborators and by Fisher. East showed that the inheritance of a number of quantitative characters in tcbacco and maize could be fully explained by the multiple factor hypothesis. Fisher carried out the integration of biometry and genetics still further.

Since the effects of many multiple factors are usually too small to be traced they cannot be individually isolated. Thus distinction between genes concerned with qualitative characters and those governing quantitative characters lies in the magnitude of their effects relative to other sources of variation. A gene with effect large enough to cause a recognisable discontinuity even in the presence of segregation at other loci and non-genetic variation can be studied by Mendelian methods, whereas a gene whose effect is not large enough to cause a discontinuity cannot be studied individually. This distinction is reflected in terms of "Major gene" and "minor gene". There are, however, all intermediate grades, genes that cannot be properly classed as major or minor. The quantitative effects observed for a given metric character could also arise as "side effects" of genes that are concerned with other processes. Because of these limitations, it is generally agreed that many of the genes are not identifiable as factors in the original sense in which the term was used. "Multiple factor" has therefore been replaced by "polygene" (proposed by Mather) in recent years. Polygenes are genes with small effect on a particular character which supplement each other's effects to produce observable quantitative changes. These quantitative effects are in some cases additive.

1.2 Evidence in Support of Multiple Factor Hypothesis

Conclusive evidence for the hypothesis that several genes with small, similar and additive effects govern the inheritance of quantitative characters was provided by E.M. East in 1916.

Flower size in tobacco is a favourable character for studies of quantitative inheritance because the size is relatively constant under a wide range of environmental conditions. East began his studies with two true breeding varieties of *Nicotiana longiflora* that differed in respect of flower length. Each variety was long inbred and therefore was homozygous at the start of experiment. East crossed these varieties and observed that the corolla length of flowers borne by the F_1 plants was intermediate to both parents. Variability observed for corolla length in F_1 generation was similar to that for both the parents. When East raised

F_2 generation, entirely different results were obtained. The F_2 generation had a wider distribution of phenotypes than either the F_1 or the parents. Although the F_2 generation cannot be expected to be immune to environmental effects it cannot be expected to be drastically sensitive to it as compared with other generations. Excess variability observed for F_2 generation could not be accounted for environmental effects alone. In this generation segregation and recombination of Mendelian genes is expected. East postulated that excess of variability in this generation originated from both these causes.

Results observed for F_1 and F_2 generations therefore conform to the Mendelian expectations. On the basis of Mendelian theory, East predicted that individuals from various parts of the phenotypic distribution of F_2 generation should produce F_3 progeny differing markedly in the mean measurements of corolla length and also the variability. In almost every case East observed that the mean value of each F_3 progeny was characteristic of its F_2 parent.

The next question was regarding the number of genes responsible for corolla length. According to Mendelian theory one individual out of four, on average, will be like either parent in genotype when one gene pair governs the inheritance. When two gene pairs are involved in inheritance, one out of 16 individuals will be like either parent in its genetic constitution. As the number of gene pairs influencing the inheritance of a character increase the probability of finding a plant in F_2 generation homozygous for all the genes decreases. In general, when n gene pairs are responsible for a trait, one individual out of 4^n will be homozygous for all the n genes. East raised 444 F_2 plants but was unable to recover parental type individuals, hence it can be concluded that more than four gene pairs governed the inheritance of corolla length.

1.3 Nuclear Basis of Inheritance

The evidence provided by East suggests that a large number of genes with small, similar and cumulative effects could explain the genetic basis of quantitative characters. Since the effect of each polygene is small and readily mimicked by non-heritable agencies it is difficult to detect the effect of individual gene. Hence, Mendelian way of analysis would not be possible to follow these genes. How then can we be sure that these genes are in truth borne of chromosomes ?

Galton showed that both the parents equally transmit hereditary factors for quantitative characters to their progeny. This equal transmission of hereditary factors by both the parents has been confirmed in several experiments involving reciprocal crosses. Reciprocal crosses do not exhibit differences, except in cases where expected, for most of the quantitative characters.

Genes located on chromosomes have two properties, viz. segregation and linkage. Although it may not be possible to show linkage between two polygenic systems governing different quantitative characters, evidence for linkage of polygenes with a major gene could be provided.

Evidence for segregation of genes governing the inheritance of metrical traits comes from relative variabilities of various generations. In case of qualitative character such as red and white flower colour of sweet peas, one expects on the basis of Mendelian laws that about 75 percent population of plants will be red and 25 percent white flowered in F_2. As compared to the parental generation and F_1, the F_2 is more variable. For quantitative characters also relatively more variability is exhibited by the F_2 generation. This variability is mainly due to segregation of genes.

Sax (1923) provided evidence in support of the linkage of genes for seed weight and seed coat colour in *Phaseolus vulgaris*. In *Drosophila melanogaster,* Mather and Harrison (1949) were able to show linkage between groups of genes governing inheritance of two quantitative characters.

1.4 Quantitative Genetics

Quantitative genetics is concerned with those differences between individuals that are of degree rather than kind, quantitative rather than qualitative. Since the inheritance of quantitative traits depends upon gene differences at many loci, the effects of which are not individually distinguishable, Mendelian ratios cannot be observed and hence Mendelian way of analysis is not appropriate. However, the genes concerned with metrical characters do follow the same laws of transmission from parents to offspring as do the genes governing the inheritance of qualitative traits. Quantitative genetics is therefore an extension of Mendelian genetics.

The nature of quantitative differences requires the measurements and not just the classification of individuals. The extension of the concepts of Mendelian genetics to understand inheritance of measurements is known as "Biometrical Genetics" or "Quantitative Genetics".

The basic theme of biometrical genetics was developed chiefly by Fisher, Haldane and Wright. Based upon their elucidations, theories and procedures were developed to understand the inheritance of quantitative attributes by several scientists. Among the prominent scientists who developed useful genetic procedures to measure various genetic parameters are Mather, Hazel, Smith, Comstock, Robinson, Hayman, Jinks, Cockerham, Kempthrone, Li, Griffing, Gamble, Eberhart, Russell. However, this list is not complete.

2

BACKGROUND

2.1 The Mendelian Population

The early geneticists rediscovered and estabilished the Mendelian principles of inheritance while attempting to understand the mechanism of heredity. They investigated the pattern of transmission of herediatry factors at family level. The criterion adopted was the similarity or dissimilarity of phenotypes between the progeny and their parents. However, geneticists are keen to learn about the behaviour of genes in the population because it is in the population of individuals that the future of many genes is decided. For example, reproductive ability of individuals carrying a given gene may depend upon fitness of this gene, frequency of this gene in the population, size of the population, genotypes of other individuals in the population and many other factors. Thus, although the genes exist within the individuals, the fate of individuals and consequently the fate of genes contained in them is strongly tied to the factors influencing the population as a whole. We therefore need to know what is population in genetic sense. What are their basic attributes? Let us see. Population, in genetic sense is not only a group of individuals but a group of sexual and cross-fertilising organisms which share a common gene pool. Genes follow the Mendelian laws of inheritance in such populations. Hence such populations have been termed by Sewall Wright as "Mendelian populations". Dobzhansky (1951) defined Mendelian population as "a reproductive community of sexual and cross-fertilising organisms which share in a common gene pool". What then is a gene pool? What is meant by sharing a common gene pool? Imagine a large random mating population and assume that all the individuals in this population produce gametes and contribute to the pool of gametes. Samples of gametes are drawn randomly from this pool and zygotes of next generation are formed. Sum total of genes contained in the reproductive gametes of a population is called the gene pool. The concept described above is sharing of a common gene pool. The genetic relationship between an entire generation and the subsequent generation is very similar to the genetic relationship between a parent and an offspring. We have used a term random mating. Natural populations are assumed to be random mating. Strictly speaking the term random mating should be applied only to those breeding systems which meet following two requirements:

(i) each member of a population has an equal chance to produce offspring, and
(ii) that any female gamete be equally likely to be fertilised by any male gamete.

2.2 Gene Frequency and Genotype Frequency

Let us assume that there are only two alleles at a locus *viz.*, A_1 and A_2. Unless stated otherwise, we shall be dealing exclusively with autosomal inheritance of diploid individuals of a large random mating population. With respect to this locus, there will be 3 genotypes in the population, namely, A_1A_1, A_1A_2 and A_2A_2. We assume here that the phenotypes of these three genotypes are easily recognisable. In order to specify the genetic constitution of such a population, we count the number of individuals belonging to each genotype. Proportion or frequency of the individuals that belong to a particular genotype is its genotype frequency. Genotype frequencies may be expressed either as proportions or percentages and hence the sum of genotype frequencies in the entire population is unity or 100. Suppose, there are 100 individuals in the population, comprising of three genotypes *viz.*, A_1A_1, A_1A_2 and, A_2A_2. If the number of individuals belonging to each of these genotypes is 25, 10 and 65 respectively, the genotype frequency may be obtained as proportion or percentage of these genotypes in this population. Thus, genotype frequencies of the three genotypes are $\frac{25}{100}$, $\frac{10}{100}$ and $\frac{65}{100}$ or 0.25, 0.10 and 0.65, respectively.

Genetic constitution of a population can also be described in terms of array of gene frequency. The latter refers to the specification of genes present at every locus and number or proportion of different alleles at each locus. Gene frequency is defined as the proportion of a given allele in the population. Since the gene frequencies are expressed in terms of proportions or percentages in a population, sum of the gene frequencies at a locus is either unity or 100. What are the frequencies of genes A_1 and A_2 in the population described in preceding paragraph? Let us find out.

We have considered a population of diploid individuals and hence each individual will bear two genes at a locus. Thus, 100 individuals contain 200 genes at A_1, A_2 locus being considered. Individuals of the genotype A_1A_1 carry two A_1 genes. The heterozygotes possess one A_1 and one A_2 gene. Hence the proportion of A_1 genes in this population is:

$$\frac{50+10}{200} \text{ or } \frac{25+5}{100} = 0.30$$

Each individual with the genotype A_2 A_2 bears two A_2 genes. Therefore, the frequency of A_2 gene in this population is:

$$\frac{130+10}{200} \text{ or } \frac{65+5}{100} = 0.70$$

Let us generalise the procedure to estimate the gene frequencies. Let the frequencies of three genotypes A_1A_1, A_1A_2 and A_2A_2 be *D*, *H* and *R* respectively, such that $D + H + R = N$. The estimate of frequency of gene $A_1\,(\hat{p})$ is then obtained as:

$$\hat{p} = \frac{2D+H}{2N} \text{ or } \frac{D+\frac{1}{2}H}{N},$$

and the estimate of frequency of gene $A_2(\hat{q})$ as:

$$\hat{q} = \frac{2R+H}{2N} \text{ or } \frac{R+\frac{1}{2}H}{N}$$

Usually, the frequencies of genotypes are given in proportions instead of actual numbers. This is particularly true when the population is large. Then $D + H + R$ will be equal to unity. The estimates of p and q are then obtained as:

$$\hat{p} = D + \frac{1}{2}H \text{ and } \hat{q} = R + \frac{1}{2}H.$$

Since the sum of gene frequencies is unity (i.e., $p + q = 1$) following relationships may be useful for estimating p and q:

$$p + q = 1$$

$$\therefore p = (1 - q)$$

and $q = (1-p)$. And by same reasoning $-p = (q - 1)$ and $-q = (p-1)$

2.3 Hardy Weinberg Law

A British mathematician, G.H. Hardy and a German physician, Dr. W. Weinberg simultaneously presented independent papers in 1908 relating to the gene frequencies in a random mating population. According to Hardy and Weinberg, a large random mating population, in the absence of migration, mutation and selection is stable with respect to both gene and genotype frequencies. There is no inherent tendency for its genetic properties to change from one generation to the next. When the gene and genotype frequencies do not change from one generation to the next, the population is said to be in "Hardy-Weinberg equilibrium". This phenomenon of genotypic equilibrium, based on stable gene frequencies, exhibited by random mating population is known as "Hardy-Weinberg Law", named after the independent discoveries of Hardy in England and Weinberg in Germany. This law is of fundamental importance in Population Genetics.

The population described in preceding paragraph will produce two kinds of gametes, namely A_1 and A_2. It can be verified that the frequency of gametes A_1 will be:

$$A_1 = \frac{2D + H}{2N} \text{ or } \frac{D + \frac{1}{2}H}{N} \text{ or } p,$$

and the frequency of gametes A_2 will be

$$A_2 = \frac{2R+H}{2N} \text{ or } \frac{R+\frac{1}{2}H}{N} \text{ or } q.$$

This relationship shows that the frequency of gamete A_1 is equal to its gene frequency.Similarly, the frequency of gamete A_2 is equal to its gene frequency.

In Mendelian population, all the individuals contribute gametes to the pool from which pairs of gametes are drawn randomly to form the zygotes of next generation (section 2.1). Random mating of the individuals is therefore equivalent to random union among their gametes. The genotype frequencies in the progeny generation are obtained as product of frequencies of uniting gametes as shown below:

		Male gametes		
		A_1	A_2	
		p	q	—Frequency
Female gametes	A_1	A_1A_1	A_1A_2	—genotype of zygote
	p	p^2	pq	
	A_2	A_1A_2	A_2A_2	
	q	pq	q^2	— frequency of zygote.

Random union of gametes results in three kinds of progeny *viz.*, A_1A_1, A_1A_2 and A_2A_2, the frequencies of these genotypes being p^2, $2pq$ and q^2, respectively. Frequency of gene A_1 in the progeny generation is given by:

$$\begin{aligned} p &= p^2 + pq \\ &= p\,(p+q), \text{ since } (p+q) = 1 \\ &= p. \end{aligned}$$

This frequency is similar to the frequency of gene A_1 in the initial parental population. The frequency of gene A_2 could be similarly derived. It is not surprising to find that the frequency of gene A_2 in the offspring generation is q.

The genotype and the gene frequencies in the offspring generation could be derived by a longer method in terms of random mating of individuals in the parental population. Let us consider a population comprising of three genotypes (A_1A_1, A_1A_2, A_2A_2) in proportions D, H and R, respectively, where $D + H + R = 1$. Random mating among the individuals in this population will reduce to six types, as shown in Table 2.1. As a matter of fact there are nine possible types of matings. However, if we combine the reciprocals, the nine mating types could be collected into six. The frequencies of the reciprocal matings are also added. Thus, the frequency of mating $A_1A_1 \times A_1A_2$ is DH. Similarly the frequency of mating $A_1A_2 \times A_1A_1$ is DH. Hence the frequency of mating type $A_1A_1 \times A_1A_2$ is 2 DH. From the knowledge of classical genetics we expect that half of the progeny from this type of mating would be A_1A_1 in genetic constitution and rest A_1A_2. Sum of the frequencies of six mating types is unity. The frequency of A_1A_1 progeny resulting from these matings is obtained by adding the frequencies of A_1A_1 progeny from different types of matings. Frequency of A_1A_1 progeny is thus $D^2 + DH + \frac{1}{4} H^2$.

TABLE 2.1: Random mating in population

Mating type	Frequency of Mating	Genotypes of the offspring and their frequency		
		A_1A_1	A_1A_2	A_2A_2
$A_1A_1 \times A_1A_1$	D^2	D^2	–	–
$A_1A_1 \times A_1A_2$	2DH	DH	DH	–
$A_1A_1 \times A_2A_2$	2DR	–	$2DR$	–
$A_1A_2 \times A_1A_2$	H^2	$\frac{1}{4} H^2$	$\frac{1}{2} H^2$	$\frac{1}{4}H^2$
$A_1A_2 \times A_2A_2$	2HR	–	HR	HR
$A_2A_2 \times A_2A_2$	R^2	–	–	R^2
Total	$(D + H + R)^2 = 1$	$(D + \frac{1}{2} H)^2$	$2 (D + \frac{1}{2}H)(R + \frac{1}{2}H)$	$(R + \frac{1}{2}H)^2$

It can be verified that it is an expansion of the term $\left(D+\frac{1}{2}H\right)^2$. It was shown that $D + \frac{1}{2}H$ is equal to p (the gene frequency of A_1), hence $\left(D+\frac{1}{2}H\right)^2$ could be expressed as p^2.

This derivation therefore suggests that:

(i) the frequency of a gene in a given generation depends upon the frequency of that gene in previous generation, if mating is random and population is large (we assume absence of migration, mutation and selection).

(ii) the genotype frequencies of a particular generation, produced by random mating among the parents, depend upon the gene frequencies in the previous generation and not upon the genotype frequencies.

If the gene and genotype frequencies of a generation, produced by random mating among the individuals in previous generation, are identical to the gene and genotype frequencies observed in previous generation which produced it, we have a reason to believe that the parental generation was in Hardy–Weinberg equilibrium. A population which is not initially in equilibrium attains equilibrium after one generation of random mating.

Let us imagine an arbitrary population in which the frequencies of genotypes A_1A_1, A_1A_2, A_2A_2 are 0.10, 0.20, 0.70, respectively. The gametic frequencies in this population (and the frequencies of genes A_1 and A_2) are:

$$A_1 = 0.1 + \frac{0.2}{2}$$
$$= 0.2$$

and
$$A_2 = 0.7 + \frac{0.2}{2}$$
$$= 0.8$$

Random union of the gametes produce three genotypes A_1A_1, A_1A_2 and A_2A_2 with frequencies 0.04, 0.32 and 0.64, respectively. Since these do not agree with parental generation, the parental generation was not in Hardy-Weinberg equilibrium. Let us call the newly produced generation as offspring generation-1. Random mating in this generation may be described in terms of random union of gametes. This generation is expected to produce two kinds of gametes. *viz.* A_1 and A_2 with frequencies 0.04 + 0.16 = 0.2 and 0.64 + 0.16 = 0.8, respectively. Random union of these gametes will produce offspring generation-2, comprising of three genotypes A_1A_1, A_1A_2, and A_2A_2 with frequencies 0.04, 0.32, 0.64, respectively. This shows that offspring generation-1 was in Hardy-Weinberg equilibrium. It can be verified that all the populations with same gene frequencies, although differing initially in their genotype frequencies, attain same genotype frequencies at equilibrium as a result of random mating. Thus, following populations will attain same genotype frequencies at equilibrium:

	Genotypes and their frequencies		
	A_1A_1	A_1A_2	A_2A_2
Population 1	0.18	0.04	0.78
Population 2	0.20	0.00	0.80
Population 3	0.01	0.38	0.61

The discussion on Hardy-Weinberg law could be summarised as:

1. In a large random mating population both the gene and genotype frequencies do not change from one generation to the next in the absence of migration, mutation and selection.
2. Genotype frequencies of the offspring generation produced by random mating among the parents are determined entirely by gene frequencies of the parental generation and not by the genotype frequencies.
3. Hardy-Weinberg equilibrium frequencies of the genotypes are attained by one generation of random mating, irrespective of initial genotype frequencies. This Hardy-Weinberg law holds true only if a few assumptions listed below are satisfied:

    (i) Population is infinitely large and mating among the individuals is random (that is, it is a panmictic population).

    (ii) There is no selection at any stage. This implies that all the genotypes contribute equally to the pool of gametes (no differential fertility) and all the zygotes resulting from random union of these gametes are equally viable (no differential viability).

(iii) There is neither immigration of individuals from other population, nor emigration from the population being considered to other population. In other words, the population is closed.

(iv) There is no differential mutation. Here it is assumed that A_1 mutates to A_2 at the same rate as A_2 mutates to A_1.

(v) Meiosis is normal.

2.3.1 Multiple Alleles

We have assumed in the preceding sections that there are only two alleles at a locus. Presence of more than two alleles at a locus is not very uncommon. Three alleles are known for coat colour of rabbits. For blood group of humans also multiple alleles are known. It would be of interest therefore to know how the gene and genotype frequencies attain Hardy-Weinberg equilibrium when multiple allelism is involved.

Direct extension of Hardy-Weinberg law to the case of multiple alleles was made by Weinberg (1909). Before we deal with this aspect, it will be better to understand the concept of gametic array and the genotypic array in a random mating population. If the offspring generation is produced by random mating in the parental generation, such that all the parents contribute equally to the pool of gametes, genotypic array of the offspring generation is given by the square of gametic array of the parental generation. For example, if p and q are the frequencies of the gametes A_1 and A_2, produced by the parental generation comprising of A_1A_1, A_1A_2, and A_2A_2 genotypes, the gametic array would be:

$$(pA_1 + qA_2)$$

The genotypic array of next generation is the square of this gametic array. Thus, the genotypic array for a single locus with two alleles would be:

$$(pA_1 + qA_2)^2$$
$$= p^2A_1A_1 + 2pq\,A_1A_2 + q^2A_2A_2$$

There are three alternative approaches to know the frequency of a genotype when multiple allelism is involved. We can adopt any one for the purpose depending upon the situations. These are:

(i) If we are interested in the genotype frequencies determined by only one of the alleles, e.g., A_1, we can consider the frequency of A_1 as p and lump the frequencies of all other alleles at that locus (e.g., $A_2, A_3, \ldots A_n$) into a single gene frequency q. The gametic array of this population would be:

$$[pA_1 + q(A_2 + A_3)].$$

It was shown in the preceding section that in random mating population the gene frequency and the gametic frequency is same. Hence the expression given above is gametic array. The genotype frequencies at equilibrium with respect to this locus (provided there is no migration, mutation and selection) would be given by the square of this gametic array. Thus,

$$[pA_1 + q(A_2 + A_3)]^2$$
$$= p^2 A_1A_1 + 2pq(A_1A_2 + A_1A_3) + q^2(A_2A_2 + A_2A_3 + A_3A_3).$$

Since the sum of p and q is unity, sum of the genotype frequencies is also unity.

(ii) Among several alleles at a locus one could be interested in two alleles, e.g. A_1 and A_2 only. It is easier to find the frequencies of genotypes involving these genes at equilibrium, by expanding the binomial expression for gametic array. Thus,

$$(q_1A_1 + q_2A_2)^2$$
$$= q_1^2 A_1A_1 + 2q_1q_2A_1A_2 + q_2^2A_2A_2,$$

where q_1 and q_2 are the frequencies of gametes (and also the genes) bearing A_1 and A_2. The sum of q_1 and q_2 is not unity because other genes at this locus are not being considered. Hence, sum of the frequencies of A_1A_1, A_1A_2, A_2A_2 genotypes will not be unity.

(iii) If our interest is in three or more alleles at a locus, the genotype frequencies at equilibrium are given by square of the gametic array, which is a multinomial expression. Thus with three genes (A_1, A_2 and A_3) whose frequencies are say p, q, r at a locus, the equilibrium frequencies, after one generation of random mating are obtained as:

$$(pA_1 + qA_2 + rA_3)^2$$
$$= p^2A_1A_1 + 2pqA_1A_2 + q^2A_2A_2 + 2prA_1A_3 + 2qrA_2A_3 + r^2A_3A_3.$$

2.3.2 Two or More Pairs of Genes

It was shown earlier that with respect to a single locus with two alleles a large random mating population attains equilibrium after one generation of random mating provided migration, mutation and selection were not operating. However, what happens when two gene pairs are involved? Does this population attain equilibrium? How many rounds of random mating would be required for this population to reach Hardy-Weinberg equilibrium? What would be the genotype frequencies at equilibrium? The attainment of equilibrium genotype frequencies in this case depends among other things upon gametic frequencies and linkage.

Let us assume that there are two alleles at each of the loci, *e.g.* A_1, A_2 and B_1 B_2. With respect to these loci, there will be $3^2 = 9$ genotypes in the population. If we assume the frequencies of genes A_1, A_2, B_1, and B_2 to be p, q, r and s respectively, the gametic array of the initial population could be expressed as:

$$(prA_1B_1 + psA_1B_2 + qrA_2B_1 + qsA_2B_2).$$

At equilibrium, the frequencies of nine genotypes would be as shown below:

		Genes at first locus			
		A_1A_1	A_1A_2	A_2A_2	
Genes	B_1B_1	p^2r^2	$2pqr^2$	q^2r^2	–frequency
at 2nd	B_1B_2	$2p^2rs$	$4pqrs$	$2q^2rs$	of genotypes
locus	B_2B_2	p^2s^2	$2pqs^2$	q^2s^2	

Population which is in equilibrium for two gene pairs considered simultaneously, will also be in equilibrium for each locus separately. From the table given above it will be seen that the sum of frequencies of 3 genotypes in 3 rows is r^2, $2rs$ and s^2. Likewise sum of the 3 genotype frequencies in the columns is p^2, $2pq$ and q^2. These are the equilibrium frequencies of genotypes B_1B_1 , B_1B_2, B_2B_2 and A_1A_1, A_1A_2, A_2A_2 respectively. In this table frequencies of nine genotypes are given which sum to unity.

Attainment of the equilibrium depends upon the equilibrium frequencies of gametes. Once the gametic frequencies attain equilibrium, genotypic frequencies also attain equilibrium values. Suppose, a population initially comprises of individuals of only two genotypes *e.g.*, $A_1A_1B_1B_1$ and $A_2A_2B_2B_2$. Individuals of the genotype $A_1A_1B_1B_1$ will produce only one kind of gametes, *viz.* A_1B_1. Similarly individuals $A_2A_2B_2B_2$ will produce gametes A_2B_2. Random mating in this population will produce three kinds of genotypes in the offspring generation. *viz.*, $A_1A_1B_1B_1$, $A_1A_2B_1B_2$ and $A_2A_2B_2B_2$. Several other genotypes will be missing. However, all the genotypes will be subsequently produced and equilibrium reached. On the other hand, if population is made up of only $A_1A_2B_1B_2$ genotype, Hardy-Weinberg equilibrium genotype frequencies will be reached after one generation of random mating, because this population produces four kinds of gametes, A_1B_1, A_2B_1, A_1B_2 and A_2B_2 in equal proportions, provided there is no linkage and there is no differential fertility. The frequencies of all the genes are equal (*i.e.*, $p = q = r = s = 0.5$) and hence produce all gametes with equal frequencies. Approach to equilibrium, considering two pairs of genes, has been described by Li (1955). Let us see how.

Let us call the gametes with the constitution A_1B_1 and A_2B_2 as in coupling and A_1B_2 and A_2B_1 in repulsion. As shown by *Li* (1955), the product of frequencies of two kinds of gametes in repulsion will be equal to the product of frequencies of gametes in coupling at equilibrium because the frequencies of genes in gametes in replusion are equal to the frequencies of genes in coupling. Thus,

$$(ps)\,(qr) = (pr)\,(qs).$$

Departure from this relationship implies that the population is not in equilibrium. For example, if the frequencies of genes A_1, A_2, B_1 and B_2 are 0.80, 0.20, 0.80, and 0.20 respectively, the frequencies of gametes A_1B_1, A_1B_2, A_2B_1 and A_2B_2 will be 0.64, 0.16, 0.16 and 0.04 respectively.

Thus,

$$A_1B_2 \times A_2B_1 = A_1B_1 \times A_2B_2$$
$$(0.16) \times (0.16) = (0.64) \times (0.04)$$
$$0.0256 = 0.0256$$

This shows that the population is in equilibrium. However, if the population is not in Hardy-Weinberg equilibrium the product (*ps*) (*qr*) will not be equal to the product (*pr*) (*qs*). The deviation (*d*) from equilibrium is therefore measured as:

$$d = (ps)\,(qr) - (pr)\,(qs).$$

If the gametes in repulsion are more frequent, the sign of *d* (for disequilibrium) will be positive. However, if the gametes in coupling are more frequent the sign of *d* will be negative. This difference between the product of frequencies of repulsion and coupling gametes will be reduced by half after each generation of random mating. If the sign of *d* is positive, half the difference will be added equally to the frequencies of two kinds of coupling gametes and subtracted from the frequency of repulsion phase gametes. On the other hand, if difference has a negative sign, half the difference will be added equally to the frequencies of two kinds of repulsion gametes and a corresponding amount subtracted equally from the frequencies of two kinds of coupling gametes. This process will continue till *d* diminishes to zero. Equilibrium is usually reached after about 4 to 5 rounds of random mating in the absence of linkage. Let us show attainment of equilibrium for two loci with an example.

Assume that the population comprises of individuals having four genotypes $A_1A_1B_1B_1$, $A_1A_1B_2B_2$, $A_2A_2B_1B_1$, and $A_2A_2B_2B_2$. The frequencies of these genotypes are say 0.70, 0.10, 0.10 and 0.10, respectively. Four kinds of gametes will be produced by this population as shown in Table 2.2.

TABLE 2.2: Showing frequencies of genotypes and the gametes produced

Genotype	Initial Frequency	Gametes produced	Frequency of Gametes
$A_1A_1B_1B_1$	0.70	A_1B_1	0.70
$A_1A_1B_2B_2$	0.10	A_1B_2	0.10
$A_2A_2B_1B_1$	0.10	A_2B_1	0.10
$A_2A_2B_2B_2$	0.10	A_2B_2	0.10

$$\begin{aligned} d &= (0.1\times 0.1) - (0.7\times 0.1) \\ &= 0.01 - 0.07 \\ &= -0.06 \end{aligned}$$

The sign of difference (d) calculated in Table 2.2 is negative, which suggests that the coupling gametes are more frequent than the gametes in repulsion. Random mating in this population will produce an offspring generation in which this difference will be halved as compared to the initial generation, *i.e.*, –0.03. Half the difference will be added equally to the frequencies of two kinds of repulsion gametes and corresponding amount deducted from the frequencies of coupling gametes produced by this offspring generation. Thus, the frequencies of gametic types A_1B_2 and A_2B_1 in offspring generation will be 0.10 + 0.03 = 0.13 each and the frequencies of gametes A_1B_1 and A_2B_2 will be 0.70–0.03 = 0.67 and 0.10 – 0.03 = 0.07, respectively.

This can be verified by preparing a checker board of random union among the gametes as shown in Table 2.3.

TABLE 2.3: Random union among the gametes A_1B_1, A_1B_2, A_2B_1 and A_2B_2 of parental generation

Gametes frequency	A_1B_1 0.70	A_1B_2 0.10	A_2B_1 0.10	A_2B_2 0.10
A_1B_1 0.70	$A_1A_1B_1B_1$ 0.49	$A_1A_1B_1B_2$ 0.07	$A_1A_2B_1B_1$ 0.07	$A_1A_2B_1B_2$ 0.07
A_1B_2 0.10	$A_1A_1B_1B_2$ 0.07	$A_1A_1B_2B_2$ 0.01	$A_1A_2B_1B_2$ 0.01	$A_1A_2B_2B_2$ 0.01
A_2B_1 0.10	$A_1A_2B_1B_1$ 0.07	$A_1A_2B_1B_2$ 0.01	$A_2A_2B_1B_1$ 0.01	$A_2A_2B_1B_2$ 0.01
A_2B_2 0.10	$A_1A_2B_1B_2$ 0.07	$A_1A_2B_2B_2$ 0.01	$A_2A_2B_1B_2$ 0.01	$A_2A_2B_2B_2$ 0.01

Frequency of the gametes A_1B_2 in the progeny generation can be calculated from the frequencies of genotypes of progeny generation shown in Table 2.3.

Thus

$$A_1A_1B_1B_2 + A_1A_2B_1B_2 + A_1A_1B_1B_2 + A_1A_1B_2B_2 +$$
$$A_1B_2 = \tfrac{1}{2}(0.07) + \tfrac{1}{4}(0.07) + \tfrac{1}{2}(0.07) + (0.01)$$
$$A_1A_2B_1B_2 + A_1A_2B_2B_2 + A_1A_2B_1B_2 +$$
$$+ \tfrac{1}{4}(0.01) + \tfrac{1}{2}(0.01) + \tfrac{1}{4}(0.01) +$$
$$A_1A_2B_1B_2 + A_1A_2B_2B_2$$
$$\tfrac{1}{4}(0.07) + \tfrac{1}{2}(0.01)$$
$$= 0.13$$

Similarly, frequencies of gametes A_1B_1 and A_2B_2 could be calculated from this table and found to be 0.67 and 0.07 respectively. This shows that half the difference is added to repulsion gametes and subtracted from coupling gametes.

At equilibrium the gametic frequencies will be:

	Gametes			
	A_1B_1	A_1B_2	A_2B_1	A_2B_2
Frequency at equilibrium	0.64	0.16	0.16	0.04

This clearly shows that the dfference d has been completely added to the frequencies of repulsion gametes and subtracted from the frequencies of coupling gametes.

2.3.3 Linkage of Genes

While describing the attainment of an equilibrium by a population it was assumed that the two loci being considered were not linked. It was mentioned in section 2.3.2 that a population made up of the individuals whose genotype is $A_1A_2B_1B_2$, attains Hardy-Weinberg equilibrium after one generation of random mating, provided that the genes at the two loci were independent in transmission. If a chromosome carries genes A_1B_1, which are tightly linked, and its homologous chromosome bears alleles A_2B_2, recombinant gametes would be rarely formed (*e.g.* A_1B_2 and A_2B_1). Hence, the population may not be able to attain equilibrium for quite some time. Reduction of half the difference after each round of random mating is expected only with independent gene pairs, otherwise the reduction of d will depend upon the extent of recombination possible between the two gene pairs. The effect of linkage is therefore to delay the attainment of equilibrium. It was pointed out in last section that at equilibrium the product of frequencies of repulsion gametes will be equal to the product of frequencies of coupling gametes. Difference between the products of frequencies of two kinds of gametes is signified by d. When linkage is involved the difference dt in any generation t is obtained as:

$$dt = (1 - c)dt - 1,$$

Where c is the recombination frequency between two loci. When $c = 0.5$ there will be independent assortment. We saw in section 2.3.2 that the difference between the frequencies of gametes in repulsion and coupling was halved, i.e. 0.03, after one generation of random mating. However, when the recombination frequency, i.e. $c = 25\%$, the difference will not be halved each generation as shown below:

$$\begin{aligned} d_1 &= (1 - 0.25) \times (0.06) \\ &= (0.75) \times (0.06) \\ &= 0.045 \end{aligned}$$

The difference is reduced by 50 per cent after each round of random mating when linkage is not involved (section 2.3.2). However, when genes are linked the rate at which difference is reduced depends upon the extent of linkage. Closer the genes are linked the longer it will take to attain equilibrium. However, equilibrium values for linked genes will not differ from those expected for genes inherited independently. The magnitude of difference d, depends upon the gametic frequencies and not upon the linkage.

2.3.4 Sex-linked Genes

In the preceding sections of this chapter it was assumed that the inheritance is autosomal. In higher animals, some insects and some plants the male and female sex is determined by the balance between autosomes and the chromosomes called the sex chromosomes. Genes borne on the sex chromosomes are called as sexlinked genes. In human beings, as well as in *Drosophila,* females bear two X chromosomes and the males possess only one X and one Y chromosome. The Y chromosome is practically inert. Hence, there will be five genotypes in the population with respect to sex-linked genes, if we assume that there are only two alleles at a locus (say A_1 and A_2). Since females have two X chromosomes, there will be three genotypes among the females, *viz.* A_1A_1, A_1A_2, A_2A_2. However, among the males there will be only two genotypes, A_1 and A_2. Males produce two kinds of gametes *viz.*, one kind carrying the X chromosome and a haploid set of autosomes and another kind possessing Y chromosome and one set of autosomes. Hence *Drosophila* males are known as heterogametic. The females produce only one kind of gamete and are therefore, known as homogametic. If we assume that the number of males and females are equal in the population, on average 1/3rd sex-linked genes will be carried by males and 2/3rd by females. (Because out of three X chromosomes, 1/3rd sex chromosomes are possessed by males and 2/3rd by females). A question that is posed is whether population attains equilibrium for sex-linked traits. If it does, then at equilibrium what are the gene and genotype frequencies in males and females?

It should be noted that with respect to sex-linked genes the population attains equilibrium. How? Let us show with an example. With respect to a single locus with two alleles there will be three genotypes among the females, *viz.* A_1A_1, A_1A_2, and A_2A_2. However, there will be only two genotypes among the males, *viz.* A_1 and A_2. Let us also assume that the frequencies of three genotypes among the females are D, H, R such that $D + H + R = 1$. The frequencies of genotypes A_1 and A_2 among the males are say W and X, respectively.

It was mentioned in section 2.3.1 that the frequencies of different genotypes in a population produced by random mating could be obtained as the square of gametic array of the parental population. Hence, we have to find the gametic array in order to know the equilibrium frequencies. We now know that the frequency of gametes bearing a particular gene in a random mating population is equal to the frequency of that gene. We are considering two alleles at a locus. Therefore, the population will produce only two kinds of gametes, *viz.*, bearing genes A_1 and A_2. We are, therefore, required to find the frequencies of genes A_1 and A_2 in the population. Frequency of gene A_1 among the females is:

$$p_f = D + \frac{1}{2}H.$$

And the frequency of this gene among the males is:

$$p_m = W.$$

The males carry 1/3rd sex-linked genes in the population and the females 2/3rd. Hence, the frequency of gene A_1 in the entire population will be

$$p = \frac{2}{3}p_f + \frac{1}{3}p_m$$

$$\text{or } \frac{1}{3}(2p_f + p_m),$$

and since $p_f = D + \frac{1}{2}H$ and $P_m = W$, p is obtained as:

$$p = \frac{1}{3}[2D + H + W].$$

In an analogous manner the average frequency of gene A_2 in the entire population is:

$$q = \frac{1}{3}[2R + H + X].$$

Gametic array of the parental population is then

$(pA_1 + qA_2)$,

and the genotypic array in the offspring generation will be:

$(pA_1 + qA_2)^2$

$= p^2 A_1A_1 + 2pq\, A_1A_2 + q^2 A_2A_2$.

These are also the equilibrium frequencies of genotypes A_1A_1, A_1A_2 and A_2A_2 among the females. At equilibrium, the frequencies of genotypes A_1 and A_2 among the males will be p and q, respectively. These equilibrium frequencies are not reached in one generation. A few rounds of random mating are required before attainment of Hardy-Weinberg equilibrium. The frequencies of genes A_1 and A_2 are indentical among the female and the male individuals of the population at equilibrium. If the frequencies of genes A_1 and A_2 are different among the males and females, the population is not in equilibrium. The equilibrium genotype frequencies are reached in an oscillating fashion, such that after one round of random mating the frequency of a gene among males increases as compared to that in the initial population, and in the following generation the frequency of the gene increases among the females and so on till the attainment of equilibrium. This point needs an explanation. Let us take an example.

Suppose the frequencies of genotypes among the females and males are as shown below:

	Females			Males	
Genotype	A_1A_1	A_1A_2	A_2A_2	A_1	A_2
Frequency	0.40	0.40	0.20	0.30	0.70

Frequency of gene A_1 among the females is then

$p_f = 0.40 + 0.20$

$= 0.60$

Frequency among the males is

$p_m = 0.30.$

Frequency of this gene in the entire population is then

$$p = \frac{1}{3}(2p_f + p_m)$$

$$= \frac{1}{3}(2 \times 0.60) + 0.30]$$

$$= \frac{1}{3}(1.50)$$

$$= 0.50$$

Since $p + q = 1$, $q = 1\text{–}0.50 = 0.50$

The gametic array of the initial population is, therefore,

$(0.50A_1 + 0.50A_2)^2$

Frequencies of the three genotypes A_1A_1, A_1A_2 and A_2A_2 among the females, at equilibrium will be:

$(0.50A_1 + 0.50A_2)^2$

$= 0.25A_1A_1 + 0.50A_1A_2 + 0.25A_2A_2.$

As pointed out in the earlier paragraphs of this section, the frequencies of two genotypes among the males, namely A_1 and A_2, will be 0.50 each i.e., equal to the frequencies of these genes at equilibrium. This equilibrium, is attained in an oscillating fashion. How? Let us see. The female individuals receive one X chromosome from their mothers and the other from their fathers. Hence, the frequency of A_1 genes among the females, after one generation of random mating, is

$$p_f = \frac{1}{2}p'_m + \frac{1}{2}p'_f \text{ or } \frac{1}{2}(p'_m + p'_f),$$

where p'_m and p'_f refer to the frequency of gene A_1 in the previous generation. On the other hand, the males receive X chromosome from their mothers only. The frequency of gene A_1 among the males after one generation of random mating is then

$p_m = P'_f$

Let us refer to the example given above to make the point clear. In the initial population, frequency of gene A_1 (and also the gametes) among the females was 0.60 (p'_f), whereas among the males it was 0.30 (p'_m). After one round of random mating, the frequency of this gene among the females will be:

$$p_f = \frac{1}{2}p'_m + \frac{1}{2}p'_f$$

$$= \frac{1}{2}(0.30) + \frac{1}{2}(0.60)$$

$$= 0.15 + 0.30$$

$$= 0.45.$$

The frequency of gene A_1 has thus reduced among the female offspring. The p_m (frequency of gene A_1 among the male offspring) will be:

$$p_m = p'_f$$

$$= 0.60.$$

This clearly shows that the frequency of gene A_1 has increased among the males. Second round of random mating will increase the frequency of gene A_1 among the females but decrease it among the males. This process continues until the population attains Hardy-Weinberg equilibrium. At equilibrium, frequency of this gene will be same in both the sexes.

We have been discussing about the gene frequencies and genotype frequencies in the preceding sections of this chapter. The reader might be wondering regarding the usefulness of these concepts. It may be pointed out that means, variances and covariances are the observable properties of population. These properties depend upon the genes and their frequencies in the population. Let us see how.

2.4 Population Mean

The value observed when a character is measured on an individual is the phenotypic value of that individual. All the observations are, therefore, based on the measurement of phenotypic values. The means, variances and covariances are also measured in terms of phenotypic value.

Now we know that the phenotype of an individual is determined by its genotype and environment surrounding it. Genotype is the particular assemblage of genes possessed by an individual. The value associated with a genotype is called genotypic value (G) and that with environment as the environmental deviation (*E*). The phenotypic value is, therefore, linearly expressed as:

$$P = G + E$$

It is assumed here that the genotype confers a certain value on individual and the environmental agencies, which include all the non-heritable agencies, cause a deviation from this value, either in the positive or in the negative direction. Hence, mean environmental deviations are zero and mean phenotypic value is equal to mean genotypic value. The population mean, therefore, refers equally to the phenotypic mean as well as to the genotypic mean. We assume that the environment remains constant from generation to generation, which implies that the phenotypic mean changes only when the genotypic mean changes.

If an inbred population is grown in several environments the mean phenotypic value of this population will represent its mean genotypic value, because the environmental deviations cancel and become zero.

We can assign genotypic values arbitrarily to various genotypes. Suppose that a population is made up of individuals with genotypes A_1A_1, A_1A_2 and A_2A_2. The origin or point of zero value is mid-way between the values of two homozygotes. The deviation of each of the homozygote from this origin or mid-point will be similar in magnitude. Let us denote the departure of A_1A_1 from midpoint by $+ a$ and that of A_2A_2 by $-a$. Here we assume that the gene A_1 tends to increase the expression of a character. Gene A_2 tends to decrease it. The value taken by the heterozygote A_1A_2 will depend upon the degree of dominance. If the genes A_1 and A_2, transmitted by a parental strains (A_1A_1, A_2A_2) do not interact, i.e. their effects are simply additive, the value of heterozygote will fall on mid-point. When heterozygote falls on mid-point we say that there is no dominance. This implies that the genotypic value of heterozygote is simple sum of the effects of genes A_1 and A_2 (Fig. 2.1). On the other hand, if gene A_1 is partially dominant to A_2, the genotypic value assumed by A_1A_2 will be in between the mid-point and A_1A_1. In this case the genotypic (phenotypic) value will deviate from the mid-point in plus direction. Departure of heterozygote from mid-point is denoted by d. Thus d measures the departure of gene effects from additivity at a locus. If gene A_2 is partially dominatnt, A_1A_2 will fall mid-way between the origin and A_2A_2. When there is complete dominance d will be equal to either $+a$ or $-a$. Overdominance results when d is greater than $+a$ or lesser than $-a$. In the absence of over-dominance, total range of expression is $2a$.

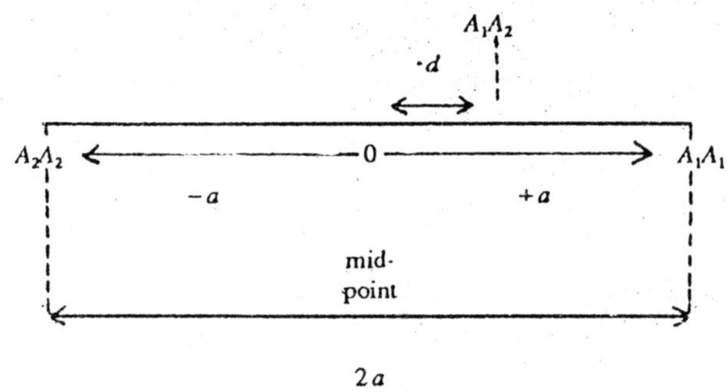

FIG. 2.1: *Population mean*

Let us now derive the population mean and see how the gene frequencies influence it. We will consider a simple situation of a single locus with two alleles viz. A_1 and A_2. With respect to this locus, there will be three genotypes, A_1A_1, A_1A_2 and A_2A_2 in the population. Frequencies of these genotypes in a large random mating population were shown to be p^2, $2pq$ and q^2, respectively. Population mean is therefore sum of the product of frequency of a genotype and its value, summation being made over all the genotypes. Sum of the genotype frequencies is unity. Hence the population mean is simply sum of (frequencies × genotypic value) over all the genotypes as shown below:

Genotype	Frequency	Value
A_1A_1	p^2	a
A_1A_2	$2pq$	d
A_2A_2	q^2	$-a$

$$\text{Population mean} = p^2a + 2pqd - q^2a$$
$$= a(p^2 - q^2) + 2pqd$$

or $\quad a\,[(p+q)\,(p-q)] + 2pqd$, since $(p+q) = 1$
$$= a\,(p-q) + 2pqd.$$

This is the genotypic as well as the phenotypic mean. Population mean has two components, *viz.* $a\,(p-q)$ which refers to the difference between the homozygotes and $2pqd$ to the heterozygote. If there is no dominance, d will be zero and consequently the population mean will be $a\,(1-2q)$ as shown below:

Genotype	Frequency	Value
A_1A_1	p^2	a
A_1A_2	$2pq$	0
A_2A_2	q^2	$-a$

$$\text{Mean} = p^2(a) + (2pq \times 0) + q^2(-a)$$
$$= p^2a - q^2a$$
$$= a(p^2 - q^2)$$
$$= a\,(p-q), \text{ and since } p = 1-q$$
$$= a\,(1-q-q)$$
$$= a\,(1-2q).$$

Population mean will be, $a\,(1-2q^2)$ if gene A_1 is completely dominant. These expressions for the population mean clearly show that in addition to the degree of dominance and difference between the values of homozygotes, population mean is influenced by the gene frequency. To make this point clear, let us take an hypothetical example. Assume that the genotypic values of A_1A_1, A_1A_2 and A_2A_2 are 16, 12 and 4, respectively. Suppose that the frequency of gene A_2 is 0.4. The population mean is then got as shown below:

Genotype	Frequency	Value
A_1A_1	0.36	16
A_1A_2	0.48	12
A_2A_2	0.16	4

The mid-point is

$$\frac{16+4}{2}=10$$

The values of a and d are therefore 16–10 = 6 and 12–10=2, respectively. Substituting these values in the expression for population mean we get

$$6\,(0.6-0.4) + 2 \times 0.6 \times 0.4 \times 2$$
$$= 6\,(0.2) + 0.96$$
$$= 1.2 + 0.96$$
$$= 2.16.$$

Since the values of a and d are obtained as deviations from mid-point (*i.e.* 10), the population mean is 10 + 2.16 = 12.16.

Now suppose that through selection the frequency of A_2 has been increased from 0.4 to 0.9. What will be the effect of rise in the frequency of gene A_2 on population mean? The population mean will be

$$6\,(0.10-0.90) + 2 \times 0.10 \times 0.90 \times 2$$
$$= 6\,(-0.80) + 4 \times 0.09$$
$$= -4.80 + 0.36$$
$$= -4.44.$$

Hence the population mean will be 10 – 4.44 = 5.56. The population mean has declined as a consequence of rise in the frequency of gene with negative effect on the character. This is how the genes influence population mean.

Now let us see what will be the population mean when several loci governing the inheritance of an attribute are taken into consideration. We assume that values of genotypes over loci are simply additive. For example, if a_A is the genotypic value of A_1A_1 and a_B that of B_1B_1, the aggregate genotypic value of $A_1A_1B_1B_1$ is $a_A + a_B$. However, reader should keep in mind that absence of non-allelic interaction which we consider here is not realistic. Effect of non-allelic interaction will be considered at the end of this chapter. If genotypic values are additive over loci, the population mean is:

$$\Sigma a_i\,(p_i - q_i) + 2\Sigma p_i q_i d_i,$$

where a_i, p_i, q_i, d_i refer to the values and gene frequencies at the ith locus. The total range of expression in this case will be 2 $\Sigma\, a$. Thus if all the genes which increase the value of a character are fixed in the population, the population mean would be $\Sigma\, a$.

2.5 Breeding Value of Genotypes

It is very well-known to the students of genetics that parents pass on their genes and not the genotypes to their offspring through the gametes. Genotypes of the offspring generation are created afresh from the genes transmitted by their parents. We, therefore, need a measure of value which refers to the genes and not to the genotypes. This measure is the "average effect of gene". This measure will permit us to assign a breeding value to the individuals, a value associated with genes carried by the individuals and transmitted to the progeny. Falconer (1960) defined average effect of a gene as "the mean deviation from population mean of individuals which received that gene from one parent, the gene received from other parent having come at random from population". To understand this concept suppose that an individual is mated randomly to a number of individuals in the population. Average deviation of genotypic values of individuals so produced from the population mean is a measure of average effect of a gene possessed by that individual.

Let us derive the average effect of genes. Assume that there are two alleles at a locus among the individuals of a large random mating population, viz. A_1 and A_2. The average effect of gene A_1 is denoted by α_1. The three genotypes, with respect to this locus in the population, will produce two kinds of gametes, *viz.* A_1 and A_2 with frequencies p and q, respectively. If the gametes produced by genotypes bearing gene A_1 unite randomly with gametes in the population, two kinds of individuals are produced, *viz.* A_1A_1 and A_1A_2 with the frequencies p and q, respectively. Why? Because, frequency of gametes A_1 in the population is p, hence, frequency of genotype A_1A_1 in the offspring generation will be p. Similarly the frequency of A_1A_2 will be q. The genotypic value of A_1A_1 is a and that of A_1A_2 is d. Mean genotypic value of the progeny is, therefore, $(pa + qd)$. Deviation of this mean genotypic value from the population mean is the average effect of gene A_1 i.e. α_1 (alpha 1). Thus:

$$
\begin{aligned}
\alpha_1 &= (pa + qd) - [a(p - q) + 2pqd] \\
&= (pa + qd) - [pa - qa + 2pqd] \\
&= pa + qd - pa + qa - 2pqd \\
&= q\,[a + d - 2pd] \\
&= q\,[a + d\,(1 - 2p)] \\
&= q[a + d\,(1 - p - p)]
\end{aligned}
$$

and since $1 - p = q$

$$\alpha_1 = q[a + d(q - p)].$$

We can derive average effect of gene A_2 in similar fashion. Average effect of A_2, *i.e.* α_2 is $-p[a + d(q - p)]$. Difference between α_1 and α_2 is $[a + d(q - p)]$ which is the average effect of gene substitution. The concept of average effect of gene substitution was given by Fisher (1930). Since α is $[a + d(q - p)]$ we can write α_1 and α_2 as $q\alpha$ as and $- p\alpha$, respectively.

Average effect of a gene is a property of a population and gene.

How useful is the concept of average effects of genes? Since parents pass on their genes to the offspring, average effect of genes of parents determine the mean genotypic value of offspring. Plant breeders usually evaluate an individual on the basis of mean performance of its progeny. Value of an individual judged by the mean value of its progeny is known as 'breeding value' of that individual. Breeding values can be defined in absolute units but it is more convenient to define it as deviation from population mean. We are considering a diploid population. Hence the breeding value of an individual defined in terms of average effect of genes is the sum of average effects of the genes it carries. Breeding values of three genotypes (A_1A_1, A_1A_2 and A_2A_2) are therefore $2q\alpha$, $\alpha(q - p)$, and $-2p\alpha$, respectively. Thus, for an homozygote, breeding value is twice the average effect of one of the genes it carries. When several loci are considered, breeding value of an individual is the sum of the breeding values over all the loci, in the absence of non-allelic interaction. The two definitions of breeding value do not agree when non-allelic interaction exists.

Because the average effects are expressed as deviations from the population mean, average breeding value in the population is zero. Thus

Genotype	Frequency	Breeding value
A_1A_1	p^2	$2q\alpha$
A_1A_2	$2pq$	$(q - p)\alpha$
A_2A_2	q^2	$-2p\alpha$

Mean breeding value

$= 2p^2q\alpha + 2pq\,(q\alpha - p\alpha) - 2pq^2\alpha$
$= 2p^2q\alpha + 2pq^2\alpha - 2p^2\,q\alpha - 2pq^2\alpha$
$= 0.$

Breeding values are sometimes referred to as additive genotype and the variance of breeding values as "additive variance".

2.5.1 Worked Example

We take the example from section 2.4, where the phenotypic values (and also the genotypic values) were 16, 12, 4 for the three genotypes, *viz.* A_1A_1, A_1A_2 and A_2A_2, respectively. The values of '*a*' and '*d*' were found to be 6 and 2, respectively. Assume that the frequency of gene A_2 is 0.4. The average effect of gene A_1 is then

$$\begin{aligned}\alpha_1 &= q[a + d\,(q - p)]\\ &= 0.4[6 + 2\,(0.4 - 0.6)]\\ &= 0.4\,[6 + 2\,(-0.2)]\\ &= 0.4\,[\,6 - 0.4]\\ &= 2.24.\end{aligned}$$

The average effect of gene A_2 is similarly found by substituting values of a, d, p and q in the expression

$$-p\,[a + d\,(q - p)]$$

Thus

$$\begin{aligned}\alpha_2 &= -\,0.6\,[6 + 2\,(0.4 - 0.6)]\\ &= -\,3.36.\end{aligned}$$

The breeding values of the three genotypes will, therefore, be:

Genotype	Breeding value
A_1A_1	4.48
A_1A_2	– 1.12
A_2A_2	– 6.72

2.6 Dominance Deviation

Non–additivity of two alleles at a locus is the cause of dominance deviation. The difference between genotypic value of a genotype and its breeding value is called as dominance deviation, provided a single locus is under consideration. Dominance deviation is the property of a population. Like the average effect of a gene, the dominance deviations are also influenced by the gene frequency.

Let us derive the dominance deviation for A_1A_1. As pointed out, dominance deviation is the difference between genotypic value of a genotype and its breeding value. The genotypic value of A_1A_1 is 'a'. However, it has not been expressed as deviation from population mean. Before subtracting the breeding value of A_1A_1 from the genotypic value we have to express genotypic value of A_1A_1 as deviation from population mean.

Thus,

$$\begin{aligned} & a - (\text{population mean}) \\ &= a - [a(p-q) + 2pqd] \\ &= a - [ap - aq + 2pqd] \\ &= a - ap + aq - 2pqd \\ &= a(1 - p + q) - 2pqd, \text{ since } 1 - p = q \\ &= a(2q) - 2pqd \\ &= 2aq - 2pqd \\ &= 2q(a - pd). \end{aligned}$$

Since the breeding value is expressed in terms of α, it will be convenient to express $2q(a - pd)$ in terms of α. We know that

$$\alpha = a + d(q - p)$$

or $$\alpha = a + dq - dp,$$

and, therefore,

$$a = \alpha - dq + dp.$$

Substituting this value for 'a' we get

$$\begin{aligned} & 2q(\alpha - dq + dp - dp) \\ &= 2q(\alpha - dq). \end{aligned}$$

Dominance deviation for A_1A_1 is then

$$\begin{aligned} & 2q(\alpha - dq) - 2q\alpha \\ &= 2q\alpha - 2q^2d - 2q\alpha \\ &= -2q^2d. \end{aligned}$$

The dominance deviations for A_1A_2 and A_2A_2 are found in similar manner. The dominance deviations for the three genotypes are given below:

Genotype	Dominance deviation
A_1A_1	$-2q^2d$
A_1A_2	$2pqd$
A_2A_2	$-2p^2d.$

Dominance deviations, therefore, depend upon gene frequency as well as d. If $d = 0$, that is, if there is no dominance, genotypic values equal the breeding values.

Similar to the breeding values, mean dominance deviations in a random mating population are equal to zero. There is no correlation between the breeding values and the dominance deviations (Kempthorne, 1957 and Falconer, 1960). This can be confirmed by multiplying breeding value, dominance deviation and the frequency of each genotype and adding the products for the three genotypes. This is zero.

2.6.1 *Worked Example*

Let us find the dominance deviations for three genotypes (section 2.5.1). The genotypic values for the three genotypes are 16, 12 and 4. These have to be expressed as deviation from population mean. In section 2.4, the population mean was found to be 12.16 Hence the genotypic values expressed as deviation from population mean will be:

Genotypes	Genotypic values	
	Original	Deviation from mean
A_1A_1	16	3.84
A_1A_2	12	–0.16
A_2A_2	4	–8.16

Dominance deviations for three genotypes are obtained as difference between their genotypic values and corresponding breeding values. Breeding values of three genotypes were calculated in section 2.5.1 Thus,

Genotype	Genotypic value	Breeding value	Dominance deviation
A_1A_1	3.84	4.48	–0.64
A_1A_2	–0.16	–1.12	0.96
A_2A_2	–8.16	–6.72	–1.44

2.7 Interaction Deviation

In sections 2.4, 2.5 and 2.6 we assumed that genes at different loci do not influence each other's effects. In other words, we assumed absence of non-allelic interaction. If we denote the genotypic value at a locus as G_A and at other locus as G_B, the aggregate genotypic value in the absence of non-allelic interaction is:

$$G = G_A + G_B.$$

However, to assume absence of non-allelic interaction is unrealistic. Hence to the expression given above we add a term I_{AB}, which represents a value ascribed to non-additivity between the loci. Thus,

$$G = G_A + G_B + I_{AB}.$$

Thus non-additivity means two things, *viz.* intra-allelic interaction within a locus (dominance) and inter-allelic interaction (epistasis).

3

GENERATION MEANS

3.1 Additive and Dominance Effects of Genes

Quantitative traits, such as yield in maize, are characterised by continuous distribution. Inheritance of such characters is governed by genes which have small, similar and cumulative effects. Non-heritable agencies also influence the phenotypic expression of these characters.

Major genes, which govern the inheritance of qualitative characters, have large effects. The effects of these genes can be separated by usual Mendelian techniques even in the presence of segregation and/or non-heritable agencies. Therefore, decision regarding the best breeding procedure can be easily taken. The choice of an appropriate breeding method for improvement of quantitative characters also depends largely on the nature of gene action. As pointed out in Chapter 2, effects of these individual genes cannot be separately measured. These genes must be considered *en masse* and statistical procedure used to obtain genetic information.

Action of the genes controlling quantitative characters can be described by the use of gene models. First attempt to construct a gene model was that of Fisher (1918). In this model he included dominance at a single locus. He stated that there may be a deviation from simple additive effects between loci, similar to dominance at one locus, if more than one locus affected a given character. He called the deviation epistacy. Fisher, Immer and Tedin (1932) used this gene model to describe gene action of any number of genes on a given character. Gene models were also developed by Comstock and Robinson (1948) and Mather (1949) to wevaluate the relative importance of additive and dominance gene effects. Epistatic effects were assumed to be negligible in these gene models.

Anderson and Kempthorne (1954), Hayman (1958) and Gamble (1962) believed that epistatic effects could be of significance for quantitative characters.

Gene model proposed by Anderson and Kempthorne (1954) was based on factorial model used in the designs of experiments. In this model the genotypic value was partitioned into additive, dominance and epistatic effects. In an attempt to assess the contribution of genic interaction to continuous variation, Hayman and Mather (1955) developed a gene model based on theory developed by Fisher *et al.* (1932) and Mather (1949). Hayman (1958) described a general procedure to estimate parameters referring to the additive, dominance, additive × additive, additive × dominance and dominance × dominance effects in addition to m. Gamble (1962), on the other hand, proposed a perfect fit solution to estimate additive, dominance, additive × additive, additive × dominance and dominance × dominance effects from the mean measurements of six generations *viz.* P_1, P_2, F_1, F_2, Bc_1 and Bc_2.

We shall follow Fisher *et al.* (1932), Mather (1949) and Mather and Jinks (1971) to describe the gene effects.

Let us begin with a simple case of an autosomal locus with two alleles, *viz.* A_1 and A_2. With respect to this locus there will be three genotypes, A_1A_1, A_1A_2 and A_2A_2. In order to describe differences among three phenotypes, two parameters are required. Mid-point between the two homozygotes is taken as origin because it does not depend upon differences among the three genotypes, but on other genotypes not under consideration and the effects of environment. Hence the mid-point reflects general circumstances of the observation. Let us assume that gene A_1 tends to increase manifestation of the character and A_2 tends to decrease it.

One parameter '*d*' represents the phenotypic difference between homozygotes and measures the extent of departure of either homozygote from the mid-point. (This parameter is similar to '*a*' which we used in chapter 2. Falconer (1960) adopted symbol '*a*' to measure half the difference between two extreme homozygotes). Thus the magnitude of deviation of A_1A_1 from the mid-point is $+d$ and that of A_2A_2, $-d$ (Fig. 2.1). The extent of departure of heterozygote A_1A_2 from the mid-point is measured by a second parameter 'h' (This is similar to parameter 'd' we adopted in Chapter 2 to measure deviation of heterozygote from mid-point). Thus the gene's contribution to additive genetic variation is proportional to 'd'. On the other hand, 'h' reflects the dominance properties of genes and, therefore, represents the contribution to non-additive variation which is unfixable. Parameter 'h' can take various values depending upon the degree of dominance. If $h = 0$, there is no dominance. If gene A_1 is completely dominant, h is equal to $+ d$. When gene A_2 is completely dominant h is equal to $-d$. With partial dominance h falls in between $\pm d$ and mid-point. Heterozygote may be superior to either of the homozygotes, a situation known as overdominance. In this case the value assumed by 'h' is greater than $+d$ or less than $-d$. Overdominance is a property shown by the two alleles when heterozygote lies outside the range of two homozygotes in genotypic value with respect to the character under consideration.

At this juncture it is useful to explain various kinds of gene effects. Genes may exhibit additivity, dominance or non-allelic interaction in their action. Genes may also act in a multiplicative fashion. However, this will be discussed elsewhere.

Simplest conception of the way genes act assumes that substitution of one allele for the other produces a plus or minus shift on the scale of measurement regardless of the genetic constitution at the other loci. This is known as additive gene action or additive gene effects. Let us explain the meaning of additivity with the help of an hypothetical example. Assume that genes at 2 loci each having two alleles, *viz.* A_1, A_2 and B_1, B_2, govern the inheritance of a character being studied. Let us also assume that the frequencies of genes are equal, *i.e.* ½ at each locus. Suppose that the observations recorded on nine genotypes are as shown in Table 3.1 (a). Genotype $A_2 A_2 B_2 B_2$ measures 2 units. If gene A_1 is substituted for A_2 in this genotype the new genotype is $A_1 A_2 B_2 B_2$. Effect of substituting A_1 for A_2 in $A_2 A_2 B_2 B_2$ is one unit. Likewise the effect of substituting A_1 for A_2 in $A_1 A_2 B_2 B_2$ is also one unit. Thus, effect of substituting A_1 for A_2 is one unit regardless of the fact whether the genotype is $A_2 A_2$ or $A_1 A_2$. Effect of substitution is also one unit when genotypes at the B_1, B_2 locus are $B_2 B_2$, $B_1 B_2$ or $B_1 B_1$. This shows that the effect of substitution of A_1 for A_2 is same irrespective of the genes present at A_1, A_2 or at B_1, B_2 locus.

Now suppose that we measure these nine genotypes for some other character and the observations are as shown in Table 3.1 (b). The value of $A_1 A_2 B_2 B_2$ is same as $A_1 A_1 B_2 B_2$ upon substitution of A_1 for A_2 in $A_2 A_2 B_2 B_2$.

TABLE 3.1: Gene effects

effects	Genotypes			Mean
	$A_2 A_2$	$A_1 A_2$	$A_1 A_1$	
(a) Additive gene effects				
$B_2 B_2$	2	3	4	3
$B_1 B_2$	3	4	5	4
$B_1 B_1$	4	5	6	5
Mean effects	3	4	5	
(b) Dominance gene effects				
$B_2 B_2$	1	2	2	1.75
$B_1 B_2$	3	4	4	3.75
$B_1 B_1$	3	4	4	3.75
Mean effects	2.50	3.50	3.50	
(c) Non-allelic interaction effects				
$B_2 B_2$	1	5	9	5
$B_1 B_2$	5	10	15	10
$B_1 B_1$	9	15	21	15
Mean effects	5	10	15	

The effect of substituting A_1 for A_2 is one unit in $A_2 A_2 B_2 B_2$, but zero unit in $A_1 A_2 B_2 B_2$. This is because gene A_1 is completely dominant to A_2. Effect of substituting A_1 for A_2 in $A_2 A_2$ is one unit irrespective of the fact whether genotype at the second locus is $B_2 B_2$, $B_1 B_2$ or $B_1 B_1$. Thus genes at second locus do not influence the substitution at first locus. The effect of substituting B_1 for B_2 is 2 units in $B_2 B_2 A_2 A_2$, however, it is zero units in $B_1 B_2 A_2 A_2$. Value of $B_1 B_2 A_2 A_2$ is same as $B_1 B_1 A_2 A_2$ and hence there is complete dominance of B_1 over B_2. This effect of substituting B_1 for B_2 is same regardless of the phases at first locus, *viz.* $A_2 A_2$, $A_1 A_2$ and $A_1 A_1$. This is an example of dominance gene effect at a locus and additivity over two loci.

In the third hypothetical model (Table 3.1c) effects of non-allelic interaction are shown. Effect of substituting gene A_1 for A_2 in $A_2A_2B_2B_2$ is 4 units, which is equal to the effect of substituting A_1 for A_2 in $A_1A_2B_2B_2$. There is thus no dominance, however, when gene A_1 is substituted for A_2 in $A_2A_2B_1B_2$ the effect is 5 units. Once again there is no dominance at A_1, A_2 locus when the phase at other locus is B_1B_2. The effect of substituting A_1 for A_2 in $A_2A_2B_1B_1$ is 6 units. But the effect of substitution is same regardless of the genotypes at A_1, A_2 locus. This model shows that the effect of gene substitution at first locus depends upon the phases at second locus. Thus this model is an example of non-allelic interaction so far as the two loci are concerned but the gene effects are additive at each of the A_1, A_2 and B_1, B_2 locus.

At the beginning of this chapter we assumed a simple situation, *i.e.* a single locus with two alleles. Quantitative traits are governed by genes at several loci. True breeding strains, therefore, possess several of these genes. Among these genes some tend to increase the phenotypic expression of character whereas others decrease it. Mean expression of true breeding strain is, therefore, expressible as

$$m + S(d+) - S(d-),$$

where $S(d+)$ is sum of the effects of genes with positive effects on the character and $S(d-)$ represents sum of the effects of genes with negative effects. For a strain with larger manifestation (we denote it by P_1) the balance of $S(d+)$ and $S(d-)$ will be positive and for P_2 it will be negative.

Difference between the mean measurements of two strains depends upon the relative distribution of genes with positive and negative effects between the strains. Suppose k genes govern the inheritance of a character. Assume that a strain with larger manifestation (P_1) carries k' alleles with negative effects and remaining, i.e. $(k-k')$ alleles, with positive effects. A strain with smaller manifestation (P_2) contains, say k' alleles with increasing and $(k-k')$ alleles with decreasing effects on the character. Mean measurements of these strains could be expressed as

$$P_1 = m + (k-k')\,d+ - (k')\,d-$$

and $$P_2 = m + (k')\,d+ - (k-k')\,d-$$

If we now assume that effects of all the genes are similar in magnitude, *i.e.* $d_a = d_b = d_c = \ldots\ldots\ldots\ldots\ldots\ldots d_k$, difference between the mean expressions of these two strains will be $2[k-2k']$ (d), as shown below:

$$\begin{aligned}\overline{P}_1 - \overline{P}_2 &= [(k - k') - (k')](d) - [(k') - (k - k')](d)\\ &= (k - k' - k')(d) - (k' - k + k')(d)\\ &= (k - k' - k' - k' + k - k')(d)\\ &= (2k - 4k')d\\ &= 2(k - 2k')d\end{aligned}$$

Mather and Jinks (1971) define $\left(\frac{k - 2k'}{k}\right)$ as r, where the value of r is a measure of gene distribution between the two strains. Said in other words, it is the measure of degree of association of genes of like effects between the parental strains. The value of r will be + 1 if all the genes with positive effects are borne by one parent and genes with negative effects by other. Value of r is zero when genes are equally dispersed between the two strains. Thus, the difference between two strain means, described above, will be $2rkd$. When genes with positive effects are present in one parent and genes with negative effects in other, *i.e.* $r = 1$, the difference between two strain means is simply $2kd$. On the other hand, if the genes are equally dispersed between two strains $r = 0$, hence difference between the means of two strains will be zero.

In the preceding paragraph it was assumed that the magnitude of effects of all the genes is same, *i.e.* $d_a = d_b = d_c = \ldots\ldots\ldots\ldots d_k$, however, this need not be so. If the degree of association of genes of like effects between the strains as well as difference in the magnitudes of gene effects are taken into consideration difference between the mean expressions of two strains, following Mather and Jinks (1971), may be written as 2 $[d]$. The deviation of a strain with larger manifestation from mid-point is then denoted by $[d]$ and that of the parent with smaller expression by $[-d]$.

By similar analogy, deviation of heterozygote from the mid-point will be $[h]$, where it is assumed that $h_a \neq h_b \neq h_c \ldots\ldots \neq h_k$. However, the mean expression of heterozygote is not influenced by r.

3.2 Mean Expressions of Generations produced by Selfing the Successive Generations derived from F$_1$, Sib-mating and Backcrossing

If the relative frequencies of three genotypes, with respect to each locus, are known with certainty for any population, expected mean expression of that population can be specified in terms of three parameters, *viz.* m, d and h (assuming absence of non-allelic interaction). Let us begin with F_2 generation obtained by selfing an F_1 with genetic constitution A_1A_2. The F_2 generation will comprise of 3 genotypes A_1A_1, A_1A_2 and A_2A_2 in proportions $\frac{1}{4}$, $\frac{1}{2}$ and $\frac{1}{4}$ respectively in the absence of differential fertility and viability. Mean measurement of F_2 generation, expressed as deviation from mid-point, will be:

$$\bar{F}_2 = \frac{1}{4}(d) + \frac{1}{2}(h) + \frac{1}{4}(-d)$$

$$= \frac{1}{4}d - \frac{1}{4}d + \frac{1}{2}h$$

$$= \frac{1}{2}h$$

Hence, it is the heterozygote which contributes to the mean expression of F_2 generation. It is half the mean expression of F_1 generation.

The F_3 generation is produced by selfing the individuals in F_2 generation. Individuals of the genotypes A_1A_1 and A_2A_2 will breed true and produce progeny with same genotype in F_3 generation. However, heterozygous individuals of F_2 generation will segregate and produce individuals similar to F_1 in the next generation, *viz.* $\frac{1}{4}A_1A_1$, $\frac{1}{2}A_1A_2$ and $\frac{1}{4}A_2A_2$. Hence, the proportions of three genotypes in the entire F_3 population will be

$$\frac{3}{8}A_1A_1, \frac{1}{4}A_1A_2, \frac{3}{8}A_2A_2$$

Contribution of this locus to the mean expression of the F_3 generation will, therefore, be

$$\bar{F}_3 = \frac{3}{8}(d) + \frac{1}{4}(h) + \frac{3}{8}(-d)$$

$$= \frac{3}{8}d - \frac{3}{8}d + \frac{1}{4}h$$

$$= \frac{1}{4}h.$$

This is half the mean expression of F_2 generation. Following Mather and Jinks (1971), therefore, expected mean of *n*th generation produced by selfing F_1 for $(n-1)$ generations is given by:

$$\overline{F}_n = m + \left(\frac{1}{2}\right)^{n-1} [h],$$

where $[h]$ is summed effect of h over all the loci as described in section 3.1 (We assume absence of non-allelic interaction at present).

If the individuals in F_1 generation are sib-mated, instead of selfing, subsequent generation so produced is not F_2 generation but it is a sib-mated progeny (S_2). The mean expression of S_2 generation is similar to $\overline{F}_2$ *i.e.* $\frac{1}{2}[h]$. However, the mean expressions of subsequent generations obtained by sib-mating are not similar to those for selfing series. For example, the mean expression of S_3 generation, obtained by sib-mating in F_2 generation, is not similar to $\overline{F}_3$, *i.e.* $\frac{1}{4}[h]$ but $\frac{1}{2}[h]$. How? Let us see. Assume a simple case of a single locus with two alleles A_1 and A_2. In F_2 generation there will be 3 genotypes, A_1A_1, A_1A_2 and A_2A_2 with frequencies $\frac{1}{4}$, $\frac{1}{2}$ and $\frac{1}{4}$, respectively. Six kinds of matings are possible among these genotypes (Table 3.2).

TABLE 3.2: Biparental mating in F_2 generation, mean and frequency of progeny

Kinds of matings	Frequency	Mean and proportion of progeny			Mean of progeny from mating
		A_1A_1	A_1A_2	A_2A_2	
$A_1A_1 \times A_1A_1$	$\frac{1}{16}$	(d)	–	–	d
$A_1A_1 \times A_1A_2$	$\frac{1}{4}$	$\frac{1}{2}(d)$	$\frac{1}{2}(h)$	–	$\frac{1}{2}(d + \text{h})$
$A_1A_1 \times A_2A_2$	$\frac{1}{8}$	–	(h)	–	h
$A_1A_2 \times A_1A_2$	$\frac{1}{4}$	$\frac{1}{4}(d)$	$\frac{1}{2}(h)$	$\frac{1}{4}(-d)$	$\frac{1}{2}(h)$
$A_1A_2 \times A_2A_2$	$\frac{1}{4}$	–	$\frac{1}{2}(h)$	$\frac{1}{4}(-d)$	$\frac{1}{2}(h - d)$
$A_2A_2 \times A_2A_2$	$\frac{1}{16}$	–	–	$(-d)$	$(-d)$

Sum of the product of frequency of mating and mean of the progeny over six mating types gives the mean expression of S_3 generation. Thus,

$$\overline{S}_3 = \frac{1}{16}(d) + \frac{1}{4}\left(\frac{1}{2}d + \frac{1}{2}h\right) + \frac{1}{8}(h) + \frac{1}{4}\left(\frac{1}{2}h\right) + \frac{1}{4}\left(\frac{1}{2}h - \frac{1}{2}d\right) + \frac{1}{16}(-d)$$

$$= \frac{1}{16}\text{d} + \frac{1}{8}\text{d} + \frac{1}{8}\text{h} + \frac{1}{8}\text{h} + \frac{1}{8}\text{h} + \frac{1}{8}\text{h} - \frac{1}{8}\text{d} - \frac{1}{16}\text{d}$$

$$= 4\left(\frac{1}{8}h\right)$$

$$= \frac{1}{2}h.$$

If several loci which influence the expression of a character are taken into consideration, $\overline{S}_3$ in the absence of non-allelic interaction is simply $\frac{1}{2}[h]$. Mean expressions of the sib-mated progenies follow a

Fibonacci series. Thus, starting with S_2 generations the mean expressions will have coefficients $\frac{1}{2}, \frac{2}{4}, \frac{3}{8}, \frac{5}{16}, \frac{8}{32}$ .... etc. for $[h]$. Following Mather and Jinks (1971), the mean expression of nth generation resulting from sib-mating subsequent to F_2 (= S_2) will be:

$$\overline{S}_n = m + f_n [h],$$

where f_n is nth term of the Fibonacci series.

Let us now consider the mean expressions of generations produced by backcrossing. Assume once again that there are only two alleles at a locus, namely A_1 and A_2. If the individuals of F_1 are crossed to the parent with larger expression, *viz.* $A_1 A_1$, the backcross generation so produced is denoted by Bc_1 or simply B_1. There will be two kinds of progeny in Bc_1 generation in equal proportions, *viz.* $\frac{1}{2} A_1 A_1$ and $\frac{1}{2} A_1 A_2$. The mean expressions of these genotypes are d and h, respectively, expressed as deviation from mid-point. Hence, contribution of this locus to the $\overline{B}c_1$, *i.e.* mean expression of Bc_1 generation, will be:

$$\frac{1}{2}d + \frac{1}{2}h, \text{ or } \frac{1}{2}(d+h)$$

By similar reasoning, the mean expression of Bc_2 generation, produced by crossing F_1 to the parent with smaller manifestation (A_2A_2) will be :

$$\frac{1}{2}h - \frac{1}{2}d$$

or

$$\frac{1}{2}(h-d).$$

These expressions will be

$$\frac{1}{2}[d] + \frac{1}{2}[h] \text{ for } \overline{B}c_1 \text{ and } \frac{1}{2}[-d] + \frac{1}{2}[h]$$

for $\overline{B}c_2$ if several loci are taken into consideration. We know that half of the progeny in either of the backcross generations will be heterozygous like the F_1, and rest, *i.e.* $\left(1-\frac{1}{2}\right)$, homozygous. Generalized expressions for expected means of backcross generations are:

$$\overline{Bc}_{n1} = m + \left[1 - \left(\frac{1}{2}\right)^n\right][d] + \left(\frac{1}{2}\right)^n [h]$$

and $$\overline{B}_{c_{n2}} = m - \left[1 - \left(\frac{1}{2}\right)^n\right][d] + \left(\frac{1}{2}\right)^n [h$$

where $\overline{Bc}_{n1}$ is mean of nth backcross to the larger parent and $\overline{Bc}_{n2}$ is the mean of nth backcross to smaller parent.

It is important to note that the mean expressions of parental and backcross generations depend upon the distribution of genes with increasing and decreasing effects between the parental strains. On the other hand, the mean expressions of progenies obtained by sib-mating and families produced by selfing the F_1 and subsequent generations are not influenced by genic distribution between the parental strains which produced them. An example will explain this point. Imagine two loci each with two alleles, *viz* A_1, A_2 and B_1, B_2. Let the genetic constitution of two parental strains be $A_1A_1B_1B_1$ and $A_2A_2B_2B_2$. The mean expressions of these strains will be $m+d_a+d_b$ and $m-d_a-d_b$, respectively, in the absence of non-allelic interaction. On the other hand, if the genotypes of parental strains are $A_1A_1B_2B_2$, and $A_2A_2B_1B_1$ the mean expressions will be $m+d_a-d_b$ and $m-d_a+d_b$ respectively. Symbol d_a referes to the departure of homozygotes A_1A_1 and A_2A_2 from their origin (mid-parental value), similarly d_b is the deviation of homozygotes B_1B_1, and B_2B_2 from their mid-parental value. (Here we assume that the effects are simply additive). Mean expression thus changes with the distribution of genes.

If one of the parental strain bears all the genes with increasing effects and the other strain possesses all the genes with decreasing effects, genes are said to be associated. On the other hand, when genes with decreasing and increasing effects are equally shared by both the parental strains, genes are said to be dispersed.

3.3. Scaling Tests

If we have the estimates of parameters, m the mid-point, $[d]$ the additive component and $[h]$ the dominance component for a given population, it is possible to calculate the expected value of mean for any generation obtained by selfing, sib-mating or backcrossing (we assume here absence of non-allelic interation). For example, in terms of these parameters, the expected mean of B_{c_1} generation, obtained by crossing F_1 to P_1 is

$$m+\frac{1}{2}[d]+\frac{1}{2}[h].$$

We know from the classical genetics that half the progency in Bc_1 generation is similar to P_1 and the rest like F_1. The mean of B_{c_1} generation could, therefore, be expressed also as

$$\overline{Bc}_1=\frac{1}{2}\overline{P}_1+\frac{1}{2}\overline{F}_1.$$

It we now substitute the expected values of $\overline{P}_1$, $\overline{F}_1$ and $\overline{Bc}_1$ in this expression we get the following relationship:

$$m+\frac{1}{2}[d]+\frac{1}{2}[h]=\frac{1}{2}(m+[d])+\frac{1}{2}(m+[h])$$

or $$m+\frac{1}{2}[d]+\frac{1}{2}[h]=\frac{1}{2}m+\frac{1}{2}[d]+\frac{1}{2}m+\frac{1}{2}[h]$$

or $$m+\frac{1}{2}[d]+\frac{1}{2}[h]=m+\frac{1}{2}[d]+\frac{1}{2}[h]$$

This relationship shows that if only the additive and dominance effects of genes are adequate to explain the inheritance of a character it is possible to find a simple relationship between the expected values of Bc_1,F_1 and P_1 generations. Such relationships could also be derived for other generations provided that the additive-dominance model is adequate, *i.e.*, non-allelic interaction is absent, there is no differential fertility and differential viability. The relationship given above could also be written as

$$2\overline{B}_{c_1}-\overline{P}_1-\overline{F}_1=0$$

In this way it is possible to test the predicted relationships between various generation means and hence test the expectation that the generation means depend only on additive and dominance effects of the genes. Several relationships between expected values of various generations have been developed by Mather (1949) to test the validity of additive-dominance model. These tests of relationships between expected values of generation means have been termed by Mather (1949) as "scaling tests". Commonly employed scaling tests are:

Test

$A \qquad 2\overline{B}_{c_1} - \overline{P}_1 - \overline{F}_1 = 0$

$B \qquad 2\overline{B}_{c_2} - \overline{P}_2 - \overline{F}_1 = 0$

$C \qquad 4\overline{F}_2 - 2\overline{F}_1 - \overline{P}_1 - \overline{P}_2 = 0$

$D \qquad 8\overline{F}_3 - 2\overline{F}_1 - 3\overline{P}_1 - 3\overline{P}_2 = 0$

These scaling tests reduce to zero, within the limits of sampling variation (because the mean measurements of the constituent generations will be subject to sampling fluctuations), if additive-dominance model is satisfactory. Now let us see how to detect the adequacy of additive-dominance model.

Means of various generations are calculated from the data recorded on experimental material. Scaling test is applied by substituting the means of generations appropriate for the chosen scaling test. For example, if mean measurements of parents, F_1 and Bc_1 generations are available, scaling test A can be peformed. It is desirable to replicate the experimental material. The scaling test equals zero, within the limits of sampling variation, when the additive-dominance model is satisfactory. However, for the reason given earlier it will deviate from zero either in plus or minus direction. To test the deviation of A from hypothetical value of zero, 't' test is applied as:

$$t_A = \frac{A - 0}{S.E_A}$$

How to calculate the standard error of A? Statistical theory tells us that variance of a sum or difference of two or more independent sample means is the sum of their variances. For example, variance of $(X - Y)$ or $(X + Y)$ is equal to variance of X plus variance of Y, *i.e.*, $\sigma^2_x + \sigma^2_y$. Now the variance of K_X, where K is a constant, is $K^2 \sigma^2_x$. Therefore, variance of scaling test A (a linear expression), is obtined as:

$$V_A = \text{Var}(2\overline{B}c_1) + \text{Var}(\overline{P}_1) + \text{Var}(\overline{F}_1),$$

$$= 4\sigma^2_{\overline{B}c1} + \sigma^2_{\overline{P}1} + \sigma^2_{\overline{F}1}.$$

Note that we need variances of $\overline{B}_{c_1}$, $\overline{P}_1$ and $\overline{F}_1$ and not the variances of Bc_1, P_1 and F_1 generations. Thus, $V_{\overline{B}c_1}$ is the variance of means of Bc_1 generation. It is calculated as

$$V_{\overline{B}c_1} = \frac{V_{Bc_1}}{n}$$

where V_{Bc1} is the variance of individuals in Bc_1 generation and n is the number of individuals on which observations were recorded in Bc_1 generation and used to calculate $\overline{Bc}_1$. The experimental families should be raised in comparable environments so that differences between the means of various generations are not biased due to non-heritable agencies, which are otherwise likely to be reflected in the estimates of $\overline{P}_1, \overline{P}_2, \overline{F}_1, \overline{F}_2, \overline{B}c_1, \overline{B}c_2$ *etc*. Variances of other scaling tests are calculated as:

$$V_B = 4\,V_{\overline{B}c2} + V_{\overline{P}2} + V_{\overline{F}1}$$

$$V_c = 16V_{\overline{F}2} + 4V_{\overline{F}1} + V_{\overline{P}1} + V_{\overline{P}2}$$

$$V_D = 64V_{\overline{F}3} + 4V_{\overline{F}1} + 9V_{\overline{P}1} + 9V_{\overline{P}2}.$$

The value observed for ratio $\frac{A}{\sqrt{V_A}}$ etc. is referred either to the '*t*' table or table of normal deviates depending upon the number of degrees of freedom involved for scaling test. The degrees of freedom for a scaling test are obtained as sum of degrees of freedom for each generation involved in a scaling test. The later is got as one less than the number of plants on which observations were recorded. Ratios calculated for *B*, *C* and *D* scaling tests are also referred to the '*t*' table or normal devitates depending upon the numbers of degrees of freedom. The null hypothesis for test of significance (H_o) is that A = 0 (or B, C, D *etc*.in place of A of the scaling tests). If the calculated '*t*' value is larger than the table value, an alternate hypothesis (H_1) that A ≠ 0, is accepted. Acceptance of latter conclusion implies that additive and dominance effects of genes are not satisfactory to explain inheritance of character being investigated.

Significance of the '*t*' test suggests two things. Firstly, the model upon which hypothesis is based is not valid. Hence, some parameter (*s*) which specify the situation should be included. Secondly, the scale upon which character has been measured is not satisfactory. Therefore, an appropriate scale must be chosen. Several assumptions involved in the scaling tests are:

(i) All the generations have been raised in comparable environments such that the estimates of mean measurements are not differentially biased by non-heritable agencies.
(ii) Only autosomal inheritance is considered. Genetical behaviour of sex-linked characters will be different from the other characters. Consequently, the proportions of genotypes expected for characters governed by autosomal genes are different from those which are sex-linked.
(iii) There is no maternal inheritance.
(iv) Non-allelic interaction is absent.
(v) There is no differential fertility and viability.

If any one of the assumptions fail the additive-dominance model will be inadequate. For example, if non-allelic interaction is also a source of variation, parameters which specify various kinds of non-allelic interactions have to be incorporated into the model. If genotype × environment interactions has influenced the generation means, it will be necessary to incorporate parameter (s) which specify the same.

A scale upon which measurements are recorded is usually chosen on the basis of convenience. It is assumed that this scale is satisfactory. However, the scale used to measure value of a character may not be satisfactory. In this situation a scale should be sought to transform the original values of data on which simple model is adequate. This aspect will be considered in section 3.4.

3.3.1 Worked Example

Sorghum variety CSV-3 was crossed to IS-9530. Six generations, *viz.* P_1, P_2, F_1, F_2, Bc_1 and Bc_2 of this cross were raised in randomised block design with two replications. Observations were recorded on days to 50 per cent flowering (Table 3.3).

TABLE 3.3 : Showing means and variances of six generations for flowering in sorghum

Generation	No. of Plants observed	Mean	Variance
P_1 (CSV-3)	20	64.825	2.154
P_2 (IS-9530)	20	53.075	7.312
F_1 (CSV-3 × IS-9530)	10	55.100	3.600
F_2	100	58.835	18.270
Bc_1 (CSV–3 × F_1)	10	63.150	18.225
Bc_2 (IS-9530 × F_1)	10	59.550	9.025

Three scaling tests applied to this data are:

$$A = 2\overline{B}c_1 - \overline{P}_1 - \overline{F}_1$$
$$= 2(63.150) - (64.825) - (55.100)$$
$$= 126.300 - 64.825 - 55.100$$
$$= 6.375$$

$$B = 2\overline{B}c_2 - \overline{P}_2 - \overline{F}_1$$
$$= 2(59.550) - (53.075) - (55.100)$$
$$= 119.100 - 53.075 - 55.100$$
$$= 10.925$$

$$C = 4\overline{F}_2 - 2\overline{F}_1 - \overline{P}_1 - \overline{P}_2$$
$$= 4\,(58.835) - 2(55.100) - (64.825) - (53.075)$$
$$= 235.340 - 110.200 - 64.825 - 53.075$$
$$= 7.240$$

From the variances given in Table 3.3. for various generations $V_{\overline{P}_1}, V_{\overline{P}2}, V_{\overline{F}1}, V_{\overline{F}2}, V_{\overline{B}c1}$ and $V_{\overline{B}c2}$ are calculated. Thus,

$$_{\overline{P}1} = \frac{V_{P1}}{n}$$

$$= \frac{2.154}{20}$$

$$= 0.1077$$

Variances of means of other generations are found likwise. Thus,

$$V_{\overline{P}2} = 0.3656 \quad V_{\overline{B}c1} = 1.8225$$

$$V_{\overline{F}1} = 0.3600 \quad V_{\overline{B}c2} = 0.9025$$

$V_{\overline{F}2} = 0.1827$

The test of significance for A scaling test will be:

$$t = \frac{A-0}{S.E._A}$$

$$= \frac{6.375}{\sqrt{[4(1.8225)+0.1077+0.3600]}}$$

$$= \frac{6.375}{2.785}$$

$$= 2.28.$$

This value is significant at five per cent level which implies that the additive-dominance model is not satisfactory. Other scaling tests are also significant which support the conclusion based on the A scaling test (Table 3.4)

TABLE 3.4: Results of 't' tests for scaling tests

Scales	Value observed	't' values
A	6.375 ± 2.785	2.28*
B	10.925 ± 2.082	5.24**
C	7.240 ± 2.199	3.29**

*, ** Significant at 5 and 1 per cent levels respectively.

As pointed out in section 3.3 there are now two alternatives, *viz.* either change the scale or find out which of the model is adequate. However, before we deal with this aspect, a general scaling test will be introduced which is known as Cavalli's Joint Scaling test. This scaling test has two distinct advantages over the scaling tests of Mather (1949). Firstly, Joint scaling test combines, very effectively, several scaling tests into one and offers a more general approach. Secondly, this test provides best possible estimates of all the parameters needed to describe differences among the means of families, in addition to the test of adequacy of additive-dominance model. If more than six generation means are available, this method also permits the estimation of parameters which specify digenic non-allelic interaction if it is present.

3.3.2 Joint Scaling Test

In the Cavalli's (1952) joint scaling test (desribed by Mather and Jinks, 1971, 1977) parameters m, $[d]$ and $[h]$ are estimated from the observed means of three or more generations. Estimates of these parameters are then used to calculate expected means which are then compared with observed means. At least three generation means are necessary for the estimation of m, $[d]$ and $[h]$. However, when only three generation means are available a perfect fit solution has to be obtained. A perfect fit solution assumes perfect agreement between observed means of the three generations and their expected means. When only three generations are available for the estimation of 3 parameters no degree of freedom is left to test the adequacy of additive-dominance model. However, with 4 or more generations to estimate m, $[d]$ and $[h]$, a χ^2 test is possible to test the adequacy of additive-dominance model. Hence, at least $n + 1$ generation means are necessary to permit a χ^2 test (n being the number of parameters to be estimated).

When more than three generation means are available to estimate three parameters a weighted least-square analysis is employed. In this approach reciprocal of variance of each of the means is used as a weight. Why should we use a least-square analysis? Since three parameters are to be estimated from more than three generation means several different relationships could be employed to calculate them. Least-square method enables precise estimation of these parameters, such that the deviations of observed from expected values are least. Why should we use weight? The means of various generations may not be known with equal precision. Hence, the means are weighted.

Let us use the data presented in Table 3.3 to estimate m, $[d]$ and $[h]$ following Cavalli (1952). The generations, observed means, coefficients of three parameters for each generation along with weights of six generations are presented in Table 3.5.

TABLE 3.5 : Generations, means, weights and coefficients for days to 50 per cent flowering in sorghum

Generations	Weights	Coefficients			Observed means
		m	[*d*]	[*h*]	
P_1	9.2850	1	1	–	64.825
P_2	2.7352	1	–1	–	53.075
F_1	2.7777	1	–	1	55.100
F_2	5.4734	1	–	0.5	58.835
Bc_1	0.5486	1	0.5	0.5	63.150
Bc_2	1.1080	1	-0.5	0.5	59.550

Weights shown in the second column of Table 3.5 are calculated as:

$$\frac{1}{\text{Variance of mean}}.$$

For example, weight for P_1 is calculated as:

$$\frac{1}{0.1077} = 9.2850.$$

Three normal equations are required to calculate three parameters, *viz.*, *m*, [*d*] and [*h*]. First equation is obtained by multiplying each element of row in the Table 3.5 by the product of weight and coefficient of *m* and adding over six generations. The weight of P_1 is 9.2850 and coefficient of *m* is 1, hence multiply each element in the row of P_1 (including the *m* itself) by 1 × 9.285 = 9.285. In similar manner each element of other rows are multiplied by the product of their weights and coefficients of *m*. Result of such a multiplication is presented in Table 3.6. Total at the end of this table gives the first normal equation.

TABLE: 3.6 : Multipilication of elements by (weight × coefficient of *m*)

	m	[*d*]	[*h*]	Observed mean
	9.2850	9.2850	–	601.9001
	2.7352	–2.7352	–	145.1707
	2.7777	–	2.7777	153.0512
	5.4734	–	2.7367	322.0274
	0.5486	0.2743	0.2743	34.6440
	1.1080	–0.5540	0.5540	65.9814
Total	21.9279	6.2701	6.3427	1322.7748

Second normal equation is obtained in similar fashion, however, coefficients of [*d*] are used for multiplication of the elements of rows instead of the coefficients of *m*. The result of such a multiplication is presented in Table 3.7.

TABLE 3.7: Showing multiplication of elements by (coefficient of [*d*] × weight)

	m	[*d*]	[*h*]	Observed mean
	9.2850	9.2850	–	601.9001
	–2.7352	2.7352	–	–145.1707
	0.2743	0.1371	0.1371	17.3220
	–0.5540	0.2770	–0.2770	–32.9907
Total	6.2701	12.4343	–0.1399	441.0607

Multiplication of each element in six rows of Table 3.5 by the product of coefficient of [*h*] and weight provides information required for third normal equation (Table 3.8). If the coefficient of a parameter in the row is zero, product will be zero and hence entire row will be deleted in the table prepared to calculate the normal equations. For example, coefficient of [*h*] is zero for P_1 and P_2, hence these rows have been deleted in Table 3.8.

TABLE 3.8 : Showing the multiplication of elements by (coefficient [*h*] × weight)

	m	[*d*]	[*h*]	Observed mean
	2.7777	–	2.7777	153.0512
	2.7367	–	1.3683	161.0137
	0.2743	0.1371	0.1371	17.3220
	0.5540	–0.2770	0.2770	32.9907
Total	6.3427	–0.1399	4.5601	364.3776

The three normal equations so derived are arranged in the matrix form:

$$\underset{J}{\begin{bmatrix} 21.9279 & 6.2701 & 6.3427 \\ 6.2701 & 12.4343 & -0.1399 \\ 6.3427 & -0.1399 & 4.5601 \end{bmatrix}} \underset{M}{\begin{bmatrix} \hat{m} \\ [\hat{d}] \\ [\hat{h}] \end{bmatrix}} = \underset{S}{\begin{bmatrix} 1322.7748 \\ 441.0607 \\ 364.3776 \end{bmatrix}}$$

Those elements of three normal equations which are obtained from the coefficients of *m*, [*d*] and [*h*] are collected in a matrix known as information matrix denoted by *J*. Parameters to be estimated *viz. m*, [*d*] and [*h*], are arranged in a column matrix of parameters, which is denoted by *M*. Elements of normal equations obtained as a result of multiplication of observed values by coefficients and weight, are arranged in a column matrix denoted by S and known as matrix of scores. Estimates of the parameters *m*, [*d*] and [*h*] are obtained as:

$$M = SJ^{-1}$$

Where J^{-1} is inverse of information matrix. The inversion of a matrix can be got in several ways. However, a method presented in Appendix I at the end of this chapter, may be convenient for use. Inversion of *J* matrix of the present example results in.

$$\begin{bmatrix} 0.102632 & -0.053378 & -0.14439 \\ -0.053378 & 0.108211 & 0.077563 \\ -0.14439 & 0.077563 & 0.422506 \end{bmatrix}$$

Inverse of *J* matrix is a variance-covariance matrix in which the diagonal elements represent variances of the estimates of parameters *m*, [*d*] and [*h*]. Now, arrange the matrices as:

$$\underset{M}{\begin{bmatrix} m \\ [d] \\ [h] \end{bmatrix}} = \underset{J^{-1}}{\begin{bmatrix} 0.102632 & -0.053378 & -0.14439 \\ -0.053378 & 0.108211 & 0.077563 \\ -0.14439 & 0.077563 & 0.422506 \end{bmatrix}} \underset{S}{\begin{bmatrix} 1322.7748 \\ 441.0607 \\ 364.3776 \end{bmatrix}}$$

Estimates of the parameters *m*, [*d*] and [*h*] are obtained as:

$$\hat{m} = (0.102632 \times 1322.7748) + (-0.053378 \times 441.0607) + (-0.14439 \times 364.3776) = 59.6036$$

$$\hat{d} = (-0.053378 \times 1322.7748) + (0.108211 \times 441.0607) + (0.077563 \times 364.3776)$$
$$= 5.3827$$

$$\hat{h} = (-0.14439 \times 1322.7748) + (0.077563 \times 441.0607) + (0.422506 \times 364.3776)$$
$$= 2.8337$$

The standard errors of the estimates of these parameters are calculated as:

$$S.E.\ \hat{m} = (0.102632)^{1/2}$$
$$= 0.3203$$

$$S.E.\ \hat{d} = (0.108211)^{1/2}$$
$$= 0.3289$$

$$S.E.\ \hat{h} = (0.422506)^{1/2}$$
$$= 0.6500$$

The test of significance revealed that the three parameters are significantly different from zero.

Chi-square test can be employed to test the adequacy of additive-dominance model because 6 generation means are available to estimate 3 parameters. If the model is satisfactory there should be a close agreement between the observed and expected means of six generations, within the limits of sampling variation. The expected values of means are obtained from the coefficients of m, $[d]$ and $[h]$ and the estimated values of these parameters. For example, the expected mean of F_2 generation is:

$$\overline{F}_2 = m + \frac{1}{2}[h]$$

$$= (59.6036) + \frac{1}{2}(-2.8337)$$

$$= 58.1867$$

Expected means of other generations are similarly calculated (Table 3.9). Summation of deviation squared × weights over six generations yields χ^2 for (6–3) = 3 degrees of freedom. The χ^2 is found to be 35.0546.

TABLE 3.9 : Observed and expected means, $(\text{deviation})^2$ and $\text{deviation}^2 \times$ weight

Generations	Means		$(\text{deviation})^2$	$(\text{deviation})^2 \times$ weight
	Observed	Expected		
P_1	64.825	64.9863	0.0260	0.2414
P_2	53.075	54.2209	1.3130	3.5913
F_1	55.100	56.7699	2.7885	7.7456
F_2	58.835	58.1687	0.4439	2.4296
Bc_1	63.150	60.8781	5.1615	2.8316
Bc_2	59.550	55.4954	16.4397	18.2151
			$\chi^2 =$	35.0546

When this value is referred to the table of χ^2 for 3 degrees of freedom probability of getting the deviations as large as these are found to be less than 0.01. Hence, the additive-dominance model is not satisfactory.

3.4 Transformation of Scale

Worked examples in sections 3.3.1 and 3.3.2 suggested that the additive-dominance model was not satisfactory to explain the inheritance of days to 50 per cent bloom in the experimental material. Inadequacy of the additive-dominance model implies that one (or more) of the assumptions upon which the model is based have not been satisfied.

Environmental agencies are likely to contribute a negligible proportion to the mean measurements of various generations provided appropriate experimental design has been adopted and various generations as well as the individuals within each generation have been raised in comparable environments. However, if the experimental material has been raised in more than one environment, genotype-environment interaction may be of some consequence. Parameters specifying interaction of genotypes with environmental agencies should, therefore, be incorporated in the model (Chapter 8).

Most of the crop species of economic importance are hermaphrodite and hence characters of interest are governed by genes borne on autosomal chromosomes.

Differences between reciprocal crosses are suggestive of maternal or cytoplasmic inheritance. Reciprocal crosses usually do not exhibit differences with respect to quantitative characters. Large part of the variation observed for metrical traits is governed by nuclear borne genes. However, for differences of some seedling characters among the sexually propagated individuals and for differences among the members of a clone cytoplasmic or maternal inheritance may be of some importance. For details reader is referred to Mather and Jinks (1971).

Differential fertility and/or viability in segregating generations may be responsible for the inadequacy of additive-dominance model. It was shown in section3.2 that the mean measurements of F_1, F_2, F_3, ...F_n generations lie on same side of mid-point (m), although with diminishing deviations from it. This is true even when non-allelic interaction is present. According to Mather and Jinks (1971) a scale should be regarded as adequate upon which the mean measurements of $F_1, F_2, F_3, ..., F_n$, fall reasonably close to but on different sides of mid-point. Differential fertility (and/or viability) may be of significance while dealing with intergeneric or interspecific crosses. However, disturbances of the kind produced by these agencies may also be encountered while handling varietal crosses.

Data recorded for any character are obtained in the form which is most convenient for measurement. Thus phenotypic values are recorded in grammes, centimetres, litres or whatever unit of measurement is most convenient. It is possible that each character has its "natural" scale, a scale upon which the biological process expressed in character works. The additive-dominance model assumes that the effects of genes involved are additive. This suggests that the total effect of all the genes, which govern the inheritance of a character, is simple sum of their individual effects. This need not be true for all the characters and even for all genes responsible for a given character. Genes may act in a multiplicative fashion such that their joint effect is a product and not the simple sum of their individual effects. The additive-dominance model will then fail for such characters.

When genes act in multiplicative fashion they form a geometric series of phenotypes such as 2, 4, 8, 16,.......representing contribution of 1, 2, 3, 4, ... active alleles, respectively. Variation observed for such characters tends to be skewed into an asymmetric curve. The mean expressions of F_1 and F_2 generations tend to be nearer to the mean measurement of one of the parents. Geometric mean of two numbers is given by square root of their product. For example, if one of the strains measures 4 units and other 9 units, mean expression of F_1 will be approximately $\sqrt{4 \times 9} = \sqrt{36} = 6$ units. Additive gene action, on the other hand, produces an arithmetic series of phenotypic values such as 2, 4, 6, 8, ... being the contributions of 1, 2, 3, 4, ... genes, respectively. Additive gene action produces a normal phenotypic distribution with mean expression of F_1 generation being intermediate to the means of two parental strains. Changing the scale may convert multiplicativity in effects to additivity in effects. Let us assume that the genotypic value of AA is Y_a and that of BB is Y_b. Aggregate value of genotype $AABB$ will be Y_aY_b if genes act in a multiplicative fashion. On the other hand, it will be $Y_a + Y_b$ if the effects of genes are additive. In terms of logarithm, product of two numbers will be the sum of their logarithmic values. Thus log (Y_a.. Y_b) will be log Ya + log Y_b . This can be explained with an example. Suppose genotypic value of *AA* is 4 units and genotypic value of *BB* is 9 units. If gene action is multiplicative the aggregate genotypic value of *AABB* would be $4 \times 9 = 36$ units rather than $4 + 9 = 13$ units. If the values are transformed to log scale, multiplicativity could be converted to additivity. Thus log 4 + log 9 = 0.602 + 0.954 = 1.556. Value of 36 on log scale is also 1.556. This shows that multiplicativity in action of genes is coverted to additivity by means of change of scale. Many relations are possible between the action of genes and phenotype which may suggest a suitable choice of scale to restore additivity in action of genes. However, it is very difficult to ascertain as to how various genes governing the inheritance of a character combine to produce their effects and whether all the genes combine their effects in similar fashion. Hence, whenever additive-dominance model fails we can transform the data empirically to a different scale in an attempt to satisfy the assumptions.

The nature of a character may sometimes suggest the choice of an appropriate scale. For example, yield of *kapas* in cotton may be thought of as a product of number of bolls per plant and weight of lint per boll. Apparently this is a multiplicative relation and suggests a log transformation to restore additivity. However, it is not necessary that transformation to log scale will satisfy the assumption of additivity of gene effects. Although the component characters appear to combine multiplicatively, genes governing the inheritance of these traits may not act in a multiplicative fashion to produce the final effect. For this reason there is no justification for drawing theoretical conclusion about physiology of gene action when a particular scale satisfies the assumption of additivity of effects of genes.

Conversion of original units, upon which measurements have been recorded, to some other units such as logarithms, reciprocals, square roots, or some other function, according to what is most appropriate for the purpose for which the data are to be used is known as transformation of scale. One scale may be suitable for one character but may not be suitable for other. Similarly a given scale may be satisfactory for an attribute in one environment but not in other. A scale may be satisfactory for one cross but not for others. A given scale may not be satisfactory for same cross in different environments.

It is necessary that original data is transformed to other scale before means, variances and other statistics are calculated. The occurrence, degree and direction of dominance also tends to change with change of scale. Likewise occurrence of non-allelic interaction is also influenced by transformation of a scale. This aspect will be explained with the help of an example.

Let us consider two loci, each with two alleles *viz.* A_1, A_2 and B_1, B_2, which influence the expression of a character. Suppose that the phenotypes of nine genotypes, with respect to these loci, are measured on an arithmetic scale (Table 3.10). It is apparent that gene A_2 is partially dominant to A_1 at all the phases of B_1, B_2 locus. However, substitution of A_1 in A_2A_2, causes a shift of 5 units, 7 units and 9 units on the scale of measurement when phases at second locus are B_2B_2, B_1B_2 and B_1B_1, respectively. This implies that B_1, B_2 locus influences the effect of gene substitution at A_1, A_2 locus. Partial dominance of B_2 over B_1 is observed at B_1, B_2 locus at all the phases of A_1, A_2. The effect of substitution of B_1 for B_2 also depends upon the phases at A_1, A_2 locus. On arithmetic scale we observed dominance and digenic non-allelic gene action.

TABLE 3.10 : Effect of scale on gene effects

	Genotypes			Choice of scale
	A_2A_2	A_1A_2	A_1A_1	
B_2B_2	4	9	16	Arithmetic
	2	3	4	Square root
	0.602	0.954	1.204	Log
B_1B_2	9	16	25	Arithmetic
	3	4	5	Square root
	0.954	1.204	1.398	Log
B_1B_1	16	25	36	Arithmetic
	4	5	6	Square root
	1.204	1.398	1.556	Log

Suppose, for some reason, the character is measured on a square-root scale. On this scale, A_1A_2 is mid-way between A_1A_1 and A_2A_2 at all the phases of B_1, B_2. Moreover, effect of substituting allele A_1 for A_2 in A_2A_2 is identical at B_2B_2, B_1B_2 and B_1B_1 phases. Similar effect is also noticed for substitution of A_1 for A_2 in A_1A_2 at all the three phase of B_1, B_2. Hence.

there is no dominance at A_1, A_2 locus and there is also no evidence of non-allelic interaction, because phases at B_1, B_2 locus do not influence the effect of substitution at A_1, A_2 locus. Similar situation is observed for B_1, B_2 locus. Only additive gene action is observed on this scale.

Lastly, assume that the character is measured on a logarithmic scale. On this scale, allele A_1 appears to be partially dominant to A_2 at B_2B_2, B_1B_2 and B_1B_1 phases. The effect of substituting A_1 for A_2 in A_2A_2 is 0.352, 0.250 and 0.194 at B_2B_2, B_1B_2 and B_1B_1 phases, respectively. The effect of substitution is largest at B_2B_2 phase unlike that observed for the arithmetic scale. Effect of substitution of B_1 for B_2 is likewise determined by phases at A_1, A_2 locus. The effect of substitution of B_1 for B_2 is largest at A_2A_2 and lowest at A_1A_1 phase. On this scale both dominance and non-allelic interaction effects are observed.

Thus, the occurrence, direction and degree of dominance as well as non-allelic interaction of genes is not an unconditional property of the genes as assumed in Mendelian genetics, but the occurrence, degree and direction of dominance and non-allelic interaction is a function of scale upon which expression of a character is measured. The choice of an appropriate scale may not enable complete elimination of effects due to non-allelic interaction, however, it can help to minimise the magnitude.

3.5 Non-allelic Interaction of Genes and Linkage

Phenotypic manifestation of genes at a locus may be influenced by genes present at other loci (section 3.4) which is known as non-allelic interaction. Since the inheritance of quantitative characters is governed by genes at several loci, non-allelic interaction of genes is not unexpected. We will restrict our discussion to interaction between genes at two loci, *i.e.*, digenic non-allelic interaction.

Let us assume a simple situation where a character is determined by genes at two loci each having two alleles, *viz.* A_1, A_2 and B_1, B_2. Nine genotypes are possible with respect to these two loci. Eight parameters are, therefore, necessary to describe differences among the phenotypic expressions of these genotypes. Two parameters are already known to us, *viz.* d_a which represents the deviation of either homozygote (A_1A_1 or A_2A_2) from the origin and h_a which measures the deviation of heterozygote A_1A_2 from the origin (section 3.2). Departure of genotypes B_1B_1 and B_2B_2

from their mid-parental value may be similarly described by a parameter d_b, and the deviation of B_1B_2 from mid-parental value by h_b. These four parameters describe the main effects of genes.

We have now to introduce parameters which specify non-allelic interactions of various kinds. When the phenotypic expression of homozygous genotype, say A_1A_1 or A_2A_2, is influenced by the homozygous genotypes (B_1B_1 or B_2B_2) at second locus, the non-allelic interaction is said to be of homozygote × homozygote or additive × additive kind. This interaction is denoted by a symbol i_{ab}. The sign of this parameter depends upon signs of main effects *i.e.*, d_a and d_b. For example, if genotype of a strain is $A_1A_1B_2B_2$, sign of i_{ab} will be negative because the sign of d_b is negative. Hence the phenotypic expression of $A_1A_1B_2B_2$ could be written as:

$$m+d_a - d_b - i_{ab}$$

If the genes at two loci do not interact then the difference between A_1A_1 and A_2A_2 will be same at B_1B_1 and B_2B_2 phases. This relationship could be expressed as:

$$A_1A_1B_1B_1 - A_2A_2B_1B_1 = A_1A_1B_2B_2 - A_2A_2B_2B_2$$
$$\text{or } A_1A_1B_1B_1 - A_2A_2B_1B_1 - A_1A_1B_2B_2 + A_2A_2B_2B_2 = 0.$$

In order to describe the additive × additive kind of non-allelic interaction for several loci, which govern the inheritance of a quantitative characters, two facts have to be kept in mind. Firstly, signs of parameters specifying additive × additive kind of digenic non-allelic interactions may differ from each other. For example, i_{ab} may be positive but i_{ac} may have a negative sign. Secondly, magnitude of each of the parameters specifying additive × additive kind of digenic non-allelic interaction may not be same. Keeping these facts in mind we prefer to write additive × additive kind of non-allelic interaction over all the loci as [i]. Parameter [i] is, therefore, sum total of additive × additive kind of digenic non-allelic interaction over all loci.

Phenotype of an homozygote at a locus may be influenced by heterozygous genotype at the second locus or *vice versa*. For instance, phenotypic expression of A_1A_1 may be influenced by genotype B_1B_2 at second locus. This kind of digenic non-allelic interaction is known as homozygote × heterozygote or additive × dominance kind, which is denoted by a symbol j_{ab} . By the same analogy, phenotypic expression of A_1A_2 may be influenced by B_1B_1 or B_2B_2 phases at second locus or *vice versa*. This kind of digenic non-allelic interaction is called as heterozygote × homozygote or dominance × additive kind. Additive × dominance kind of digenic non-allelic interaction implies that the superiority or inferiority of an heterozygote or homozygote does not depend solely on its genetic constitution but also upon the genic phase at other locus. If several loci influencing the expression of a metric character are taken into consideration, the homo × hetero and hetero × homo kinds of digenic non-allelic interactions may be treated as one and denoted by a symbol [j], where [ ] suggests that the signs and magnitudes of additive × dominance (or dominance × additive) kind of interactions may not be same and it is the algebraic sum of all increments.

Third kind of digenic non-allelic interaction could be identified when phenotypic expression of heterozygote at one locus is influenced by heterozygous genotype at second locus. This digenic non-allelic interaction belongs to heterozygote × heterozygote or dominance × dominance kind. Phenotype of A_1A_2 for example, may be influenced by genotype B_1B_2 at the second locus or *vice versa*. This kind of non-allelic interaction is described by a parameter l_{ab}. Dominance × dominance kind of digenic non-allelic interaction is denoted by [l] when several loci are taken into consideration. [l] like the [i] and [j] takes into consideration differences in the signs as well as magnitudes of digenic non-allelic interactions, and is algebraic sum of all l increments.

Now we have six parameters to specify various kinds of gene effects, *viz*. m, [d], [h], [i], [j] and [l]. We have followed Hayman and Mather (1955) and Mather and Jinks (1971, 1977 and 1980) in the use of these symbols. Gamble (1962) on the other hand, used m, [a], [d], [aa], [ad] and [dd] to describe mid-parental value or constant, additive, dominance, additive × additive, additive × dominance, and dominance × dominance gene effects, respectively. Thus symbols [d], [h], [i], [j] and [l] of Mather and Jinks (1971) could be regarded as equivalent to Gamble's (1962) [a], [d], [aa], [ad] and [dd], respectively.

Phenotype of any generation, produced by either selfing or back crossing or sib-mating series, could be described in terms of these parameters. For example, phenotypes of $A_1A_1B_1B_1$ and $A_2A_2B_2B_2$ could be described, in the absence of digenic non-allelic interaction as:

$$A_1A_1B_1B_1 = m + d_a + d_b$$

and $A_2A_2B_2B_2 = m - d_a - d_b$

If the genes manifest non-allelic interaction, phenotypes could be expressed as:

$$A_1A_1B_1B_1 = m + d_a + d_b + i_{ab}$$
$$A_2A_2B_2B_2 = m - d_a - d_b + i_{ab}$$

Sign of parameter i_{ab} associated with $A_2A_2B_2B_2$ is positive because the product of two negatives is positive, *e.g.*, $-d_a \times (-d_b) = +i_{ab}$.

If several loci are taken into consideration, mean measurements of strains with larger (P_1) and smaller (P_2) manifestations could be expressed as:

$$\overline{P}_1 = m + [d] + [i]$$

and $\overline{P}_2 = m - [d] + [i]$

Mean phenotypic expression of F_1 produced by crossing P_1 and P_2 could be written as:

$$\overline{F}_1 = m + [h] + [l].$$

It was pointed out in section 3.2 that the mean expressions of true breeding parental lines and backcross generations are influenced by the distribution of genes between the parental lines. This is true in the presence of digenic non-allelic interaction also. For example, the mean expressions of $A_1A_1B_2B_2$ and $A_2A_2B_1B_1$ would be :

$$A_1A_1B_2B_2 = m + d_a - d_b - i_{ab}$$

and $A_2A_2B_1B_1 = m - d_a + d_b - i_{ab}$

However, mean expression of F_1 generation produced by crossing these parental lines will not differ from the one given above because the sign of $[h]$ does not depend upon association or dispersion of genes between the parental lines, like $[d]$.

The coefficients associated with parameters specifying three kinds of digenic non-allelic interactions are simple to find. For example, mean of Bc_1 generation ($A_1A_1B_1B_1 \times A_1A_2B_1B_2$) in the absence of digenic non-allelic interaction is:

$$m + \frac{1}{2}d_a + \frac{1}{2}d_b + \frac{1}{2}h_a + \frac{1}{2}h_b$$

However, if digenic non-allelic interaction is present $\overline{Bc}_1$ will be:

$$m+\frac{1}{2}d_a+\frac{1}{2}d_b+\frac{1}{2}h_a+\frac{1}{2}h_b+\frac{1}{4}i_{ab}+\frac{1}{4}j_{ab}+\frac{1}{4}j_{ba}+\frac{1}{4}l_{ab}$$

Coefficients of interaction parameters are the products of coefficients of main parameters. Mean expressions of Bc_1 and Bc_2 generations, when digenic non-allelic interaction is present, could be expressed as:

$$\overline{Bc}_1 = m+\frac{1}{2}[d]+\frac{1}{2}[h]+\frac{1}{4}[i]+\frac{1}{4}[j]+\frac{1}{4}[l]$$

$$\overline{Bc}_2 = m-\frac{1}{2}[d]+\frac{1}{2}[h]+\frac{1}{4}[i]-\frac{1}{4}[j]+\frac{1}{4}[l]$$

These expressions account for association or dispersion of genes between the parental lines, in addition to differences in the magnitudes and signs of gene effects over several loci.

When digenic non-allelic interaction is present, two things should be kept in mind, namely

(i) if there is a parameter $[d]$ in the mean expression of a generation, there may be a parameter $[i]$, and
(ii) if there are $[h]$ and $[d]$ in the mean expression of a generation there may be $[j]$ and $[l]$ components as well.

Mean expression of F_2 generation, in the presence of digenic non-allelic interaction, is:

$$m+\frac{1}{2}[h]+\frac{1}{4}[l].$$

Mid-point in section 3.1 was described as mean of two homozygous parental strains. This definition does not hold good if digenic non-allelic interaction is present. Why? Let us see.

Let us take a simple case of two loci each having two alleles, *viz.* A_1, A_2 and B_1, B_2. There will be four true breeding strains with respect to these loci, *viz.* $A_1A_1B_1B_1$, $A_2A_2B_2B_2$, $A_1A_1B_2B_2$ and $A_2A_2B_1B_1$. A cross capable of segregating for both gene pairs could be initiated by crossing either $A_1A_1B_1B_1$ with $A_2A_2B_2B_2$ or $A_1A_1B_2B_2$ with $A_2A_2B_1B_1$. Mid-parental value of the cross $A_1A_1B_1B_1 \times A_2A_2B_2B_2$ is

Genotype	Phenotype
$A_1A_1B_1B_1$	$m + d_a + d_b + i_{ab}$
$A_2A_2B_2B_2$	$m - d_a - d_b + i_{ab}$

$$\text{mid parental value} = \frac{m+d_a+d_b+i_{ab}+m-d_a-d_b+i_{ab}}{2}$$

$$= m + i_{ab}$$

Mid-parental value of the cross $A_1A_1B_2B_2 \times A_2A_2B_1B_1$ is $m - i_{ab}$.

Mid-parental value of neither cross is m. However, these two crosses will produce true breeding genotypes $A_1A_1B_1B_1$, $A_1A_1B_2B_2$, $A_2A_2B_1B_1$ and $A_2A_2B_2B_2$ in equal proportions by prolonged inbreeding, provided the two gene pairs are independently inherited. Mean expressions of these true breeding strains is m since the d_a, d_b and i_{ab} cancel as shown below:

Genotype	Phenotype
$A_1A_1B_1B_1$	$m + d_a + d_b + i_{ab}$
$A_1A_1B_2B_2$	$m + d_a - d_b - i_{ab}$
$A_2A_2B_1B_1$	$m - d_a + d_b - i_{ab}$
$A_2A_2B_2B_2$	$m - d_a - d_b + i_{ab}$
mean	m

According to Mather and Jinks (1971) mid-points is "the mean of inbred population derived from a cross between two true breeding lines". This definition of m is satisfactory whether digenic non-allelic interaction is present or absent.

Following Mather and Jinks (1971) non-allelic interaction may be broadly classified into two types, *viz.* complementary and duplicate. When the signs of $[h]$ and $[l]$ are in same direction the digenic non-allelic interaction is said to be of complementary type. On the other hand, when the signs of $[h]$ and $[l]$ are opposite the digenic non-allelic interaction is referred to as duplicate type.

Metrical characters are predominantly governed by nuclear-borne genes. Hence polygenes exhibit effect of linkage. Mean expressions of non-segregating generations, such as the true breeding parental strains and F_1 between them, do not reflect the effects of linkage. However, mean expressions of F_2 and subsequent generations are influenced by linkage. How? Let us see.

Suppose, two true breeding parental strains are $A_1A_1B_1B_1$ and $A_2A_2B_2B_2$ in genetic constitution. Assume that genes at two loci *viz.* A_1, A_2 and B_1, B_2, are linked and that the recombination frequency is p (= 1 – q). Also assume that digenic non-allelic interaction is involved in the inheritance of character being studied. The genetic constitution of F_1 of these strains will be A_1B_1/A_2B_2. This F_1 will produce four kinds of gametes, *i.e.*, A_1B_1, A_1B_2, A_2B_1 and A_2B_2. Among these gametic types, A_1B_1 and A_2B_2 are parental whereas A_1B_2 and A_2B_1 are recombinant. Frequency of recombinant gametes will be p. And the frequency of parental types will be q (= 1 – p). Two kinds of recombinant gametes will be produced in equal proportion, *i.e.*, pA_1B_2 and pA_2B_1. Frequencies of parental type gametes will be qA_1B_1 and qA_2B_2. Random union of these gametes will result in nine genotypes (Tables 3.11 and 3.12). Let us assume that the frequencies of four kinds of gametes among the male and female individuals of the population are equal. Mean expression of F_2 generation could be obtained as sum of the product of frequency × phenotype (in terms of m, d_a, d_b, i_{ab}, h_a, h_b, l_{ab} parameters) over nine genotypes. The mean of the F_2 generation will be as shown below, if the genes are in coupling phase:

$$m+\frac{1}{2}h_a+\frac{1}{2}h_b+\frac{1}{2}(1-2p)i_{ab}+\frac{1}{2}(1-2pq)l_{ab}$$

TABLE 3.11: Random union of F_1 gametes, genotypes in F_2 and their frequencies

		Male gametes and frequency			
		A_1B_1 1/2q	A_1B_2 1/2p	A_2B_1 1/2p	A_2B_2 1/2q
Female gametes and frequency	A_1B_1 1/2q	$A_1A_1B_1B_1$ 1/4q^2	$A_1A_1B_1B_2$ 1/4pq	$A_1A_2B_1B_1$ 1/4pq	$A_1A_2B_1B_2$ 1/4q^2
	A_1B_2 1/2p	$A_1A_1B_1B_2$ 1/4pq	$A_1A_1B_2B_2$ 1/4p^2	$A_1A_2B_1B_2$ 1/4p^2	$A_1A_2B_2B_2$ 1/4pq
	A_2B_1 1/2p	$A_1A_2B_1B_1$ 1/4pq	$A_1A_2B_1B_2$ 1/4p^2	$A_2A_2B_1B_1$ 1/4p^2	$A_2A_2B_1B_2$ 1/4pq
	A_2B_2 1/2q	$A_1A_2B_1B_2$ 1/4q^2	$A_1A_2B_2B_2$ 1/4pq	$A_2A_2B_1B_2$ 1/4pq	$A_2A_2B_2B_2$ 1/4q^2

TABLE 3.12: Genotypes, frequency of genotypes and phenotypes in F_2 generation

Genotypes	Frequency	Phenotypes
$A_1A_1B_1B_1$	$1/4q^2$	$m + d_a + d_b + i_{ab}$
$A_1A_1B_1B_2$	$1/2pq$	$m + d_a + h_b + j_{ab}$
$A_1A_1B_2B_2$	$1/4p^2$	$m + d_a - d_b - i_{ab}$
$A_1A_2B_1B_1$	$1/2pq$	$m + h_a + d_b + j_{ba}$
$A_1A_2B_1B_2$	$1/2p^2 + 1/2q^2$	$m + h_a + h_b + l_{ab}$
$A_1A_2B_2B_2$	$1/2pq$	$m + h_a - d_b - j_{ba}$
$A_2A_2B_1B_1$	$1/4p^2$	$m - d_a + d_b - i_{ab}$
$A_2A_2B_1B_2$	$1/2pq$	$m - d_a + h_b - j_{ab}$
$A_2A_2B_2B_2$	$1/4q^2$	$m - d_a - d_b + i_{ab}$

However, when the genes are linked in repulsion in the parental strains, mean expression of F_2 will be

$$m+\frac{1}{2}h_a+\frac{1}{2}h_b-\frac{1}{2}(1-2p)i_{ab}+\frac{1}{2}(1-2pq)l_{ab}$$

It should be apparent from the mean expression of F_2 given above that in the absence of non-allelic interaction $\overline{F}_2$ will be $m+\frac{1}{2}h_a+\frac{1}{2}h_b$. Thus, linkage has no effect on the mean expression of F_2 generation in the absence of non-allelic interaction. It can be shown that the mean expressions of generations produced by selfing series are not influenced by linkage in the absence of non-allelic interaction. However, when non-allelic interaction is present, effect of linkage on mean expression depends upon the strength of linkage, *i.e.*, *p*.

3.5.1 Estimation of Components of Means

It was mentioned in section 3.3 that significance of *t* values for scaling tests and/or χ^2 for joint scaling test suggests inadequacy of the simple additive-dominance model. In some cases choice of an appropriate scale could be helpful to obtain a satisfactory fit. Nevertheless, when inadequacy is due to digenic or higher order non-allelic interaction, it is desirable to incorporate parameters specifying non-allelic interactions of various kinds and to attempt to find the adequacy of model. Let us assume a simple situation of digenic non-allelic interaction which is satisfactory in most of the cases.

Hayman (1958), Gamble (1962) and Mather and Jinks (1971) proposed procedures to obtain the estimates of six parameters.

Hayman (1958) developed a general method to estimate *m, d, h, i, j* and *l* from mean measurements of six or more generations. In the matrix form estimates of six parameters could be obtained as:

$$Y = C_1X_1 + C_2X_2,$$

where Y is the vector (see Appendix I) of observed generation means, C_1 and C_2 are matrices comprising of coefficients of *m, d, h* and *i, j, l*, respectively, expected for each generation mean, X_1 and X_2 refer to the column vectors consisting of parameters *m,d, h* and *i, j, l*, respectively, to be estimated. If E is the diagonal matrix of error variances corresponding to six generation means, estimates of six parameters are obtained as:

$$\left[\frac{\hat{X}_1}{\hat{X}_2}\right] = \hat{X} = (C'E^{-1}C)^{-1}CE^{-1}Y,$$

Where C' is the transpose of C matrix. Error variances of estimated parameters are computed as:

$$V(\hat{X}) = (C'E^{-1}C)^{-1}$$

With more than six generations for the estimation of six parameters, a χ^2 test is possible to detect adequacy of six parameter model. Procedure proposed in section 3.3 is used to calculate χ^2 when Cavalli's (1952) least square analysis is followed. Hayman (1958) described a general procedure to calculate χ^2 as:

$$\chi^2 = Y'E^{-1}Y - Y'E^{-1}CX,$$

where Y' is is the transpose of column matrix Y. Six parameter model is not adequate if the probability of finding χ^2 value is low. When χ^2 is significant for three parameter model, attempt is made to fit a six parameter model. However, inadequacy of six parameter model may be due to one or more of the following reasons:

(i) Trigenic or higher order non-allelic interaction,

(ii) Some of the assumptions have not been satisfied. For example, genotype × environment interaction might be involved in the inheritance of character being investigated. It is, therefore, necessary to incorporate parameter specifying this interaction in the model,

(iii) Linkage between the two pairs of interacting genes.

As pointed out in section 3.3.2, when six generations are available to estimate six parameters, a perfect fit solution is desired. Means of six generations, *viz.* P_1, P_2, F_1, F_2, Bc_1 and Bc_2 could be used to estimate six parameters following a perfect fit solution given by Hayman (1958). The solutions are:

$$\hat{m} = \overline{F}_2$$

$$[\hat{d}] = \overline{B}c_1 - \overline{B}c_2$$

$$[\hat{h}] = 2\overline{B}c_1 + 2\overline{B}c_2 - 4\overline{F}_2 + \overline{F}_1 - \frac{1}{2}\overline{P}_1 - \frac{1}{2}\overline{P}_2$$

$$[\hat{i}] = 2\overline{B}c_1 + 2\overline{B}c_2 - 4\overline{F}_2$$

$$[\hat{j}] = \overline{B}c_1 - \frac{1}{2}\overline{P}_1 - \overline{B}c_2 + \frac{1}{2}\overline{P}_2$$

$$[\hat{l}] = \overline{P}_1 + \overline{P}_2 + 2\overline{F}_1 + 4\overline{F}_2 - 4\overline{B}c_1 - 4\overline{B}c_2$$

Variances of the estimates of these parameters are obtained as linear combinations of error variances of generation means used to compute various parameters. For example

$$V_{\hat{j}]} = V_{\overline{B}c_1} + \frac{1}{4}V_{\overline{P}_1} + V_{\overline{B}c_2} + \frac{1}{4}V_{\overline{P}_2}$$

Significant departure of the estimate of parameters, *i.e.*, m, $[d]$, $[h]$ and so on from zero is tested by a 't' test, as described for scaling tests in section 3.3

Perfect fit solutions to estimate six parameters, proposed by Gamble (1962) are similar to those suggested by Hayman (1958). Mather and Jinks (1971), however, proposed a different set of perfect fit solutions. Reader should note that in Hayman's (1958) solution $\overline{F}_2$ is taken as an estimate of m, whereas Mather and Jinks (1971) have given a different solution. Perfect fit solutions proposed by Mather and Jinks (1971) are:

$$\hat{m} = \frac{1}{2}\overline{P}_1 + \frac{1}{2}\overline{P}_2 + 4\overline{F}_2 - 2\overline{B}c_1 - 2\overline{B}c_2$$

$$[\hat{d}] = \frac{1}{2}\overline{P}_1 - \frac{1}{2}\overline{P}_2$$

$$[\hat{h}] = 6\overline{B}c_1 + 6\overline{B}c_2 - 8\overline{F}_2 - \overline{F}_1 - 1\frac{1}{2}\overline{P}_1 - 1\frac{1}{2}\overline{P}_2$$

$$[\hat{i}] = 2\overline{B}c_1 + 2\overline{B}c_2 - 4\overline{F}_2$$

$$[\hat{j}] = 2\overline{B}c_1 - \overline{P}_1 - 2\overline{B}c_2 + \overline{P}_2$$

$$[\hat{l}] = \overline{P}_1 + \overline{P}_2 + 2\overline{F}_1 + 4\overline{F}_2 - 4\overline{B}c_1 - 4\overline{B}c_2$$

Steps involved in the computation of standard errors of these parameters are similar to those described for Hayman's (1958) estimates of parameters. For example

$$V_{\hat{d}]} = \frac{1}{4}V_{\overline{P}_1} + \frac{1}{4}V_{\overline{P}_2}$$

3.5.2 *Worked Example*

Data provided in Table 3.3 are used to obtain the estimates of six parameters. In section 3.3.1 and 3.3.2, three parameter model was found to be unsatisfactory. Various generations, their means and variances are presented again in Table 3.13. Estimates of the six parameters along with their standard errors will be calculated for days to flowering by three methods presented in the last section

TABLE 3.13: Means, variances of means for days to flowering in sorghum

Generations	No. of plants	Mean	Variance of mean
P_1	20	64.825	0.1077
P_2	20	53.075	0.3656
F_1	10	55.100	0.3600
F_2	100	58.835	0.1827
B_{c1}	10	63.150	1.8225
B_{c2}	10	59.550	0.9025

Following Mather and Jinks (1971) the estimates of m, $[d]$, $[h]$, $[i]$, $[j]$ and $[l]$ are calculated as:

$$\hat{m} = \frac{1}{2}\overline{P}_1 + \frac{1}{2}\overline{P}_2 + 4\overline{F}_2 - 2\overline{B}c_1 - 2\overline{B}c_2$$

$$= \frac{1}{2}(64.825) + \frac{1}{2}(53.075) + 4(58.835) - 2(63.150) - 2(59.550)$$

$$= 48.890$$

$$[\hat{d}] = \frac{1}{2}\overline{P}_1 - \frac{1}{2}\overline{P}_2$$

$$= \frac{1}{2}(64.825) - \frac{1}{2}(53.075)$$

$$= 5.875$$

$$[\hat{h}] = 6\overline{B}c_1 + 6\overline{B}c_2 - 8\overline{F}_2 - \overline{F}_1 - 1\frac{1}{2}\overline{P}_1 - 1\frac{1}{2}\overline{P}_2$$

$$= 6\,(63.150) + 6\,(59.550) - 8\,(58.835) - 55.100$$

$$-1\frac{1}{2}(64.825) - 1\frac{1}{2}(53.075)$$

$$= 33.570$$

$$[\hat{i}] = 2\overline{B}c_1 + 2\overline{B}c_2 - 4\overline{F}_2$$

$$= 2\,(63.150) + 2\,(59.550) - 4\,(58.835)$$

$$= 10.060$$

$$[\hat{j}] = 2\overline{B}c_1 - \overline{P}_1 - 2\overline{B}c_2 + \overline{P}_2$$

$$= 2\,(63.150) - 64.825 - 2\,(59.550) + 53.075$$

$$= -4.550$$

$$[\hat{l}] = \overline{P}_1 + \overline{P}_2 + 2\overline{F}_1 + 4\overline{F}_2 - 4\overline{B}c_1 - 4\overline{B}c_2$$

$$= 64.825 + 53.075 + 2\,(55.100) + 4\,(58.835)$$

$$-4\,(63.150) - 4\,(59.550)$$

$$= -27.360$$

The standard errors of these parameters are calculated as:

$$S.E._{\hat{m}} = \left(\frac{1}{4}V_{\overline{P}_1} + \frac{1}{4}V_{\overline{P}_2} + 16V_{\overline{F}_2} + 4V_{\overline{B}c_1} + 4V_{\overline{B}c_2}\right)^{\frac{1}{2}}$$

$$= \left[\frac{1}{4}(0.1077) + \frac{1}{4}(0.3656) + 16(0.1827) + 4(1.8225) + 4(0.9025)\right]^{\frac{1}{2}}$$

$= 3.7338$

$$S.E._{[\hat{d}]} = \left(\frac{1}{4}V_{\bar{P}_1} + \frac{1}{4}V_{\bar{P}_2}\right)^{\frac{1}{2}}$$

$$= \left[\frac{1}{4}(0.1077) + \frac{1}{4}(0.3656)\right]^{\frac{1}{2}}$$

$= 0.3439$

$$S.E._{[\hat{h}]} = \left(36V_{\bar{B}c_1} + 36V_{\bar{B}c_2} + 64V_{\bar{F}_2} + V_{\bar{F}_1} + 2\frac{1}{4}V_{\bar{P}_1} + 2\frac{1}{4}V_{\bar{P}_2}\right)^{\frac{1}{2}}$$

$= [36(1.8225) + 36\ (0.9025) + 64\ (0.1827) + 0.3600$

$$+2\frac{1}{4}(0.1077) + 2\frac{1}{4}(0.3656)\Big]^{\frac{1}{2}}$$

$= 10.5459$

$$S.E._{[\hat{i}]} = \left(4V_{\bar{B}c_1} + 4V_{\bar{B}c_2} + 16V_{\bar{F}_2}\right)^{\frac{1}{2}}$$

$$= [4(1.8225) + 4(0.9025) + 16(0.1827)]^{\frac{1}{2}}$$

$= 3.7179$

$$S.E._{[\hat{j}]} = (4V_{\bar{B}c_1} + V_{\bar{P}_1} + 4V_{\bar{B}c_2} + V_{\bar{P}_2})^{\frac{1}{2}}$$

$= [4\ (1.8225) + 0.1077 + 4\ (0.9025) + 0.3656]^{\frac{1}{2}}$

$= 3.3724$

$$S.E._{[\hat{l}]} = \left(V_{\bar{P}_1} + V_{\bar{P}_2} + 4V_{\bar{F}_1} + 16V_{\bar{F}_2} + 16V_{\bar{B}c_1} + 16V_{\bar{B}c_2}\right)^{\frac{1}{2}}$$

$= [0.1077 + 0.3656 + 4(0.3600) + 16(0.1827)$

$+16(1.8225) + 16\ (0.9025]^{\frac{1}{2}}$

$= 6.9596$

Significance of the parameters is tested by a 't' test. For example, 't' test for $[\hat{h}]$ is:

$$t = \frac{[\hat{h}] - 0}{SE_{[\hat{h}]}}$$

$$= \frac{33.570}{10.5459} = 3.1832$$

When this value is referred to the t table it is found to be highly significant. Hence the $[\hat{h}]$ is significantly different from zero.

Estimates of the six parameters were also calculated following Gamble (1962). These estimates along with their standard errors are presented in Table 3.15

Cavalli's (1952) least square analysis will be described in details. Generation means, weights and coefficients of parameters given in Table 3.14 are used to calculate six normal equations. As described in section 3.3.2 the first step to obtain normal equation is to multiply each element of six rows in Table 3.14 by weight × coefficient of m in each row. Result of such a multiplication is presented below. Summation of all entries in seven columns gives the first normal equation (total at the end of the table).

TABLE 3.14 Generations, means, coefficients of parameters and weights for days to flowering in sorghum

Generation	Weight	Coefficients of						Observed mean
		m	$[d]$	$[h]$	$[i]$	$[j]$	$[l]$	
P_1	9.2850	1	1	–	1	–	–	64.825
P_2	2.7352	1	-1	–	1	–	–	53.075
F_1	2.7777	1	–	1	–	–	1	55.100
F_2	5.4734	1		0.5	–	–	0.25	58.835
B_1	0.5486	1	0.5	0.5	0.25	0.25	0.25	63.150
B_2	1.1080	1	-0.5	0.5	0.25	-0.25	0.25	59.550

Coefficient of m × weight

	m	$[d]$	$[h]$	$[i]$	$[j]$	$[l]$	Observed means
	9.2850	9.2850	–	9.2850	–	–	601.9001
	2.7352	–2.7352	–	2.7352	–	–	145.1707
	2.7777	–	2.7777	–	–	2.7777	153.0512
	5.4734	–	2.7367	–	–	1.3683	322.0274
	0.5486	0.2743	0.2743	0.1371	0.1371	0.1371	34.6440
	1.1080	–0.5540	0.5540	0.2770	–0.2770	0.2770	65.9814
Total	21.9279	6.2701	6.3427	12.4343	–0.1399	4.5601	1322.7748

Other normal equations are obtained in an analogous manner. However, the coefficients of $[d]$, $[h]$, $[i]$, $[j]$ and $[l]$ are used in place of coefficients of m as described above to get 2nd, 3rd, 4th, 5th, and 6th normal equations. The procedure is described below:

Coefficient of [d] × weight

	m	$[d]$	$[h]$	$[i]$	$[j]$	$[l]$	Observed mean
	9.2850	9.2850	–	9.2850	–	–	601.9001
	–2.7352	2.7352	–	–2.7352	–	–	–145.1707
	0.2743	0.1371	0.1371	0.0685	0.0685	0.0685	17.3220
	–0.5540	0.2770	–0.2770	–0.1385	0.1385	–0.1385	–32.9907
Total	6.2701	12.4343	–0.1399	6.4798	0.2070	– 0.0700	441.0607

Coefficient of $[h]$ × weight

	m	$[d]$	$[h]$	$[i]$	$[j]$	$[l]$	Observed mean
	2.7777	–	2.7777	–	–	2.7777	153.0512
	2.7367	–	1.3683	–	–	0.6841	161.0137
	– 0.2743	0.1371	0.1371	0.0685	0.0685	0.0685	17.3220
	– 0.5540	–0.2770	0.2770	0.1385	–0.1385	0.1385	32.9907
Total	6.3427	–0.1399	4.5601	0.2070	–0.0700	3.6688	364.3776

Coefficient of [*i*] × weight

	m	[*d*]	[*h*]	[*i*]	[*j*]	[*l*]	Observed mean
	9.2850	9.2850	–	9.2850	–	–	601.9001
	2.7352	–2.7352	–	2.7352	–	–	145.1707
	0.1371	.0.0685	0.0685	0.0342	0.0342	0.0342	8.6610
	0.2770	–0.1385	0.1385	0.0692	–0.0692	0.0692	16.4953
Total	12.4343	6.4798	0.2070	12.1236	-0.0350	0.1034	772.2271

Coefficient of [*j*] × weight

	m	[*d*]	[*h*]	[*i*]	[*j*]	[*l*]	Observed mean
	0.1371	0.0685	0.0685	0.0342	0.0342	0.0342	8.6610
	–0.2770	0.1385	–0.1385	–0.0692	0.0692	–0.0692	–16.4953
Total	–0.1399	0.2070	–0.0700	–0.0350	0.1034	–0.0350	-7.8343

Coefficient of [*l*] × weight

	m	[*d*]	[*h*]	[*i*]	[*j*]	[*l*]	Observed mean
	2.7777	–	2.7777	–	–	2.7777	153.0512
	1.3683	–	0.6841	–	–	0.3420	80.5068
	0.1371	0.0685	0.0685	0.0342	0.0342	0.0342	8.6610
	0.2770	–0.1385	0.1385	0.0692	–0.0692	0.0692	16.4953
Total	4.5601	–0.0700	3.6688	0.1034	–0.0350	3.2231	258.7143

The six normal equations so obtained are arranged in a matrix form as:

$$\begin{bmatrix} 21.9279 & 6.2701 & 6.3427 & 12.4343 & -0.1399 & 4.5601 \\ 6.2701 & 12.4343 & -0.1399 & 6.4798 & 0.2070 & -0.0700 \\ 6.3427 & -0.1399 & 4.5601 & 0.2070 & -0.0700 & 3.6688 \\ 12.4343 & 6.4798 & 0.2070 & 12.1236 & -0.0350 & 0.1034 \\ -0.1399 & 0.2070 & -0.0700 & -0.0350 & 0.1034 & -0.0350 \\ 4.5601 & -0.0700 & 3.6688 & 0.1034 & -0.0350 & 3.2231 \end{bmatrix}$$

$$J$$

$$\begin{bmatrix} \hat{m} \\ [\hat{d}] \\ [\hat{h}] \\ [\hat{i}] \\ [\hat{j}] \\ [\hat{l}] \end{bmatrix} = \begin{bmatrix} 13.22.7748 \\ 441.0607 \\ 364.3776 \\ 772.2271 \\ -7.8343 \\ 258.7143 \end{bmatrix}$$

$$M \qquad\qquad S$$

Estimates of six parameters are obtained as:

$$M = SJ^{-1}$$

Hence an inverse of matrix J is required. It may be obtained by any method given in matrix algebra or following the method given in Appendix I. The inverse of matrix J in the present example is

$$\begin{bmatrix} 12.9200 & -0.0646 & -36.0263 & -12.8107 & -3.2348 & 23.0990 \\ -0.0646 & 0.1180 & 0.1953 & 0.0005 & -0.2353 & -0.1306 \\ -36.0263 & 0.1953 & 103.1228 & 35.6892 & 9.7515 & -67.4368 \\ -12.8107 & 0.0005 & 35.6892 & 12.8150 & 3.3643 & -22.8738 \\ -3.2348 & -0.2353 & 9.7515 & 3.3643 & 11.2723 & -6.5135 \\ 23.0990 & -0.1306 & -67.4368 & -22.8738 & -6.5135 & 45.0450 \end{bmatrix}$$

Estimates of six parameters are calculated as described in section 3.3.2.The estimates and their standard errors are presented in Table 3.15. It is apparent from the table that estimates of *m*, [*d*], [*h*], [*j*] and [*l*] differ some what from one method to another. This is expected because Cavalli's (1952) method is a weighted analysis. Hayman (1958) and Gamble (1962) have taken $\overline{F}_2$ as a constant (m), whereas Cavalli (1952) and Mather and Jinks (1971) have used a different criterion for estimation of mid-parental value. However, results of these three methods suggest that additive effects, additive × additive and dominance × dominance kinds of non-allelic interaction effects are responsible for the inheritance of days to 50 per cent flowering. If Gamble's (1962) results are ignored for some time. it seems that dominance effects predominantly govern the inheritance of this attribute because estimates of [h] are not only highly significant but considerably larger than [d] in magnitude. Magnitude of dominance × dominance kind of non-allelic interaction is also larger than either [d] or [i]. The signs of [l] are, however, negative in all the methods which suggest that dominance at some of the loci is in negative direction, *i.e.*, towards early flowering. The components of means, therefore, suggest that non-additive gene effects are more important for this attribute. Since the sign of [l] in all the methods is opposite to that of [h], the non-allelic interaction is of duplicate type.

These analyses revealed that only five components of means were significant (with the exception of Gamble's 1962 method in which dominance effect was also non-significant). Hence, a five parameter model could be fitted to the data following Cavalli's (1952) least square method and remaining one degree of freedom used to test the adequacy of five parameter model (m, [d], [h], [i] and [l]). This is expected to increase the precision of estimates. Estimates of five parameters so obtained are presented in Table 3.16 along with estimates of six parameters for comparison.

It is clear from Table 3.16 that the estimates of five parameters have improved as compared with those of six parameter model. The standard errors have also improved. Since six generation means have been employed to estimate five parameters. one degree of freedom is available for a χ^2 test. The observed and expected means of six generations. the deviations *(O–E)*, and other information required for calculation of χ^2 is presented in Table 3.17.

TABLE 3.15: The six components of means calculated by 3 methods for days to flower in sorghum

Parameter	Method adopted		
	Mather & Jinks (1971)	Cavalli (1952)	Gamble (1962) (and also Hayman, 1958)
$\hat{m}$	48.890** ± 3.733	43.195** ± 3.594	58.835** ± 7.670
$[\hat{d}]$	5.875** ± 0.343	6.198** ± 0.343	3.600* ± 1.650
$[\hat{h}]$	33.570** ± 10.545	44.002** ± 10.154	6.210 ± 3.781
$[\hat{i}]$	10.060** ± 3.717	10.848** ± 3.579	10.060** ± 3.717
$[\hat{j}]$	–4.550 ± 3.372	–4.907 ± 3.357	–2.275 ± 1.686
$[\hat{l}]$	–27.360** ± 6.959	–34.240** ± 6.711	–27.360** ± 6.959

*, ** Significant at 5 and 1 per cent levels, respectively.

TABLE 3.16: Showing estimates of components of means for days to 50 per cent flowering in sorghum

Parameters	Estimates of components of mean	
	6 Parameter model	5 Parameter model
$\hat{m}$	43.195** ± 3.594	43.393** ± 3.4646
$[\hat{d}]$	6.198** ± 0.343	5.7935** ± 0.3364
$[\hat{h}]$	44.002** ± 10.154	49.0395** ± 9.7354
$[\hat{i}]$	10.848** ± 3.579	15.4468** ± 3.4388
$[\hat{j}]$	–4.907 ± 3.357	–
$[\hat{l}]$	–34.240** ± 6.711	–37.6729** ± 6.4282

*,** Significant at 5 and 1 per cent levels, respectively,

When referred to the table of chi-square for one degree of freedom, probability of getting a value as large as 3.83804 is found to be between 0.05 to 0.01, which suggests that the five parameter model is satisfactory for days to 50 per cent flowering.

Magnitude of the estimate of dominance effects is considerably larger than the estimate of additive effects as well as additive × additive effects (Table 3.16). Dominance effects, therefore, seem to be more important for this attribute. Estimate of parameter specifying dominance

× dominance type of non-allelic interaction is also larger in magnitude than either the $[\hat{d}]$ or $[\hat{i}]$. Hence, this digenic non-allelic interaction is also important for days to flowering. Sign of the estimate of $[l]$ is opposite to that of $[h]$. Non-allelic interaction is, therefore, of duplicate type. Parameter specifying dominance × dominance type of non-allelic interaction has a negative sign which implies that this non-allelic interaction tends to induce early flowering. Although, additive and additive × additive gene effects are significant for attribute being investigated, non-additive gene effects appear to overpower them. For this reason a breeding procedure which could exploit this kind of gene action would be appropriate for improvement. Biparental mating or recurrent selection generate more heritable variation. In the present situation biparental mating or recurrent selection followed by conventional selection method appears to be the appropriate breeding plan.

Table 3.17: Showing observed and expected means, (deviation)^2 and (deviation)^2 × weight for six generations in sorghum

Generation	Mean		Deviation	(deviation)^2	(deviation)^2 × weight
	Observed	Expected			
P_1	64.825	64.631	0.1940	0.03764	0.34949
P_2	53.075	53.044	0.0310	0.00096	0.00263
F_1	55.100	54.757	0.3430	0.11765	0.32680
F_2	58.835	58.492	0.3430	0.11765	0.64395
B_{C1}	63.150	65.250	-2.1000	4.41000	2.41933
B_{C2}	59.550	59.457	0.0930	0.00865	0.09584
				χ^2	3.83804

3.6 Components of Heterosis

Breeders of crop species usually observe that the mean performance of F_1 generation, produced by crossing two genetically diverse genotypes, is superior than the mean performance of better parent. This phenomenon is known as heterosis. Heterosis is defined as the amount by which mean performance of F_1 exceeds better parent (heterobeltiosis) or mid-parent (relative heterosis). This phenomenon has been exploited in several crops like maize, sorghum, rice, cotton, pearl millets and vegetable crops such as tomato. As a consequence, production of these crops been elevated considerably.

An hypothesis was proposed that joint action of favourable combinations of genes at different loci could be responsible for heterosis. Results of the experiments conducted by Jinks (1954, 1956) indicated that F_1 generations of crosses, for which non-allelic interaction was important, were in general superior in their performance as compared with the F_1s of those crosses for which additive-dominance model was adequate. These results, therefore, suggested that non-allelic interaction was an important cause of heteroses.Jinks and Jones (1958) proposed a procedure which enabled assessment of the role of various components of generation means in the determination of heterosis.

Since the mean expressions of various generations are expressible in terms of three parameters (m, $[d]$ and $[h]$) or six parameters (m, $[d]$, $[h]$, $[i]$, $[j]$ and $[l]$), depending upon the absence or presence of digenic non-allelic interaction, expected magnitude of heterosis can also be described in terms of these parameters. This provides a basis to assess relative importance of components of generation means in the determination of heterosis. Appropriate breeding procedure could then be developed to exploit various kinds of gene effects.

Heterosis may be positive or negative. For example, when grain yield of the F_1 generation is superior than that of the better parent (P_1), heterosis assumes a positive sign. On the other hand, when the means of characters like flowering time or days required for maturity are lesser than the earlier parent (P_2), heterosis assumes a negative sign. If, however, this character is measured in terms of rate of growth, heterosis would be positive.

When additive-dominance model is satisfactory to explain the inheritance of a character, $\overline{F_1}$ and $\overline{P_1}$ could be expressed as:

$$\overline{F_1} = m + [h]$$
$$\overline{P_1} = m + [d]$$

Therefore, the expected magnitude of heterosis is given by

$$\overline{F_1} - \overline{P_1} = (m + [h]) - (m + [d])$$
$$= m + [h] - m - [d]$$
$$= [h] - [d]$$

For positive heterosis to occur, $[h]$ must be positive and greater in magnitude than $[d]$. Negative heterosis is measured as $\overline{F}_1 - \overline{P}_2$. Therefore, expected magnitude of heterosis is given by

$$\overline{F}_1 - \overline{P}_2 = (m+[h]) - (m+[-d])$$
$$= m + [h] - m - [-d]$$
$$= [h] - [-d]$$

Negative heterosis is likely to occur and occur with large magnitude if the sign of $[h]$ is negative and its value smaller than $[-d]$.

Thus whenever additive-dominance model is adequate, heterosis will occur if $\pm$ $[h]$ is larger in magnitude than $[d]$. For $[h]$ to be greater than $[d]$ one or both of the following conditions should be satisfied:

(i) h must be greater than d at some or all the loci, *i.e.*, there should be superdominance or overdominance at some or all the loci.

(ii) r, which is a measure of distribution of genes of like effects, should be less than unity and approaching zero. In other words, genes should be dispersed between the parental strains rather than associated in two parents. This will result in smaller value of $[d]$ than $[h]$. Then partial or complete dominance at some or all loci will be sufficient to produce heterosis.

Heterosis will occur with large magnitude if in addition to these two conditions, direction of dominance is in same direction *i.e.*, dominance is unidirectional. In this way magnitude of $[h]$ will not reduce. Balancing of dominance in positive and negative directions may lead to $[h] = 0$.

Nature of gene action responsible for heterosis will determine the breeding procedure to be employed for exploitation of heterosis. Dispersion of genes between the parents and overdominance are two probable causes of heterosis.

Role of dispersion could be explained with an arbitrary example using a simple model. Suppose four genes A, B, C, and D each add four units to a given character. On the other hand, each of the four genes a,b,c and d, add only one unit to the same character. Also assume that there is complete dominance of A over a (and likewise for B, C and D genes). A highly heterotic (heterobeltiosis) hybrid could be produced by crossing two genotypes, say *AABBccdd* and *aabbCCDD*. Phenotypic values of parents would be 20 units each while the F_1 would measure 32 units. F_1 with same genetic constitution could be produced by crossing genotypes *AABBCCDD* and *aabbccdd*. However, the F_1 (*AaBbCcDd*) would not exhibit heterobeltiosis.

Selection of segregates with high values and also with low values from the cross *AABBccdd* and *aabbCCDD*, would result in true breeding lines similar to or exactly like *AABBCCDD* and *aabbccdd*. Upon crossing these high and low value lines, F_1 would be produced which will not exhibit heterobeltiosis. This shows that heterosis observed in the first case was due to dispersion of genes between the parents. Such an evidence was obtained by Jayasekara and Jinks (1976) and Pooni and Jinks (1981) in favour of dispersion of genes for *Nicotiana rustica*.

When dispersion of genes is responsible for heterosis, true breeding varieties could be produced in case of self-pollinated crops which are as superior as F_1 in performance, but farmers could retain part of the produce as seed for next season. Similar suggestion was also given by Smith (1952).

On the other hand, when overdominance is involved, its efficient exploitation by the plant breeder could be through development of a hybrid variety. Hybrid seed is relatively costlier and farmers have to purchase fresh F_1 seed every year for sowing.

However, Gardner (1963) was of the view that the overdominance observed in maize was probably due to repulsion phase linkages of genes in parents because in later segregating generations the magnitude of average degree of dominance declined considerably.

When additive-dominance model is not satisfactory for an attribute and digenic non-allelic interaction is suggested, means of F_1, P_1 and P_2 are expressed as:

$$\overline{F}_1 = m + [h] + [l]$$

$$\overline{P}_1 = m + [d] + [i]$$

and $$\overline{P}_2 = m - [d] + [i]$$

Therefore, expected value of positive heterosis in terms of these parameters is got as:

$$\bar{F}_1 - \bar{P}_1 = m + [h] + [l] - m - [d] - [i]$$
$$= [h] + [l] - [d] - [i]$$

For positive heterosis to occur and to occur with larger magnitude, ([*h*] + [*l*]) should be positive and larger than ([*d*] + [*i*]). For parental strain with larger expression [*d*] will not be negative. However, [*i*] may be negative or positive. The sign of either [*h*] or [*l*] may be negative, but the be sign of ([*h*] + [*l*]) should not be negative and the magnitude should not be smaller than ([*d*] + [*i*]). Expected value of negative heterosis, in terms of these parameters is obtained as:

$$\bar{F}_1 - \bar{P}_2 = ([h] + [l]) - ([-d] + [i])$$

For negative heterosis to occur and to occur with greater magnitude ([*h*] + [*l*]) should be negative and larger in magnitude than ([–*d*] +[*i*]). However, either [*h*] or [*l*] may be positive or negative.

In the presence of digenic non-allelic interaction heterosis can arise in many ways. But it is more likely to arise, and arise with greater magnitude if one or both of the following conditions are satisfied:

(i) Signs of [*l*] and [*h*] should be in same direction, i.e., the digenic non-allelic interaction should be of complementary kind.

(ii) Two or more pairs of genes showing digenic non-allelic interaction should be dispersed between the two parental strains. When the genes are dispersed between the parental strains magnitude of [*d*] as well as [*i*] will be smaller.

A genetic model was proposed by Jinks and Jones (1958) to evaluate the relative importance of non-allelic interaction for the occurrence and magnitude of heterosis. When 28 crosses of *Nicotiana rustica* were raised for three years, they observed that only those crosses consistently manifested considerable heterosis for three years for which the simple additive-dominance model was not satisfactory. In their opinion non-allelic interaction played predominant role in the occurrence and magnitude of heterosis. Jinks and Jones (1958) measured heterosis as deviation of $\bar{F}_1$ from $\bar{P}_1$. However, according to them $\bar{P}_1$, $\bar{P}_2$ and $\bar{F}_1$ could be expressed as:

$$\overline{P_1} = m + [d] + [i] - \frac{1}{2}[j] + \frac{1}{4}[l]$$

$$\overline{P_2} = m - [d] + [i] + \frac{1}{2}[j] + \frac{1}{4}[l]$$

and $$\overline{F_1} = m + [h] + \frac{1}{4}[l]$$

According to Jinks and Jones (1958) expected value of heterosis will have four components as:

$$[h] - [i] \left| [d] + \frac{1}{2}[j] \right|$$

In their opinion expected heterosis, on the basis of estimated components of mean measurements, will be

$$\left| [h] - [i] \right| - \left| [d] - \frac{1}{2}[j] \right|$$

Where $|\quad|$ denotes absolute value without taking signs into consideration. Expected heterosis in various situations is calculated as:

$$[h] - [i] - [d] + \frac{1}{2}[j]$$

when $[h] > [i]$ and $[d] > \frac{1}{2}[j]$,

as $$[h] - [i] + [d] - \frac{1}{2}[j]$$

when [d] is less than $\frac{1}{2}[j]$,

as $$-[h] + [i] - [d] + \frac{1}{2}[j]$$

when $[h] < [i]$ and $[d] > \frac{1}{2}[j]$,

and as $-[h]+[i]+[d]-\frac{1}{2}[j]$

when $[d]<\frac{1}{2}[j]$.

Method advocated by Hayman (1958) should be adopted for computation of estimates of six parameters. These estimates are then used to find the expected value of heterosis. If the perfect fit solution given by Mather and Jinks (1971, 1977) or the Cavalli's (1952) weighted least square method is used to calculate the six parameters, the expected value of heterosis will be given by:

$$([h] + [l]) - ([d] + [i])$$

When the additive-dominance model is satisfactory, expected heterosis is calculated as $[h] - [d]$, which should be in close agreement with observed heterosis. However, when additive-dominance model is not adequate, six parameter model is fitted assuming digenic non-allelic interaction. These components of generation means are then employed to calculate value of expected heterosis. Close agreement between observed and expected heterosis then implies that non-allelic interaction is also important for heterosis. Relative magnitudes of the components of heterosis then indicate which gene effect is predominant determinant of heterosis. For example, if additive effects and additive × additive effects (following Mather and Jinks, 1971) are significant and larger in magnitude than the estimates of $[h]$ and $[l]$, former gene effects are largely responsible for determination of heterosis. Selection of genotypes as good as F_1 hybrid is possible when additive gene effects determine heterosis. On the other hand, non-additive gene effects could be exploited through F_1 hybrids.However, development of F_1 hybrids for commercial planting could be a useful proposition only when the magnitude of heterosis is considerably large,hybrid seed production is relatively simple and not a costly affair.

Comstock and Robinson (1948) proposed that linkage may bias the average degree of dominance. According to them genes linked in repulsion could result in apparent overdominance or pseudo-overdominance.

Although linkage does not influence the mean expressions of non-segregating generations, such as P_1, P_2 and F_1 (section 3.5), it does influence the magnitude of heterosis as well as the components of heterosis. This point will be clear with the help of an example. Assume that a character is governed by two loci each with two alleles, *viz* A_1, A_2 and B_1, B_2. Also assume that genes A_1 and B_1 increase the expression of a character. If the genes are linked in repulsion, genotypes and phenotypes of P_1 and P_2 will be:

Parents	Genotype	Means
P_1	$A_1A_1B_2B_2$	$m + d_a - d_b - i_{ab}$
P_2	$A_2A_2B_1B_1$	$m - d_a + d_b - i_{ab}$

If we also assume that $m = 0$ and $d_a = d_b = h_a = h_b = i_{ab} = l_{ab} = 1$ unit, mean measurements of both the parental strains will be -1. The genotype of F_1 produced by crossing these strains will be $A_1A_2B_1B_2$ and the mean expression will be:

$$m + h_a + h_b + l_{ab}$$

Since $h_a = h_b = l_{ab} = 1$ mean value of F_1 will be 3 units. Heterosis measured as deviation of $\overline{F}_1$ from $\overline{P}_1$ is, therefore,

$$\overline{F}_1 - \overline{P}_1 = m + h_a + h_b + l_{ab} - m - d_a + d_b + i_{ab}$$

$$= h_a + h_b + l_{ab} - d_a + d_b + i_{ab}$$

which equals four units. This is how repulsion phase linkage causes an upward bias in dominance. In the present example, overdominance observed is really pseudo-overdominance. As the linkages break and recombinations take place, degree of dominance declines in subsequent generations.

3.6.1 Worked Example

Data provided for days to 50 per cent flowering for sorghum presented in Table 3.3 will be used. Since the method described by Mather and Jinks (1971) will be followed, estimates in the second column of Table 3.14 will be used to calculate the expected heterosis.

Observed heterosis is

$\overline{F}_1 - \overline{P}_2 = 55.100 - 53.075$
$= 2.025$

The expected heterosis is got as

$([h] + [l]) - (-[d] + [i])$
$= [\,33.570 + (-27.360)] - [(-5.875) + 10.060]$
$= 33.570 - 27.360 + 5.875 - 10.060$
$= 2.025$

There is a perfect agreement between observed heterosis and expected heterosis. Components of heterosis make it clear that although the magnitudes of [*h*] and [*l*] are larger than either [*d*] or [*i*], magnitude of heterosis is very low because the signs of [*h*] and [*l*] are opposite to each other. In other words, the non-allelic interaction is of duplicate type. It was pointed out in preceding paragraphs that for heterosis to occur with greater magnitude non-allelic interaction should be of complementary type besides other requirements.

Let us calculate expected value of heterosis from the components of means estimated following Hayman (1958)/Gamble (1962). We need estimates of *h*, *i*, *d* and 1/2*j* which are 6.21,10.06, 3.60 and –2.275, respectively. Expected value of heterosis may be obtained as:

$$-[h]+[i]-[d]+\frac{1}{2}[j],$$

because magnitude of [*h*] is less than [*i*] and $[d] > \frac{1}{2}[j]$ (Jinks and Jones 1958). Thus, expected heterosis is

$-6.21 + 10.06 - 3.60 + 2.275$
$= 2.525$

Once again there is a close agreement between observed and expected heterosis. It appears that additive × additive epistatic type of non-allelic interaction is more important for the manifestation of heterosis than either the dominance effects or additive × dominance effects (latter two are in fact non-significant).

APPENDIX I

A rectangular array of numbers enclosed by a pair of brackets as:

$$\begin{bmatrix} 1 & 3 & 1 \\ 2 & 1 & 4 \\ 4 & 7 & 6 \end{bmatrix}$$

and subject to certain rules of operations is called a matrix. Individual numbers in the matrix are known as elements of matrix. A matrix of m rows and n columns is said to be of $m \times n$ order. If $m = n$, the matrix is said to be square matrix of order n or an n square matrix. The element in ith row and jth column of matrix A is usually denoted by aij or Aij. The diagonal elements of a square matrix (such as the one shown above) are the elements Aii = 1, 2,......, n. A square matrix whose elements $aij \neq 0$, for $i < j$, is called upper triangular. Thus matrix shown below is an upper triangular matrix.

$$\begin{bmatrix} a_{11} & a_{12} & a_{13} \\ 0 & a_{22} & a_{23} \\ 0 & 0 & a_{33} \end{bmatrix}$$

A *diagonal matrix* is a square one in which the elements not on the diagonal are zero. For example, matrix shown below is a diagonal matrix.

When, elements $a_{11} = a_{22} = a_{33}$ ..... $a_{nn} = k$ [such as shown below (*a*)], the diagonal matrix is known as *scalar matrix*. However, if k is 1, the matrix is called the Identity matrix (I), such as shown in (*b*).

$$\begin{bmatrix} 6 & 0 & 0 \\ 0 & 6 & 0 \\ 0 & 0 & 6 \end{bmatrix} \qquad \begin{bmatrix} 1 & 0 & 0 \\ 0 & 1 & 0 \\ 0 & 0 & 1 \end{bmatrix}$$

(*a*) (*b*)

Any matrix with a single row is called the row matrix or also vector of a vector matrix. For example, [1, 2, 3,] is a row matrix. A matrix with a single column is called the column matrix or also a vector of vector matrix.

The matrix of the order $m \times n$ obtained by interchanging the rows and columns of an $m \times n$ matrix A is called "Transpose" of A and is denoted by A' (A transpose). For example, transpose of

$$A = \begin{bmatrix} 1 & 3 & 1 \\ 2 & 1 & 4 \\ 4 & 7 & 6 \end{bmatrix} \text{ is } \quad A' = \begin{bmatrix} 1 & 2 & 4 \\ 3 & 1 & 7 \\ 1 & 4 & 6 \end{bmatrix}$$

Note that element aij in the ith row and jth column of A stands in jth row and ith column of A'

Addition of Matrices

Two matrices A and B can be added only if they have same dimensions. The sum of these matrices results in another matrix with similar dimensions. For example,

$$(A + B)_{ij} = C_{ij} = A_{ij} + B_{ij}$$

In other words,

$$\begin{bmatrix} 1 & 2 \\ 3 & 4 \end{bmatrix} + \begin{bmatrix} 2 & -3 \\ 5 & -6 \end{bmatrix} = \begin{bmatrix} 3 & -1 \\ 8 & -2 \end{bmatrix}$$

$$\text{A} \quad + \quad \text{B} \quad = \quad \text{C}$$

Subtraction

Subtraction of matrices is possible under same circumstances as addition, *i.e.*

$$(A - B)_{ij} = C_{ij} = A_{ij} - B_{ij}$$

Thus,

$$\begin{bmatrix} 1 & 2 \\ 3 & 4 \end{bmatrix} - \begin{bmatrix} 2 & -3 \\ 5 & -6 \end{bmatrix} = \begin{bmatrix} -1 & 5 \\ -2 & 10 \end{bmatrix}$$

$$\text{A} \quad - \quad \text{B} \quad = \quad \text{C}$$

Multiplication of Matrices

We can multiply matrix A by B on right side, if B has same number of rows as the columns in A. The resulting matrix AB shall have rows of matrix A and columns of B. For example,

$$\underset{A}{\begin{bmatrix} 3 & 1 \\ 2 & 4 \end{bmatrix}} \times \underset{B}{\begin{bmatrix} 2 \\ 5 \end{bmatrix}} \begin{matrix} (3\times2)+(1\times5)= \\ (2\times2)+(4\times5)= \end{matrix} \underset{AB}{\begin{bmatrix} 11 \\ 24 \end{bmatrix}}$$

Thus AB, has two rows and one column.

Inverse of a Matrix

If A and B are square matrices such that $AB = BA = I$, then B is called inverse of A and we write $B = A^{-1}$ (B equals A inverse). The B matrix has also A as its inverse and we write $A = B^{-1}$. For example,

$$\begin{bmatrix} 1 & 2 & 3 \\ 1 & 3 & 3 \\ 1 & 2 & 4 \end{bmatrix} \begin{bmatrix} 6 & -2 & -3 \\ -1 & 1 & 0 \\ -1 & 0 & 1 \end{bmatrix} = \begin{bmatrix} 1 & 0 & 0 \\ 0 & 1 & 0 \\ 0 & 0 & 1 \end{bmatrix} = I$$

where each matrix in the product is inverse of other. Inverse is not possible for every matrix.

Doolittle Method

Although inverse can be obtained in several ways, Doolittle method is given here for ready reference. This method will permit calculation of partial and multiple correlations, and is also useful in path analysis. The method will be illustrated for data provided in section 3.3.2. The J matrix in this section is symmetrical about the diagonal. Write the elements of J matrix on left hand side as shown in Table 3.18. The J matrix is a 3×3 matrix. We need a matrix, which when multiplied with J matrix will yield an identity matrix. Hence, on right hand side we enter a 3×3 identity matrix. Fourth step is to rewrite step 1. Fifth step involves division of each element of row of 4th step by first element of 4th step, *i.e.*, 21.9279. This results in unity in first column on left hand side.

To get the elements in sixth row, write row 2 as shown below:

12.4343	–0.1399	0	1

Multiply each element of 4th row leaving the first element (*i.e.*, 21.9279) by the second element in 5th row. Thus,

6.2701	6.3427	1	0	0
× 0.2859				
1.7926	1.8133	0.2859	0	0

Subtract the products from the elements of second row given above. Thus,

12.4343	–0.1399	0	1	0
–1.7926	–1.8133	–0.2859	0	0
10.6417	–1.9532	–0.2859	1	0

TABLE 3.18: Dollittle method

Steps	Left hand side			Right hand side		
1.	21.9279	6.2701	6.3427	1	0	0
2.	–	12.4343	–0.1399	0	1	0
3.	–	–	4.5601	0	0	1
4.	21.9279	6.2701	6.3427	1	0	0
5.	1	0.2859	0.2892	0.0456	0	0
6.	–	10.6417	–1.9532	–0.2859	1	0
7.	–	1	–0.1835	–0.0268	0.0939	0
8.	–	–	2.3674	–0.3416	0.1835	1
9.	–	–	1	–0.1442	0.0775	0.4224
10.				0.10252	–0.05332	–0.14429
11.				–0.05332	0.10812	0.07751
12.				–0.14429	0.07751	0.4224

Enter the balance in 6th row from 2nd column onwards. Divide each element of 6th row by 10.6417 including itself. This results in unity at second position also in row 7.

In order to get eighth row, write elements of 3rd row as:

4.5601	0	0	1

From these elements of 3rd row, subtract the sum of two products, for which the first product is obtained by multiplying each element of 4th row (from 3rd column onwards) by 0.2892 and second product is got by multiplying each element of 6th row (from 3rd column onwards) by –0.1835. Thus,

	6.3427	1	0	0
	× 0.2892			
	1.8343	0.2892	0	0
and	–1.9532	–0.2859	1	0
	× –0.1835			
	0.3584	0.0524	–0.1835	0
and	1.8343	0.2892	0	0
	+ 0.3584	0.0524	–0.1835	0
	2.1927	0.3416	–0.1835	0

Subtraction of this sum from elements of third row yields the 8th row. Hence,

4.5601	0	0	1
– 2.1927	–0.3416	0.1835	0
2.3674	–0.3416	0.1835	1

Divide each element of 8th row by 2.3674 including itself to get ninth row. Thus, we get unity in all the three columns on left hand side.

Now we are equipped to get inverse of the J matrix. We shall now operate only on right hand side. Summation of the products of elements of first column commencing from 4th row as shown below yields first element of first column and first row of J^{-1}. Thus

$$(1 \times 0.0456) + (-0.2859 \times -0.0268)$$
$$+ (-0.3416 \times -0.1442)$$
$$= 0.1025208$$

The second diagonal element of this matrix is got by summation of product of the terms in second column starting from 6th row onwards. Thus

$$(1 \times 0.0939) + (0.1835 \times 0.0775) = 0.10812.$$

To get the last figure of diagonal, multiply the elements in third column, starting from 8th row onwards. Thus

$$(1 \times 0.4224) = 0.4224$$

The second element in the first row of J^{-1} matrix is got as shown below:

$$(-0.3416 \times 0.0775) + (-0.2859 \times 0.0939) = -0.05332$$

Since the matrix is symmetrical about the diagonal, it is also the second element of first column.

To get the third element of first row (and also the first column), perform the following operation:

$$(-0.3416 \times 0.4224) = -0.14429$$

Lastly, we need third element of second row, which is also the 2nd element of third row. To get it, multiply 0.1835 with 0.4224. It is 0.07751.

This is how we get an inverse of a symmetrical square matrix.

4

COMPONENTS OF HERITABLE VARIANCES AND COVARIANCES

4.1 Genotypic Variance

Plant breeding is known as an art and science of improving genetic pattern of plants in relation to their economic use. In the process of improvement, desirable plants are continuously being selected from genetically variable populations. Breeders know it well that selection can act effectively only on heritable differences and that selection cannot create variability. Variability is, therefore, a key factor which determines the amount of progress expected from selection.

In Chapter 2, it was shown that phenotypic value measured on an individual, is made up of genotypic value and environmental deviation. Variation of phenotypic values is, therefore, determined by variance attributable to genotypic values and environmental deviations. And since the genotypic values are composed of breeding values, dominance deviations and interaction deviations, genotypic variance is made up of variances of these components. Variation of breeding values is known as additive genetic variance, whereas variances of dominance deviations and interaction deviations are referred to as dominance variance and interaction variance, respectively.

The primary object of measuring phenotypic variation is to partition it into components attributable to different causes. It is the relative magnitude of these components which determines the genetic properties of populations, particularly the extent to which various relatives resemble each other. Thus, when a breeder selects plants from F_2 population, he desires that progeny descending from these selections should resemble their F_2 parents. The degree to which progeny will resemble and continue to resemble the parents is determined by relative amounts of additive and non-additive (comprising of dominance and interaction variance) components which make up genotypic variance. Let us therefore, examine how various components determine the genotypic variance. However, before this we should also look at the complications caused by relationship between genotypes and environmental agencies.

It is many times implicitly assumed that all the genotypes are associated with same amount of environmental variance. However, this is not a correct notion. For example, when inbred lines of maize and their F_1 hybrids are grown over environments (may be several locations and/ or several seasons or years), it is observed that inbred lines exhibit relatively more variation than F_1 s. Since all the individuals within each inbred line and F_1 are genetically alike (except for a rare mutation), variation within the lines is entirely environmental in origin. This shows that environmental variance may depend upon genotypes being observed.

Second complication is that genotype and environment may be correlated. Usually it is believed that genotypic values and environmental deviations are independent of each other, *i.e.*, there is no correlation between these values. However, this is not true. For example, in dairies cows which give more milk yield are given more and better feed than other cows. Thus better phenotypes are correlated with better environment. And since ability to give more milk is partly a property of genotype, it is the genotypic value which is related to environmental agencies. When genotypic values and environmental deviations are correlated, phenotypic variance can be linearly expressed as:

$$\sigma^2_p = \sigma^2_g + \sigma^2_e + 2\ \text{Cov}\ (ge),$$

where σ^2_p, σ^2_g, σ^2_e are phenotypic, genotypic and environmental variances, respectively and Cov(*ge*) refers to the covariances of genotypic values with environmental deviations. And since correlation between genotypic values and environmental deviations is obtained as:

$$r_{ge} = \frac{\text{Cov}\,(ge)}{\sigma_g . \sigma_e},$$

Covariance (*ge*) could be expressed as $r_{ge} . \sigma_g . \sigma_e$. Substitution of this expression for Cov(*ge*) in the linear expression for phenotypic variance gives us:

$$\sigma^2_p = \sigma^2_g + \sigma^2_e + 2\,(r_{ge}\ .\ \sigma_g\ .\ \sigma_e).$$

However, if proper experimental design is chosen and experimental population randomised, correlation between genotypic values and environmental deviations will be taken care of.

Third complication is the interaction between different genotypes and environmental agencies. When a breeder plants several genotypes over a number of locations to evaluate their performance, he finds very often that a specific change in the location does not have similar effects on different genotypes. For example, as shown in the following table genotype *A* gives 20 grammes grain/plant in *X* location and *B* gives 18 grammes. However, in location *Y* it is the *B* genotype which is superior. Interaction is absent when a specific change in the environment has similar effects on different genotypes.

		Genotypes		
		A	*B*	*C*
Environments	*X*	20	18	16
	Y	18	21	20

Interaction between genotypes and environments, when present, gives rise to an additional component of variance *viz.* σ^2_{ge}. This component can be isolated and measured only when genotypes are grown in several environments (such as several locations and/or several years). This aspect is discussed in Chapter 8. In normal circumstances, therefore, variance due to genotype-environment interaction, since it cannot be separately measured, is best regarded as part of environmental variance. However, one should keep in mind that when it is not separated, estimate of genotypic variance is biased.

4.2 Components of Genotypic Variance in Random Mating Population

To start with, let us consider a simple case of a single locus with two alleles, *viz.* A_1 and A_2. With respect to this locus there will be three genotypes in the population. As pointed out in the preceding section, genotypic variance is made up of additive, dominance and interaction variance. For the time being let us assume that interaction variance is absent. In order to derive expectations for additive and dominance variance we need the frequencies, breeding values and dominance deviations of three genotypes. Since breeding values and dominance deviations are expressed as deviation from population mean, variance is obtained as sum of (frequency × value) over 3 genotypes. Correction for mean is not required.

4.2.1 *Additive Genetic Variance*

Additive genetic variance is the variance of breeding values. Breeding value of an individual was defined in section 2.5 as sum of the average effects of genes it carries, summation being made over pair of alleles at each locus and over all loci. It was also pointed out in this section that the mean genotypic value of progeny is determined by average effects of genes transmitted by parents. Additive genetic variance, therefore, determines degree of resemblance between parents and offspring. Additive genetic variance is the chief cause of resemblance between relatives, and also the chief determinant of observable genetic properties of the population. This component of genotypic variance is, therefore, of much importance to the breeders.

The genotypes, frequencies of genotypes, breeding values and squares of breeding values required to derive the additive genetic variance (σ^2_A) are given in Table 4.1

TABLE 4.1: Breeding values of three genotypes and frequencies of genotypes

Genotypes	Frequency	Breeding value	(Breeding value)^2
A_1A_1	p^2	$2q\alpha$	$4q^2\alpha^2$
A_1A_2	$2pq$	$(q-p)\alpha$	$(q\alpha - p\alpha)^2$
A_2A_2	q^2	$-2p\alpha$	$4p^2\alpha^2$

From Table 4.1, additive genetic variance is derived as:

$$\begin{aligned}
\sigma^2_A &= p^2 (4q^2\alpha^2) + 2pq (q\alpha - p\alpha)^2 + q^2 (4p^2\alpha^2) \\
&= 4p^2q^2\alpha^2 + 2pq^3\alpha^2 - 4p^2q^2\alpha^2 + 2p^3q\alpha^2 + 4p^2q^2\alpha^2 \\
&= 2pq^3\alpha^2 + 2p^3q\alpha^2 + 4p^2q^2\alpha^2 \\
&= 2pq\alpha^2 (p^2 + q^2 + 2pq)
\end{aligned}$$

and since $(p^2 + 2pq + q^2) = (p + q)^2 = (1)^2$,

$$\sigma^2_A = 2pq\alpha^2$$

In this expression α is the average effect of gene substitution, which is $[a + d (q - p)]$. Hence σ^2_A can be expressed as:

$$2pq\ [a + d (q - p)]^2$$

4.2.2 *Dominance Variance*

Dominance variance is variation of dominance deviations. Information required for deriving dominance variance of a random mating population, which has attained equilibrium, is presented in Table 4.2.

TABLE 4.2: Genotypes, frequencies of genotypes and dominance deviations

Genotypes	Frequency	Dominance deviation	(Dominance deviation)^2
A_1A_1	p^2	$-2q^2d$	$4q^4d^2$
A_1A_2	$2pq$	$2pqd$	$4p^2q^2d^2$
A_2A_2	q^2	$-2p^2d$	$4p^4d^2$

Dominance variance is then got as:

$$\begin{aligned}
\sigma^2_D &= p^2(4q^4d^2) + 2pq (4p^2q^2d^2) + q^2 (4p^4d^2) \\
&= 4p^2q^4d^2 + 8p^3q^3d^2 + 4p^4q^2d^2 \\
&= 4p^2q^2d^2 (q^2+2pq + p^2),
\end{aligned}$$

and since $(p^2 + 2pq + q^2)$ is equal to unity,

$$= 4\ p^2q^2d^2.$$

4.2.3 *Interaction Variance*

Contribution of interaction variance to the genotypic variance of random mating population is not yet very well understood. Reader is referred to

Kempthorne (1957) for deeper insight into this subject.

Interaction variance is the variance of interaction deviations. Interaction between two, three....., several loci may contribute to the interaction deviations. Interaction involving larger number of loci contribute relatively little to the genotypic variance. Hence we will restrict our discussion to the digenic non-allelic interaction. Interaction between two loci may involve interaction of breeding values or dominance deviations. There are thus three kinds of interactions involving two loci. Interaction variance arising from interaction between breeding values is additive × additive variance (σ^2_{AA}). Variation can also arise due to interaction between breeding value and dominance deviation, which is called as the additive × dominance kind. Lastly, dominance deviations at the two loci may interact giving rise to dominance × dominance variance (σ^2_{DD}). Thus interaction variance (σ^2_I) is made up of:

$$\sigma^2_{AA} + \sigma^2_{AD} + \sigma^2_{DD}$$

Genotypic variance is, therefore, made up of following components:

$$\sigma^2_g = \sigma^2_A + \sigma^2_D + \sigma^2_{AA} + \sigma^2_{AD} + \sigma^2_{DD}$$

4.3 Gene Frequencies and Components of Genotypic Variance

Gene frequencies influence not only population mean but also breeding values, dominance deviations and interaction deviations (Chapter 2). It is, therefore, not surprising to find that gene frequencies also govern the magnitude of components of genotypic variance, *i.e.*, σ^2_A, σ^2_D and σ^2_I. Degree of dominance also determines the composition of genotypic variance. Let us see how.

Let us begin with a situation where there is no dominance, *i.e.*, A_1A_2 falls on mid-point. Where there is no dominance, d will be zero. Genotypic variance of the population is, therefore, $2pqa^2$ (because when $d = 0$, $4p^2q^2d^2$, which is dominance variance, is zero). If we assume that deviation of either homozygote (A_1A_1 or A_2A_2) from mid-parental value (*i.e.*, a) is 4, values assumed by the genotypic variance (which is also the additive genetic variance, because dominance variance is zero) at various frequencies of genes could be obtained by substituting values of p, q and a in the following expression

$$\sigma^2_g = 2pqa^2.$$

For example, σ^2_g (and also the σ^2_A) at $p = 0.80$ is got as:

$$2 \times 0.80 \times 0.20 \times 4^2$$
$$= 2 \times 0.16 \times 16$$
$$= 32 \times 0.16$$
$$= 5.12$$

Magnitudes of σ^2_g (and also σ^2_A) for three frequencies of gene A_2 (*i.e.*, q) have been calculated and presented in Table 4.3.

TABLE 4.3: Magnitude of σ^2_g (and also σ^2_A) at various gene frequencies

Gene Frequency		Magnitude of σ^2_A (= σ^2_g)
p	q	
0.80	0.20	5.12
0.50	0.50	8.00
0.30	0.70	6.72

Table 4.3 reveals that additive genetic variance is maximum when $p = q = 0.50$.

Let us consider another situation where A_1A_2 is equal to A_1A_1, *i.e.*, there is complete dominance of gene A_1 over A_2. When dominance is present, genotypic variance is made up of two components, *viz.* additive and dominance variance. When dominance is complete, σ^2_g is maximum when $q = 0.75$. However, component due to dominance variance will be maximum when $p = q = 0.50$. On the other hand, σ^2_A will be maximum when $q = 0.75$. This will be clear with the help of an example. Suppose, $d = a = 4$ units. Magnitudes of σ^2_A and σ^2_D could be calculated by substituting values of a, d, p and q in the following expression:

$$2pq\ [a + d\,(q - p)]^2 + 4p^2q^2d^2$$

Magnitudes of additive, dominance and genotypic variance at various gene frequencies have been calculated and presented in Table 4.4.

TABLE 4.4: Magnitudes of σ^2_A, σ^2_D and σ^2_g at various frequencies of gene A_2 (q) and A_1 (p), assuming complete dominance of gene A_1 ($d = a = 4$)

Gene Frequencies		Magnitudes of		
p	q	σ^2_A	σ^2_D	σ^2_g
0.90	0.10	0.1152	0.5184	0.6336
0.80	0.20	0.8192	1.6384	2.4576
0.70	0.30	2.4192	2.8224	5.2416
0.60	0.40	4.9152	3.6864	8.6016
0.50	0.50	8.0000	4.0000	12.0000
0.40	0.60	11.0592	3.6864	14.7456
0.30	0.70	13.1712	2.8224	15.9936
0.20	0.80	13.1072	1.6384	14.7456
0.10	0.90	9.3312	0.5184	9.8496

Lastly, imagine a situation where A_1A_2 is superior than A_1A_1, *i.e.*, there is overdominance. When degree of dominance is in overdominance range, *i.e.*, $d > +a$, genotypic variance will attain maximum value when $p = q = 0.50$ and dominance variance will also be maximum when $p=q= 0.50$. On the other hand, σ^2_A will be zero when $p = q = 0.50$. Additive genetic variance has maximum values when either $q = 0.15$ or $q = 0.85$. When $a = 0$ and $d = 4$, it can be confirmed that values of σ^2_A, σ^2_D and σ^2_g are as shown inTable 4.5 at various frequencies of gene A_2 (*i.e.*, q).

TABLE 4.5: Showing influence of gene frequencies on σ^2_A, σ^2_D and σ^2_g when $a = 0$, and $d = 4$

Gene Frequency		Magnitudes of		
p	q	σ^2_A	σ^2_D	σ^2_g
0.85	0.15	1.9992	1.0400	3.0392
0.75	0.25	1.5000	2.2464	3.7464
0.50	0.50	0.0000	4.0000	4.0000
0.25	0.75	1.5000	2.2464	3.7464
0.15	0.85	1.9992	1.0400	3.0392

Additive genetic variance, when referred to a random mating population, does not imply that gene effects are necessarily additive. Expression for additive variance is $2pq\ [a + d\,(q - p)]^2$ which includes d, denoting departure of heterozygote from mid-point. Hence only when $d = 0$, additive variance can arise from genes acting in additive fashion (in the absence of non-allelic interaction).

4.4 Environmental Variance

In Section 2.4 it was mentioned that environmental deviations which determine phenotypic values embrace effects attributable to all kinds of non-genetic sources. Environmental variance is variation of environmental deviations. Differences in the fertility levels of plots, moisture contents of soil, seasonal fluctuations, *etc.* contribute to this component of variation. There are several other causes in addition to these which contribute to the environmental variation but are difficult to be eliminated by choice of appropriate experimental designs. For example, weight of bolls on the same cotton plant exhibit variation which could be attributed to developmental causes. Although some environmental variation can be reduced by proper experimentation its total elimination is an impossibility.

4.5 Components of Genotypic Variation in Populations Derived by Controlled Crossing

Fisher, Immer and Tedin (1932) developed genetic theory to describe heritable components of variances of several kinds of populations produced by controlled crossing. These ideas were further elaborated by Mather (1949) and Mather and Jinks (1971, 1977 and 1982). In the preceding section of this chapter, notations used by Falconer (1960) were adopted. Since we shall be dealing now with populations developed by controlled crossing, notations of Mather and Jinks (1971) will be followed.

In what follows, we will restrict ourselves to the generations developed by selfing F_1 and subsequent generations or through biparental mating or by backcrossing. Initially non-allelic interaction will be disregarded. However, subsequently the consequences of non-allelic interaction and linkage will be considered.

Variation of quantitative characters exhibited by true breeding strains and F_1 generation obtained by crossing these strains is entirely non-heritable in origin. It could be ascribed to environmental agencies. On the other hand, variation observed for F_2 generation is heritable as well as non-hertiable in origin. In Chapter 3, three parameters were introduced to describe various generation means. What is the heritable variation of F_2 generation in terms of these parameters ? Let us derive. Let us consider a simple situation of a single locus with two alleles, *viz.* A_1 and A_2. With respect to this locus 3 genotypes in F_2 generation would be A_1A_1, A_1A_2 and A_2A_2 in proportions $\frac{1}{4}, \frac{1}{2}$ and $\frac{1}{4}$, respectively. Contribution of this locus to the mean of this generation would be:

$$\frac{1}{4}(d)+\frac{1}{2}(h)+\frac{1}{4}(-d)$$

$$=\frac{1}{2}(h).$$

Contribution of this locus to the heritable variation of F_2 generation can be got in the usual way, *i.e.*, squaring the values, multiplying the squared values by their frequencies and summation of products over three genotypes from which correction factor is subtracted. Correction factor is square of mean because sum of frequencies is unity (hence the total and mean are identical). Thus, heritable variation of F_2, V'_{F_2} is

$$=\frac{1}{4}(d)^2+\frac{1}{2}(h)^2+\frac{1}{4}(-d)^2-\left(\frac{1}{2}h\right)^2$$

$$=\frac{1}{4}d^2+\frac{1}{2}h^2+\frac{1}{4}d^2-\frac{1}{4}h^2$$

$$=\frac{1}{2}d^2+\frac{1}{4}h^2.$$

In the absence of non-allelic interaction, contribution of several loci, which influence the expression of character to V'_{F_2} will be

$$\frac{1}{2}S(d^2)+\frac{1}{4}S(h^2).$$

If we denote $S(d^2)$ and $S(h^2)$ by D and H, respectively, heritable variation of F_2 generation can be expressed as

$$\frac{1}{2}D+\frac{1}{4}H.$$

To this expression should be added the environmental component of variance (E). The total phenotypic variation of F_2 generations is, therefore:

$$V_{F_2} = \frac{1}{2}D+\frac{1}{4}H+E$$

The component D depends upon $S\,(d^2)$ or the sum of squared deviations of either homozygote from mid-point at each of the locus being considered. Hence this kind of variation is fixable. Fixable variation enables evolution of true breeding strains in self-pollinated crops. For example, if genotype $A_1A_1B_1B_1$ is superior, a variety could be easily developed for cultivation with this genotype in self-pollinated crops. Fixation of genotypes is not easy and practicable in case of cross-pollinated crops. Since the term H is a function of $S\,(h^2)$, which is the sum of departure of heterozygote at each locus from corresponding mid-parental value, variation of this kind is unfixable. For example, if genotype $A_1A_2B_1B_2$ is superior than either $A_1A_1B_1B_1$ or $A_2A_2B_2B_2$ by virtue of dominance, it may not be possible to fix this genotype. This genotype will segregate in subsequent generations and superior performance exhibited by heterozygote will dissipate. Such a variation could be best exploited (and this is especially true for overdominance) by developing F_1 hybrids for commercial planting, provided the cost of hybrid seed production is not high, seed production is easy and the magnitude of heterosis is also large to compensate for extra cost involved in hybrid seed production.

Variation observed for F_2 generation is a result of one round of segregation in the course of gamete formation by F_1 generation. Hence, Mather and Jinks (1971) denote variation of F_2 generation by V_{1F2}. Significance of this notation will be understood in the later part of this chapter.

Generations subsequent to F_2 could be produced either by selfing the plants in F_2 or through sib-mating. Let us describe heritable variation of generation produced by selfing the plants in F_2 generation, *i.e.*, F_3. Selfing of genotypes A_1A_1 and A_2A_2 in F_2 generation will produce progenies with similar genotypes. However, upon selfing individuals with genotype A_1A_2, genes A_1 and A_2 will segregate and hence produce genotypes A_1A_1, A_1A_2 and A_2A_2 in proportions ¼, ½ and ¼ respectively. With respect to this locus, therefore, genetic constitution of F_3 generation will be:

F_2 *parents*					
Genotype	A_1A_1		A_1A_2		A_2A_2
Frequency	¼		½		¼
F_3 *progeny*					
Genotype	A_1A_1	A_1A_1	A_1A_2	A_2A_2	A_2A_2
Frequency (Family-wise)	¼	½(¼	½	¼)	¼
Frequency in the entire population	3/8		¼		3/8

Contribution of this locus to the sum of squares is:

$$\frac{3}{8}(d)^2 + \frac{1}{4}(h)^2 + \frac{3}{8}(-d)^2$$

$$= \frac{3}{8}d^2 + \frac{1}{4}h^2 + \frac{3}{8}d^2$$

$$= \frac{3}{4}d^2 + \frac{1}{4}h^2.$$

After subtracting the correction factor, which is square of mean of F_3 generation (because it is also the total), we get heritable variation of F_3 generation. Thus

$$V_{F3} = \frac{3}{4}d^2 + \frac{1}{4}h^2 - \left(\frac{1}{4}h\right)^2$$

$$= \frac{3}{4}d^2 + \frac{1}{4}h^2 - \frac{1}{16}h^2$$

$$=\frac{3}{4}d^2+\frac{3}{16}h^2$$

When several loci, which influence the expression of a character, are considered V_{F3}, in in the absence of non-allelic interaction, will be:

$$\frac{3}{4}S(d^2)+\frac{3}{16}S(h^2)$$

or $$\frac{3}{4}D+\frac{3}{16}H.$$

This heritable variation of F_3 generation has two components, *viz.* variance of means of F_3 progeny families (*i.e.*, V_{1F3} or $_{\bar{F}_3}V_{\bar{F}3}$) and mean variance of F_3 progeny families (i.e., V_{2F3} or $\bar{V}_{F3}$). Let us now derive variance of means of F_3 families,. Initially V_{1F3} will be derived with respect to a single locus with two alleles (A_1 and A_2). It is obtained after deducting correction factor (square of F_3 mean) from sum of squares of means of F_3 progeny families,. Thus V_{1F3} is :

$$\left[\frac{1}{4}(d)^2+\frac{1}{2}\left(\frac{1}{2}h\right)^2+\frac{1}{4}(-d)^2\right]-\left(\frac{1}{4}h\right)^2$$

$$=\frac{1}{4}d^2+\frac{1}{2}\left(\frac{1}{4}h^2\right)+\frac{1}{4}d^2-\frac{1}{16}h^2$$

$$=\frac{1}{2}d^2+\frac{1}{8}h^2-\frac{1}{16}h^2$$

$$=\frac{1}{2}d^2+\frac{1}{16}h^2.$$

This heritable variation of means of F_3 families could be expressed as $\frac{1}{2}D+\frac{1}{16}H$, when several loci governing the inheritance of a character are taken into consideration. This assumes absence of non-allelic interaction.

Individuals with genotypes A_1A_1 and A_2A_2 when selfed in F_2 generation, produce progenies with genotypes similar to parents and hence these families do not contribute to the mean heritable variation of F_3. However, genotypes A_1A_2 segregate upon selfing and give rise to progenies with genotypes A_1A_1, A_1A_2 and A_2A_2. Heritable variation of this family is, therefore, similar to V_{1F2} *i.e.* $\frac{1}{2}d^2+\frac{1}{4}h^2$. Mean variance of F_3 is obtained by taking into consideration proportions of different families as shown below:

Genotypes in F_2	Frequency in F_2	Family variance in F_3
A_1A_1	$\frac{1}{4}$	0
A_1A_2	$\frac{1}{2}$	$\frac{1}{2}d^2+\frac{1}{4}h^2$
A_2A_2	$\frac{1}{4}$	0

$$V_2F_3=\frac{1}{4}(0)+\frac{1}{2}\left[\frac{1}{2}d^2+\frac{1}{4}h^2\right]+\frac{1}{4}(0)$$

$$=\frac{1}{4}d^2+\frac{1}{8}h^2.$$

When several loci involved in the inheritance are considered V_{2F3} could be expressed as:

$$\frac{1}{4}D+\frac{1}{8}H.$$

Mean expression of each F_3 family is based on number of individuals in the family, say *n*. Therefore, heritable variance of means of F_3 families is subject to sampling variance equal to $1/n$th the mean variance of F_3 families.

Like the F_2 generation, non-heritable variation also contributes to the variance of F_3 means and mean variance of F_3. But the contribution of non-heritable variation to V_{1F3} and V_{2F3} will not be alike. Why? Let us see.

Individuals within a family exhibit non-heritable variation which, following Mather and Jinks (1971), may be denoted by E_1. Non-heritable variation of family means may be denoted by E_2. Since the mean of each family is based on *n* individuals, E_2 will be usually less than E_1. Moreover, if differences in environment between individuals belonging to different families are similar to differences in environment between two individuals within a family, E_2 will be only $\frac{1}{n}E_1$ in magnitude. This situation can be secured by appropriate design of experiment. However, where individuals belonging to same family share a common environment, E_2 may exceed $\frac{1}{n}E_1$. This necessitates subdivision of non-heritable variation in a different manner. Let E_w and E_b represent the non-heritable variation within family and between family, respectively. Then $E_1 = E_w$. Since environmental variation of a family is subject to sampling variation based on n individuals in each family, $E_2 = E_b + \frac{1}{n}(E_w)$. Thus, V_{1F3} and V_{2F3} could be expressed as:

$$V_{1F_3} = \frac{1}{2}D + \frac{1}{16}H + E_2, \left(\text{Since } E_2 = E_b + \frac{1}{n}V_{2F_3}\right)$$

$$= \frac{1}{2}D + \frac{1}{16}H + E_b + \frac{1}{n}V_{2F_3} \text{ and}$$

$$V_{2F_3} = \frac{1}{4}D + \frac{1}{8}H + E_1, (\text{Since } E_1 = E_w),$$

$$= \frac{1}{4}D + \frac{1}{8}H + E_w.$$

Environmental variation of true breeding parental strains and F_2 is simply denoted by E. However, it is in fact E_w. Hence V_{1F2} is

$$\frac{1}{2}D + \frac{1}{4}H + E_w.$$

Starting with F_2, heritable variation of any generation (n) produced by selfing could be obtained, following Mather and Jinks (1971), as:

$$V_{jFn} = \left(\frac{1}{2}\right)^j D + \left(\frac{1}{2}\right)^{2n-j-1} H$$

where j is the rank, being number of rounds of recombination instrumental in affecting the statistic measuring the differences among the individuals. For example, variation of means of F_3 progeny families is of rank 1, because variation of means of F_3 families arises from one round of recombination among genes at the time of gametogenesis in F_1 generation. However, mean variation of F_3 progeny families is a result of two rounds of recombination among the genes, *viz.* one at gametogenesis in F_1 and another in F_2.

Advanced segregating generation is also produced by biparental mating of individuals in F_2 generation. It is designated as S_3. Like the heritable variation of F_3 generation, variance of S_3 generation has two components, *viz.* variance of means of S_3 families $\left(V_{\bar{S}_3}\ or\ V_{1S_3}\right)$ and mean variance of the S_3 families $\left(\bar{V}_{S_3}\ \text{or}\ V_{2S_3}\right)$. Total variation of S_3 generation, however, is not identical with total variation of F_3 generation. With respect to a single locus with two alleles (A_1 and A_2) $V_{\bar{S}3}$ is similar to V_{1F2}, *i.e.*, $\frac{1}{2}d^2+\frac{1}{4}h^2$. If several loci which influence the character are taken into consideration, $V_{\bar{S}3}$ would be $\frac{1}{2}D+\frac{1}{4}H$. Let us derive the heritable component of V_{1S3}. For a single locus with two alleles, *viz.* A_1 and A_2, there will be three kinds of genotypes in F_2 and hence 6 kinds of biparental matings (Table 4.6).

TABLE 4.6: Biparental mating in F_2, frequency of matings, means of progenies and variance of S_3 progeny families

Matings	Frequency of matings	Mean of S_3 progeny	Variance of S_3 progeny family
$A_1A_1 \times A_1A_1$	$\frac{1}{16}$	d	0
$A_1A_1 \times A_1A_2$	$\frac{1}{4}$	$\frac{1}{2}(d+h)$	$\frac{1}{4}(d-h)^2$
$A_1A_1 \times A_2A_2$	$\frac{1}{8}$	h	0
$A_1A_2 \times A_1A_2$	$\frac{1}{4}$	$\frac{1}{2}h$	$\frac{1}{2}d^2+\frac{1}{2}h^2$
$A_1A_2 \times A_2A_2$	$\frac{1}{4}$	$\frac{1}{2}(h-d)$	$\frac{1}{4}(d+h)^2$
$A_2A_2 \times A_2A_2$	$\frac{1}{16}$	$-d$	0

The heritable variance of means of S_3 families is obtained in usual manner from the means of progeny families. Thus :

$$V_{1S3}=\left[\frac{1}{16}(d)^2+\frac{1}{4}\left(\frac{1}{2}d+\frac{1}{2}h\right)^2+\frac{1}{8}(h)^2+\frac{1}{4}\left(\frac{1}{2}h\right)^2\right.$$

$$\left.+\frac{1}{4}\left(\frac{1}{2}h-\frac{1}{2}d\right)^2+\frac{1}{16}(-d)^2\right]-\left(\frac{1}{2}h\right)^2$$

$$=\frac{1}{4}d^2+\frac{1}{16}h^2$$

The correction factor is square of the total of S_3 family means (the total is also the overall mean of S_3 generation because sum of frequencies is unity).

When several loci which influence the inheritance of a character are taken into consideration V_{1S3} may be expressed as:

$$\frac{1}{4}D+\frac{1}{16}H.$$

Mean variance of the S_3 progeny families can be obtained from last column of Table 4.6 by weighting the variance of each progeny family. Thus V_{2S3} will be

$$\frac{1}{4}d^2+\frac{3}{16}h^2.$$

When several loci are taken into consideration, V_{2S3} will be:

$$\frac{1}{4}D+\frac{3}{16}H.$$

The two components of V_{S3} will also include environmental components similar to those shown for V_{1F3} and V_{2F3}. Hence,

$$V_{1S_3}=\frac{1}{4}D+\frac{1}{16}H+E_2$$

$$=\frac{1}{4}D+\frac{1}{16}H+E_b+\frac{1}{n}V_{2S3}$$

and $$V_{2S_3}=\frac{1}{4}D+\frac{3}{16}H+E_w.$$

Let us now examine the variation of progeny families obtained by backcrossing. Initially we will assume a simple case of single locus having two alleles, namely A_1 and A_2. It will be assumed that gene A_1 has a positive effect on the expression of an attribute. If heterozygote is backcrossed to A_1A_1, two kinds of progeny families appear in Bc_1 generation, *viz.*, $\frac{1}{2}A_1A_1$ and $\frac{1}{2}A_1A_2$. The genotypic values associated with A_1A_1 and A_1A_2 expressed as deviation from mid-parental value are d and h, respectively. The mean of Bc_1 generation was shown in section 3.2 to be $\frac{1}{2}(d+h)$. Hence the heritable variance of Bc_1 generation ($V_{Bc\,1}$) will be sum of squares minus correction factor, Thus,

$$V_{Bc_1} = \frac{1}{2}(d)^2 + \frac{1}{2}(h)^2 - \left(\frac{1}{2}d + \frac{1}{2}h\right)^2$$

$$= \frac{1}{4}(d-h)^2.$$

By similar reasoning, heritable variance of Bc_2 generation will be $\frac{1}{4}d^2 + \frac{1}{2}dh + \frac{1}{4}h^2$ or $\frac{1}{4}(d+h)^2$. It is apparent that heritable variation of Bc_2 generation is larger than $V_{Bc\,1}$ when dominance is present. This enhanced variance of Bc_2 generation can be attributed to the term dh. Because of of this term d^2 and h^2 (additive and dominance variance) cannot be separately estimated in either Bc_1 or Bc_2. When sereral loci are considered, heritable variance of Bc_1 and Bc_2 could be expressed, in the absence of non-allelic interaction, as: $V_{Bc_1} = \frac{1}{4}D - \frac{1}{2}F + \frac{1}{4}H$ and $V_{Bc_2} = \frac{1}{4}D + \frac{1}{2}F + \frac{1}{4}H$. Here F is equal to S (dh). Although it is not possible to separate the additive and dominance components of heritable variances from either V_{Bc1} or $V_{Bc\,2}$, summed heritable variances of two backcrosses enable separate estimation of additive and dominance variance components because $V_{Bc\,1} + V_{Bc\,2}$ is $\frac{1}{2}D + \frac{1}{2}H$.

In addition to the heritable components, $V_{BC1} + V_{BC2}$ will also include the environmental component of variance. Thus $V_{BC\,1} + V_{BC\,2}$ is $\frac{1}{2}\mathrm{D} + \frac{1}{2}\mathrm{H} + 2E$.

Heritable variation of a random mating population was described in Section 4.2 to comprise of

$$S2pq\,[a + d\,(q - p)]^2 + S4p^2q^2d^2,$$

in the absence of non-allelic interaction. Mather (1949) used symbols d and h instead of a and d, respectively adopted by Falconer (1960). While describing the components of genotypic variance of random mating population Mather and Jinks (1971) symbolised the additive and dominance components as D_R and H_R, respectively. According to them D_R and H_R are:

$$D_R = S4pq\,[d + h\,(q - p)]^2$$

and $$H_R = S16p^2q^2h^2.$$

From these expressions it becomes evident that additive genetic variance (D_R) of random mating population will be equal to additive variance (D) of selfing series only when $p = q = \frac{1}{2}$ or $h = 0$. Expansion of D_R shows that it has following four components:

$$S4pqd^2 + S4pqh^2 - S16p^2q^2h^2 - S8pq\,(p - q)dh.$$

where $S4pqd^2 = D$, $S4pqh^2 = H_1$, $S16p^2q^2h^2 = H_2 = H_R$ and $S8pq\,(p-q)dh = F$.

When $p = q = \frac{1}{2}$, $H_R = H_2 = H_1$ and $F = 0$. We will discuss more about these in Chapter 6.

4.5.1 *Non-allelic Interaction and Genotypic Variance*

In the preceding sections we have tacitly assumed absence of non-allelic interaction. Contribution of gene pairs at various loci to the heritable variation will be additive, as we have assumed, only if gene pairs are independent both in inheritance and action. Independence in action implies that the increment added to a character by substitution of one allele for the other at a locus is not influenced by genes at other loci. This is not always true. Due attention should, therefore, be paid to the influence of non-allelic interaction on heritable variation.

Variation observed for true breeding strains and F_1 obtained by crossing two such strains is non-heritable in origin. We shall, therefore, begin with F_2 generation. Unless otherwise mentioned, linkage will be assumed to be absent (*i.e.*, genes inherited independently of each other). Let us assume that a quantitative character is governed by two loci each with two alleles, *viz.* A_1, A_2 and B_1, B_2. Variance of F_2 generation resulting from hybridisation of $A_1A_1B_1B_1$ and $A_2A_2B_2B_2$ could be expressed, in the absence of digenic non-allelic interaction, as:

$$\frac{1}{2}d_a^2 + \frac{1}{2}d_b^2 + \frac{1}{4}h_a^2 + \frac{1}{4}h_b^2 .$$

However, if non-allelic interaction is present, heritable variation of F_2 generation can be derived from Table 4.7.

TABLE 4.7: Showing genotypes, phenotypic values* and frequencies of offspring in F_2 generation of a cross $A_1A_1B_1B_1 \times A_2A_2B_2B_2$

	Genotypes			
	A_2A_2	A_1A_2	A_1A_1	
	$\frac{1}{4}$	$\frac{1}{2}$	$\frac{1}{4}$	Frequency
B_2B_2	$A_2A_2B_2B_2$	$A_1A_2B_2B_2$	$A_1A_1B_2B_2$	Genotype
$\frac{1}{4}$	$\frac{1}{16}$	$\frac{1}{8}$	$\frac{1}{16}$	Frequency
	$-d_a - d_b + i_{ab}$	$h_a - d_b - j_{ba}$	$d_a - d_b - i_{ab}$	Value
B_1B_2	$A_2A_2B_1B_2$	$A_1A_2B_1B_2$	$A_1A_1B_1B_2$	
$\frac{1}{2}$	$\frac{1}{8}$	$\frac{1}{4}$	$\frac{1}{8}$	
	$-d_a + h_b - j_{ab}$	$h_a + h_b + l_{ab}$	$d_a + h_b + j_{ab}$	
B_1B_1	$A_2A_2B_1B_1$	$A_1A_2B_1B_1$	$A_1A_1B_1B_1$	
$\frac{1}{4}$	$\frac{1}{16}$	$\frac{1}{8}$	$\frac{1}{16}$	
	$-d_a + d_b - i_{ab}$	$h_a + d_b + j_{ba}$	$d_a + d_b + i_{ab}$	

* Expressed as deviation from mid-parental value.

Contribution of these two loci to the sum of squares of F_2 generation will be:

$$\frac{1}{16}(-d_a - d_b + i_{ab})^2 + \frac{1}{8}(h_a - d_b - j_{ba})^2 + \frac{1}{16}(d_a - d_b - i_{ab})^2 +$$

$$\frac{1}{8}(-d_a + h_b - j_{ab})^2 + \frac{1}{4}(h_a + h_b + l_{ab})^2 + \frac{1}{8}(d_a + h_b + j_{ab})^2 +$$

$$\frac{1}{16}(-d_a + d_b - i_{ab})^2 + \frac{1}{8}(h_a + d_b + j_{ba})^2 + \frac{1}{16}(d_a + d_b + i_{ab})^2.$$

After subtracting correction factor from this sum of squares we get the heritable variance of F_2 (V_{IF2}). Thus V_{IF2} is:

$$\frac{1}{2}\left(d_a + \frac{1}{2}j_{ab}\right)^2 + \frac{1}{2}\left(d_b + \frac{1}{2}j_{ba}\right)^2 + \frac{1}{4}\left(h_a + \frac{1}{2}l_{ab}\right)^2 +$$

$$\frac{1}{4}\left(h_b + \frac{1}{2}l_{ab}\right)^2 + \frac{1}{4}(i_{ab})^2 + \frac{1}{8}(j_{ab})^2 + \frac{1}{8}(j_{ba})^2 + \frac{1}{16}(l_{ab})^2.$$

In the absence of non-allelic interaction, heritable variance of F_2 generation was described in terms of d_a^2, d_b^2 and h_a^2, h_b^2. However, in the presence of digenic non-allelic interaction, components d^2_a and d^2_b have been replaced by $\left(d_a + \frac{1}{2}j_{ab}\right)^2$ and $\left(d_b + \frac{1}{2}j_{ba}\right)^2$, respectively. Similarly components of dominance variance, *viz.* h_a^2 and h_b^2, have been replaced by $\left(h_a + \frac{1}{2}l_{ab}\right)^2$ and $\left(h_b + \frac{1}{2}l_{ab}\right)^2$, respectively. In addition to these changes in the additive and dominance components of heritable variance of F_2, components representing various kinds of non-allelic interactions are also present in pure form, *viz.* $(i_{ab})^2$, $(j_{ab})^2$, $(j_{ba})^2$ and $(l_{ab})^2$. The coefficients for interaction components are found as product of coefficients of main factors. For example, $(i_{ab})^2$ is an interaction variance of additive × additive kind. Since coefficients of both the additive components are $\frac{1}{2}$, coefficient of this interaction variance is $\frac{1}{2} \times \frac{1}{2} = \frac{1}{4}$. If same principle is extended to several loci which influence the inheritance of the character, V_{IF2} can be expressed as $\frac{1}{2}D+\frac{1}{4}H+I$, provided we redefine D and H as $S\left(d_a+\frac{1}{2}S_{ja\cdot}\right)^2$ and $S\left(h_a+\frac{1}{2}S_{la\cdot}\right)^2$, respectively. The term I in this generation is composed of $\frac{1}{4}S(i)^2+\frac{1}{8}S(j)^2+\frac{1}{16}S(l)^2$. Since V_{F2} includes non-heritable component, also add E_w to V_{IF2}.

This concept can be extended to F_3 generation. If two loci govern the inheritance of a character, heritable variance of F_3 generation will be:

$$\frac{3}{4}d_a^2+\frac{3}{4}d_b^2+\frac{3}{16}h_a^2+\frac{3}{16}h_b^2,$$

in the absence of non-allelic interaction. When digenic non-allelic interaction is involved, V_{F3} will be:

$$\frac{3}{4}\left(d_a+\frac{1}{4}j_{ab}\right)^2+\frac{3}{4}\left(d_b+\frac{1}{4}j_{ba}\right)^2+\frac{3}{16}\left(h_a+\frac{1}{4}l_{ab}\right)^2+$$

$$\frac{3}{16}\left(h_b+\frac{1}{4}l_{ab}\right)^2+\frac{9}{16}\left(i_{ab}\right)^2+\frac{9}{64}\left(j_{ab}\right)^2+\frac{9}{64}(j_{ba})^2+\frac{9}{256}(l_{ab})^2.$$

It is interesting to note that in the F_3 generation d^2_a and d^2_b have been replaced by $\left(d_a+\frac{1}{4}j_{ab}\right)^2$ *and* $\left(d_b+\frac{1}{4}j_{ba}\right)^2$, respectively. Similarly h_a^2 and h_b^2 have been replaced by (ha + ¼ l_{ab}) and (ha + ¼ l_{ab}) respectively. In the presence of digenic non-allelic interaction, compositions of additive and dominance components of genotypic variance have changed. Moreover, the coefficients associated with j_{ab} and j_{ba} have changed from generation to generation. Same is the case for l_{ab} associated with h_a and h_b. It can be verified that coefficient associated with j_{ab} and j_{ba} will be $\frac{1}{8}$ in F_4 generation. Same will be true for l_{ab} associated with h_a and h_b.

When non-allelic interaction is not present, heritable variation of means of F_3 progeny families will be:

$$\frac{1}{2}d_a^2+\frac{1}{2}d_b^2+\frac{1}{16}h_a^2+\frac{1}{16}h_b^2.$$

If digenic non-allelic interaction is present the heritable variance of means of F_3 progeny families (V_{1F3}) will be:

$$\frac{1}{2}\left(d_a+\frac{1}{4}j_{ab}\right)^2+\frac{1}{2}\left(d_b+\frac{1}{4}j_{ba}\right)^2+\frac{1}{16}\left(h_a+\frac{1}{4}l_{ab}\right)^2+$$

$$\frac{1}{16}\left(h_b+\frac{1}{4}l_{ab}\right)^2+\frac{1}{4}(i_{ab})^2+\frac{1}{32}(j_{ab})^2+\frac{1}{32}(j_{ba})^2+\frac{1}{256}(l_{ab})^2.$$

With several genes governing the expression of a metric character, V_{1F3} will be:

$$\frac{1}{2}D+\frac{1}{16}H+I,$$

provided we redefine D as $S\left(d_a+\frac{1}{4}S_{ja}\cdot\right)^2$, H as $S\left(h_a+\frac{1}{4}Sl_a\cdot\right)$ and I as $\frac{1}{4}S(i)^2+\frac{1}{32}S(j)^2+\frac{1}{256}S(l)^2$.

Since $V_{F3}=V_{1F3}+V_{2F3}$, V_{2F3} could be got as a difference between V_{F3} and V_{1F3}. Thus V_{2F3} will be:

$$\frac{1}{4}\left(d_a+\frac{1}{4}j_{ab}\right)^2+\frac{1}{4}\left(d_b+\frac{1}{4}j_{ba}\right)^2+\frac{1}{8}\left(h_a+\frac{1}{4}l_{ab}\right)^2+$$

$$\frac{1}{8}\left(h_b+\frac{1}{4}l_{ab}\right)^2+\frac{5}{16}(i_{ab})^2+\frac{7}{64}(j_{ab})^2+\frac{7}{64}(j_{ba})^2+\frac{1}{32}(l_{ab})^2.$$

It should be clear to the reader that leaving apart the pure forms of interaction variance components (I), the constitutions of D and H tend to change when digenic non-allelic interaction is operative. Additive component includes a term which specifies additive × dominance interaction, and hence when digenic non-allelic interaction is present estimate of additive variance is bound to be biased upward or downward depending upon the sign and magnitude of additive × dominance interaction parameter. Dominance variance is not only composed of terms based on h^2 but includes a parameter specifying dominance × dominance interaction. Magnitude of dominance variance, therefore, depends upon the sign and magnitude of dominance × dominance kind of digenic non-allelic interaction.

Proceeding to the biparental families, it can be shown that composition of additive and dominance variances, in the presence of digenic non-allelic interaction, is similar to that for V_{IF2}. Assuming a simple situation of two loci, each with two alleles, *viz.* A_1, A_2 and B_1, B_2, it can be confirmed that V_{S3} is:

$$\frac{1}{2}\left(d_a+\frac{1}{2}j_{ab}\right)^2+\frac{1}{2}\left(d_b+\frac{1}{2}j_{ba}\right)^2+\frac{1}{4}\left(h_a+\frac{1}{2}l_{ab}\right)^2+$$

$$\frac{1}{4}\left(h_b+\frac{1}{2}l_{ab}\right)^2+\frac{1}{4}(i_{ab})^2+\frac{1}{8}(j_{ab})^2+\frac{1}{8}(j_{ba})^2+\frac{1}{16}(l_{ab})^2.$$

The heritable variance of means of S_3 progeny families (V_{1S3}), in the absence of non-allelic interaction, could be expressed as:

$$\frac{1}{4}d_a^2+\frac{1}{4}d_b^2+\frac{1}{16}h_a^2+\frac{1}{16}h_b^2.$$

When non-allelic interaction exists, the composition of d_a^2, d_b^2 in V_{1S3} changes to that shown for V_{F2}. Similarly the composition of h_a^2, h_b^2 changes to $\left(h_a+\frac{1}{2}l_{ab}\right)^2$ and $\left(h_b+\frac{1}{2}l_{ab}\right)^2$, respectively. Moreover pure forms of digenic non-allelic interaction parameters will also be present. Thus V_1s_3 will be:

$$\frac{1}{4}\left(d_a+\frac{1}{2}j_{ab}\right)^2+\frac{1}{4}\left(d_b+\frac{1}{2}j_{ba}\right)^2+\frac{1}{16}\left(h_a+\frac{1}{2}l_{ab}\right)^2+$$

$$\frac{1}{16}\left(h_b+\frac{1}{2}l_{ab}\right)^2+\frac{1}{16}(i_{ab})^2+\frac{1}{64}(j_{ab})^2+\frac{1}{64}(j_{ba})^2+\frac{1}{256}(l_{ab})^2$$

Since $V_{S3}=V_{1S3}+V_{2S3}$, $V_{2S3}=V_{S3}-V_{1S3}$. Thus, V_{2S3} will be:

$$\frac{1}{4}\left(d_a+\frac{1}{2}j_{ab}\right)^2+\frac{1}{4}\left(d_b+\frac{1}{2}j_{ba}\right)^2+\frac{3}{16}\left(h_a+\frac{1}{2}l_{ab}\right)^2+$$

$$\frac{3}{16}\left(h_b+\frac{1}{2}l_{ab}\right)^2+\frac{3}{16}(i_{ab})^2+\frac{7}{64}(j_{ab})^2+\frac{7}{64}(j_{ba})^2+\frac{15}{256}(l_{ab})^2$$

The coefficients associated with pure forms of digenic non-allelic interaction parameters for second rank variances, such as V_{2F3}, V_{2S3}, *etc.* cannot be obtained as a product of coefficients of corresponding main factors, like the rank one variances.

We shall now consider variances of the generations obtained by backcrossing F_1 to either of the true breeding parental strains. It was shown in section 3.5 that the mean expressions of backcross generations are influenced by distribution of genes between the parental strains. Although we are not taking into consideration the linkage of genes, distribution of genes between the parental strains cannot be neglected while deriving heritable variances of backcrosses. The heritable variance of summed backcrosses, *viz.* $V_{BC1} + V_{BC2}$, following Mather and Jinks (1980), will be:

$$\frac{1}{2}\left(d_a + \frac{1}{2} j_{ab} \mp \frac{1}{2} j_{ba}\right)^2 + \frac{1}{2}\left(d_b \mp \frac{1}{2} j_{ab} + \frac{1}{2} j_{ba}\right)^2 +$$

$$\frac{1}{2}\left(h_a \mp \frac{1}{2} i_{ab} + \frac{1}{2} l_{ab}\right)^2 + \frac{1}{2}\left(h_b \mp \frac{1}{2} i_{ab} + \frac{1}{2} l_{ab}\right)^2 +$$

$$\frac{1}{8}(i_{ab} \pm l_{ab})^2 + \frac{1}{8}(j_{ab} \pm j_{ba})^2$$

in the presence of digenic non-allelic interaction. In this expression upper signs refer to the genes in association whereas the lower signs refer to the genes in dispersion. The summed heritable variances of Bc_1 and Bc_2 depend for their magnitude not only upon the signs and magnitudes of digenic non-allelic interaction parameters, like the heritable variances of F_2, F_3, S_3, *etc.* but also upon the distribution of genes between parents. Unlike the variances of F_2, F_3, S_3, *etc.* the additive component of $V_{Bc1} + V_{Bc2}$ is associated with both j_{ab} and j_{ba}. Similarly, dominance variance is clubbed not only with dominance × dominance interaction component but also a parameter specifying additive × additive interaction. Even the interaction term i_{ab} is not pure, but is coupled with l_{ab}.

It was pointed out in section 3.5 that non-allelic interaction may be classified into two broad categories, *viz.* complementary and duplicate. Signs of [l] and [i] will be similar in direction to [h] if interaction is of complementary type. In addition, the sign of [j] will be positive when non-allelic interaction is complementary (Mather and Jinks, 1977). Since parameters j and l are coupled with additive and dominance variances, respectively, additive and dominance components of genotypic variance will be biased upwards when non-allelic interaction is of complementary type. On the other hand, sign of [j] will be negative and the signs of [l] and [i] opposite to [h], when non-allelic interaction is of duplicate type.

Hence the magnitudes of additive and dominance variances of F_2, F_3, F_4, S_3, S_4, *etc.* will be reduced when duplicate type of non-allelic interaction is present. Nevertheless, increasing or decreasing effect of non-allelic interaction is also a function of strength of interaction.

4.5.2 *Linkage and Heritable Variation*

In section 4.5.1 consequences of non-independence of genes in action were described. Contribution of gene pairs at various loci to the heritable variation is additive only if genes are independent in inheritance and independent in action. What is meant by independence in inheritance? Suppose a character is governed by genes at two loci, each having two alleles, *viz.* A_1, A_2 and B_1, B_2. If alleles A_1 and A_2 are equally likely to be transmitted from parents to offspring with a given allele, say B_1 at other locus, genes are said to be independent in their inheritance. This is possible when genes are not tightly linked. Linkage does not affect the frequencies with which either allele A_1 or A_2 is recovered in the segregating population (so also alleles B_1 and B_2 at other locus). However, linkage tends to influence the proportion in which combinations of two genes at different loci are recovered. Proportion in which combinations of two genes appear, *e.g.* A_1B_1, A_1B_2, A_2B_1 and A_2B_2 in the present case, is a function of recombination frequency p (= $1-q$).

Mean expressions of true breeding parental strains and the F_1 resulting from their hybridisation are not influenced by linkage (section 3.5). Since, these generations do not exhibit heritable variation, let us start with F_2 generation in order to understand the effect of linkage on heritable variation. In what follows we assume absence of non-allelic interaction.

Let us assume a simple situation where the inheritance of a metric trait is governed by two loci, each having two alleles, *viz.* A_1, A_2 and B_1, B_2. Let us also assume that the recombination frequency between these gene pairs is p (= $1-q$). If we cross two inbreds $A_1A_1B_1B_1$ and $A_2A_2B_2B_2$ (genes in coupling phase), genetic constitution of F_1 will be A_1B_1/A_2B_2. Four kinds of gametes produced by F_1 will be A_1B_1, A_2B_2, A_1B_2 and A_2B_1, provided that linkage is not very tight. Gametes A_1B_1 and A_2B_2 are parental types and A_2B_1 and A_1B_2 recombinant or non-parental types. Since, the total frequency of recombinant gametes will be p, proportion of each of the two kinds, *viz.* A_1B_2 and A_2B_1, will be $\frac{1}{2}p$. By similar analogy the proportion of parental type gametes will be $\frac{1}{2}q$ each. Random union of these gametes will give rise to F_2 generation (Table 4.8). The heritable variation of F_2 generation derived in usual manner will be:

$$\frac{1}{2}[d_a^2 + d_b^2 + 2(1-2p)d_a d_b] + \frac{1}{4}[h_a^2 + h_b^2 + 2(1-2p)^2 h_a h_b]$$

TABLE 4.8: Showing genotypes, frequencies and phenotypes* of individuals in F_2 when linkage is considered

	Gametes and frequency			
	A_1B_1 $\frac{1}{2}q$	A_1B_2 $\frac{1}{2}p$	A_2B_1 $\frac{1}{2}p$	A_2B_2 $\frac{1}{2}q$
A_1B_1 $\frac{1}{2}q$	$A_1A_1B_1B_1$ $\frac{1}{4}q^2$ $d_a + d_b$	$A_1A_1B_1B_2$ $\frac{1}{4}pq$ $d_a + h_b$	$A_1A_2B_1B_1$ $\frac{1}{4}pq$ $h_a + d_b$	$A_1A_2B_1B_2$ $\frac{1}{4}q^2$ $h_a + h_b$
A_1B_2 $\frac{1}{2}p$	$A_1A_1B_1B_2$ $\frac{1}{4}pq$ $d_a + h_b$	$A_1A_1B_2B_2$ $\frac{1}{4}p^2$ $d_a - d_b$	$A_1A_2B_1B_2$ $\frac{1}{4}p^2$ $h_a + h_b$	$A_1A_2B_2B_2$ $\frac{1}{4}pq$ $h_a - d_b$
A_2B_1 $\frac{1}{2}p$	$A_1A_2B_1B_1$ $\frac{1}{4}pq$ $h_a + d_b$	$A_1A_2B_1B_2$ $\frac{1}{4}p^2$ $h_a + h_b$	$A_2A_2B_1B_1$ $\frac{1}{4}p^2$ $-d_a + d_b$	$A_2A_2B_1B_2$ $\frac{1}{4}pq$ $-d_a + h_b$
A_2B_2 $\frac{1}{2}q$	$A_1A_2B_1B_2$ $\frac{1}{4}q^2$ $h_a + h_b$	$A_1A_2B_2B_2$ $\frac{1}{4}pq$ $h_a - d_b$	$A_2A_2B_1B_2$ $\frac{1}{4}pq$ $-d_a + h_b$	$A_2A_2B_2B_2$ $\frac{1}{4}q^2$ $-d_a - d_b$

*Expressed as deviation from mid-parental value.

When the genes are linked, additive component of V_{1F2} contains in addition to d^2_a and d^2_b a term involving recombination value.

Likewise dominance variance comprises of a term referring to recombination in addition to h^2_a and h^2_b. When genes are independent in inheritance, *i.e.* $p = \frac{1}{2}$, heritable variation of F_2 will reduce to

$\frac{1}{2}d^2_a + \frac{1}{2}d^2_b + \frac{1}{4}h^2_a + \frac{1}{4}h^2_b$ (because when $p = \frac{1}{2}$, term $1-2p$ will be zero). On the other hand, with tight linkage ($p = 0$) V_{1F2} would be:

$$\frac{1}{2}[d_a^2 + d_b^2 + 2d_a d_b] + \frac{1}{4}[h_a^2 + h_b^2 + 2h_a h_b]$$

$$= \frac{1}{2}[d_a + d_b]^2 + \frac{1}{4}[h_a + h_b]^2.$$

When the genes are tightly linked, the two genes appear to act as one. Even if recombination takes place, frequency of recombinant gametes will be very low. Hence the recovery of such recombinants is difficult.

If the two genes are linked in repulsion phase V_{1F2} will appear as:

$$\frac{1}{2}[d_a^2 + d_b^2 - 2(1-2p)d_a\, d_b] + \frac{1}{4}[h_a^2 + h_b^2 + 2(1-2p)^2\, h_a\, h_b].$$

The sign of $d_a d_b$ changes with the phase of linkage. However, the sign of $h_a h_b$ remains unchanged irrespective of linkage phase. When genes are linked, magnitude of additive variance depends upon the sign and value of $d_a d_b$ in addition to the extent of recombination frequency. The magnitude of dominance variance similarly depends upon p as well as the magnitude and the sign of $h_a h_b$. The sign of $h_a h_b$ is not determined by linkage phase but by the positive and negative signs of h_a and h_b (*i.e.* direction of dominance at each locus). When the signs of h_a and h_b are in same direction, gene effects are said to be reinforcing each other (Mather and Jinks, 1971, 1977). On the other hand, when h_a and h_b have opposite signs, effects are said to be in opposition to each other. Hence, when h_a and h_b are in opposition, sign of $h_a h_b$ is negative and if magnitude of $h_a h_b$ is larger than ($h^2_a + h^2_b$), magnitude of dominance variance will be reduced. Opposition *vs.* reinforcement results from physiological reasons as opposed to repulsion and coupling which is a mechanical phenomenon resulting when two or more genes are located on same chromosome. Heritable variance of F_2 generation (V_{1F2}) can be expressed as:

$$\frac{1}{2}D + \frac{1}{4}H$$

when genes are linked, provided we redefine D as:

$[d^2_a + d^2_b \pm 2(1-2p)d_a d_b]$ and H as $[h^2_a + h^2_b + 2(1-2p)^2 h_a h_b]$.

Heritable variance of means of F_3 progeny families can also be described using these definitions. Thus V_{1F3} is:

$$\frac{1}{2}[d_a^2 + d_b^2 \pm 2(1-2p)d_a d_b] + \frac{1}{16}[h_a^2 + h_b^2 + 2(1-2p)^2 h_a h_b].$$

Nevertheless, second rank variance of this generation, *i.e.* V_{2F3}, will differ from these compositions for additive and dominance variance. Following Mather and Jinks (1971), V_{2F3} can be expressed as:

$$\frac{1}{4}[d_a^2 + d_b^2 + 2(1-2p)^2 d_a d_b] +$$

$$\frac{1}{8}[h_a^2 + h_b^2 + 2(1-2p)^2 (1-2p+2p^2) h_a h_b].$$

The composition of D and H in V_{1S3} and V_{2S3} will be as shown below:

$$V_{1S3} = \frac{1}{4}[d_a^2 + d_b^2 + 2(1-2p)d_a d_b] + \frac{1}{16}[h_a^2 + h_b^2 + 2(1-2p)^2 h_a h_b]$$

and $$V_{2S3} = \frac{1}{4}[d_a^2\, d_b^2 \pm 2(1-2p)^2 d_a d_b] +$$

$$\frac{3}{16}[h_a^2 + h_b^2 + 2(1-2p)^2 (1-2p+2p^2) h_a h_b].$$

Rank 2 variances can be written in terms of D and H in the presence of linkage, provided they are redefined as:

$$D = [d^2_a + d^2_b \pm 2(1-2p)^2 d_a d_b]$$

and $$H = [h^2_a + h^2_b + 2(1-2p)^2 (1-2p+2p^2) h_a h_b].$$

The compositions of additive and dominance components of heritable variances appear to change from rank to rank in the presence of linkage. "Rank being the number of occasions on which recombination has had opportunity to affect the differences that the statistic in question is measuring" (Mather and Jinks, 1971).

The heritable portion of summed backcross variances will have different constitution in the presence of linkage than the one considered in preceding paragraphs. Let us continue with hypothetical genetic situation of a single locus with two alleles, *viz.* A_1 , A_2 and B_1 , B_2. If F_1 $(A_1A_2B_1B_2)$ is backcrossed to $A_1A_1B_1B_1$ (P_1) and $A_2A_2B_2B_2$ (P_2) frequencies of resulting progenies and genotypes will be as shown in Table 4.9.

TABLE 4.9: Genotypes, frequencies and genotypic values of backcross progenies

Gametes in parents	Gametes and frequencies in F_1				
	A_1B_1	A_1B_2	A_2B_1	A_2B_2	
	$\frac{1}{2}q$	$\frac{1}{2}p$	$\frac{1}{2}p$	$\frac{1}{2}q$	
$A_1B_1(P_1)$	$\frac{1}{2}q$	$\frac{1}{2}p$	$\frac{1}{2}p$	$\frac{1}{2}q$	Frequency
	$A_1A_1B_1B_1$	$A_1A_1B_1B_2$	$A_1A_2B_1B_1$	$A_1A_2B_1B_2$	Genotype
	$d_a + d_b$	$d_a + h_b$	$h_a + d_b$	$h_a + h_b$	
$A_2B_2(P_2)$	$\frac{1}{2}q$	$\frac{1}{2}p$	$\frac{1}{2}p$	$\frac{1}{2}q$	
	$A_1A_2B_1B_2$	$A_1A_2B_2B_2$	$A_2A_2B_1B_2$	$A_2A_2B_2B_2$	
	$h_a + h_b$	$h_a - d_b$	$-d_a + h_b$	$-d_a - d_b$	

Summed heritable variance of backcross generations in the presence of linkage will, therfore, be:

$$\frac{1}{2}[d_a^2 + d_b^2 + 2(1-2p)d_ad_b] + \frac{1}{2}[h_a^2 + h_b^2 + 2(1-2p)h_ah_b].$$

When the genes are linked in repulsion phase in parental strains, sign of $2(1-2p)d_ad_b$ will be negative. Magnitudes of components of heritable summed backcross variances, therefore, depend upon the strength of linkage (p) as well as upon signs and magnitudes of d_ad_b and h_ah_b. In addition to the intrinsic sign of d_ad_b, coupling/repulsion phase will also determine its sign. On the other hand, reinforcement *vs.* opposition will determine the sign of h_ah_b.

If we consider several loci which govern the expression of a character, linkage will have maximum influence on the variances when all the genes are linked in coupling phase and the effects of genes are reinforcing each other (leading to positive sign of $h_a h_b$, $h_a h_c$, *etc.*). Although linkage may in fact be present, its effect on the variance of character being measured may not be perceptible because of cancellation of effects. The cancellation or balancing of the effects can result from some genes being in coupling and some in repulsion phases as well as from opposition and reinforcement phenomenon.

As shown previously, heritable variation of F_2 generation, in the absence of linkage (*i.e.*, $p = \frac{1}{2}$), will be $\frac{1}{2}d_a^2 + \frac{1}{2}d_b^2 + \frac{1}{4}h_a^2 + \frac{1}{4}h_b^2$ and mean heritable variance of F_3 generation will be $\frac{1}{4}d_a^2 + \frac{1}{4}d_b^2 + \frac{1}{8}h_a^2 + \frac{1}{8}h_b^2$. In the absence of linkage, V_{1F2} will be twice that of V_{2F3}. Test of linkage is, therefore, test of homogeneity of D and H over statistics of different ranks. It was shown in section 3.3 that scaling tests can detect the presence of non-allelic interaction. Nevertheless, linkage can be detected with difficulty through analysis of means. Second degree statistics, such as V_{1F2}, V_{2F3}, provide a convenient test for detection of linkage.

4.6 Resemblance Between Relatives

In our own race it is common to observe resemblance between close relatives. Resemblance between relatives is also observed in higher plants. For example, in F_2 generation of a cross between red and white flowered sweet peas, about 75 per cent plants resemble the red parent and 25 per cent look like the white parent with respect to flower colour. Resemblance is thus a property of qualitative characters. Relatives resemble each other either because of genetic factors or due to the influence of environment. In sweet peas, 75 per cent plants in F_2 look like red parent because they possess gene or genes similar to their parent. An individual plant may be high-yielding like its high-yielding parent because of desirable genes possessed by it or due to favourable environment around it. Only a progeny test can discriminate between these two causes of resemblance.

For quantitative characters also resemblance may be observed between various sorts of relatives. In the segregating material generated as a result of hybridisation betwen a high-yielding and a low-yielding genotype, a range of variation can be observed for this character. If large progeny is raised some plants could be identified which closely resemble either of the parents. Others will differ in degree of resemblance. Degree to which relatives resemble, is a property of a character, some characters show more resemblance, some less.

In order to determine the degree of resemblance between relatives, measurements are made on phenotypes. Since phenotype is determined by genotype and environmental agencies, degree of resemblance is also determined by these agencies.

Phenotypic variance was shown in section 4.1 to be determined by genotypic variance and the environmental variance, *i.e.*, $\sigma^2{}_p = \sigma^2 g + \sigma^2{}_e$ (assuming absence of correlation and interaction between genotype and environmental agencies). These are the causal components of phenotypic variance. In order to measure the degree of resemblance between relatives, phenotypic variation is partitioned in a different manner. Suppose we have F_3 progenies, each descending from different F_2 plants. Total variation of individuals in F_3 generation ($\sigma^2{}_T$) will comprise of two components, *viz.* variation of individuals within each family ($\sigma^2{}_w$) and of variation of means of families ($\sigma^2{}_b$). We may call these components as within family variation and between family variation. These are the observational components of phenotypic variance. If individuals within each of the family are alike, within family variance will be negligible. For a given amount of total variance, therefore, between family variance will be large. On the other hand, if individuals within each family manifest less resemblance with each other, within family variance will be relatively larger. Thus greater the resemblance of individuals within each family, greater will be the variance of family means (σ_b^2). The degree of resemblance between relatives measured as covariance, and distinctness of groups of relatives from each other, measured as variance, are really the same thing. Thus the ratio:

$$t = \frac{\sigma_b^2}{\sigma_b^2 + \sigma_w^2},$$

which is an intra-class correlation (t) and can be used to measure the degree of resemblance between relatives.

Resemblance betwen relatives can be expressed as correlation or regression. In the case of offspring and parent relationship, it is desirable to measure the degree of resemblance in terms of regression of offsprings on their parents. On the other hand, while dealing with full-sibs, correlation among individuals is a better measure of degree of resemblance. In any case, a new property of pouplation, *viz*, covariance, has to be determined. Phenotypic covariance is determined by genotypic covariance and environmental covariance. We shall deal only with the former. As will be shown subsequently, genotypic covariance of relatives is determined largely by additive genetic variance and in some cases by dominance variance also (neglecting for the time being interaction variance as a cause of resemblance). Hence, phenotypic resemblance can be translated into genetic components of variance such as σ^2_A and σ^2_D. For this reason geneticists are interested to measure the degree of resemblance between relatives.

Expectations for genetic covariance between relatives of various sorts have been derived by Kempthorne (1957), Falconer (1960) and Mather and Jinks (1971,1977). Reader should refer to these works for details.

We will examine, a few relationships such as offspring and one parent, half-sibs, offspring and mid-parent and full-sibs, which will be required in connection with various mating designs.

4.6.1 *Covariance Between Relatives in a Random Mating Population*

Initially we will deduce the covariance between relatives of various kinds in a random mating population, which has attained Hardy-Weinberg equilibrium. Since our discussion will centre around genetic causes of resemblance, we have to find covariance between genotypic values of the relatives.

(i) Offspring and One Parent: We have to deduce the covariance of genotypic value of one parent and mean genotypic value of their offspring which has resulted from random mating of a parent with number of individuals in the population. It was shown in section 2.6 that the genotypic value of an individual is made up of breeding value and

dominance deviations (we shall assume that non-allelic interaction is absent. However, role of this component will be discussed at the end of this section). What will be the mean genotypic value of the offspring? Let us find out.

Assume a single locus with two alleles, *viz.* A_1 and A_2. With respect to this locus, there will be three kinds of genotypes in the population, *viz.* A_1A_1, A_1A_2 and A_2A_2, in proportions p^2, $2pq$ and q^2, respectively. If individuals of the genotype A_1A_1 are mated randomly to a number of individuals in the population, two kinds of progeny will be produced, *viz.* A_1A_1 and A_1A_2 in proportions p and q, respectively (section 2.5). Mean of this progeny, expressed as deviation from population mean, is the average effect of gene A_1 carried by the parent A_1A_1, which is half the breeding value of parent. Mean genotypic value of the progeny resulting from random mating of one individual with a number of individuals in the population is, therefore, equal to half the breeding value of parent. If we denote breeding value and dominance deviation by *BV* and *DD*, respectively, then we have to derive covariance of $\frac{1}{2}$(BV) with ($BV + DD$). Since the sum of genotype frequencies is unity, covariance is simply the sum of cross products. Thus,

$$\text{Cov}_{op} = \frac{1}{2}(BV).(BV + DD)$$

$$= \frac{1}{2}(BV)^2 + \frac{1}{2}(BV \cdot DD).$$

Breeding values and dominance deviations are not correlated (section 2.6) and, therefore, $\frac{1}{2}(BV \cdot DD)$ is zero. If we consider several loci which influence the inheritance of metric trait being investigated, the covariance of mean of offspring and one parent would be $\frac{1}{2}S(BV)^2$. This is also the variance of breeding values because sum of genotype frequencies is unity. Variance of breeding values is known as additive genetic variance. Hence, covariance of offspring with one parent in equal to $\frac{1}{2}\sigma^2_A$.

This covariance could be derived in a different manner. With respect to a single locus with two alleles, A_1 and A_2, there will be three genotypes A_1A_1, A_1A_2 and A_2A_2 in the population at equilibrium. Frequencies of these genotypes will be p^2, $2pq$ and q^2, respectively. It was shown in chapter 2 that breeding values of these genotypes in terms of α would be $2q\alpha$, $(q-p)\alpha$ and $-2p\alpha$, respectively. We have to derive covariance of genotypic value of one parent with mean genotypic value of its progeny. Mean genotypic value of progeny is half the breeding value of its common parent (chapter 2.) These values are given in Table 4.10. Since mean genotypic values of offspring are given in terms of α it is desirable to express genotypic values of parents also in terms of *alpha.* Genotypic values of genotypes A_1A_1, A_1A_2 and A_2A_2 were derived in terms of α in Chapter 2. Information required to deduce covariance of offspring with one parent is presented in Table 4.10. Covariance of offspring with one parent (Cov_{op}) is then obtained as:

$$p^2(2q\alpha-2q^2d)(q\alpha)+2pq[q\alpha-p\alpha+2pqd]\left(\frac{1}{2}q\alpha-\frac{1}{2}p\alpha\right)+$$

$$q^2(-2p\alpha-2p^2d)(-p\alpha),$$

$$=(2p^2q\alpha-2p^2q^2d)(q\alpha)+[2pq^2\alpha-2p^2q\alpha+4p^2q^2d]$$

$$\left(\frac{1}{2}q\alpha-\frac{1}{2}p\alpha\right)+(-2pq^2\alpha-2p^2q^2d)(-p\alpha),$$

$$=2p^2q^2\alpha^2-2p^2q^3\alpha d+pq^3\alpha^2-2p^3q^2\alpha^2+2p^2q^3\alpha d$$

$$+p^3q\alpha^2+2p^3q^2\alpha d+2p^3q^2\alpha^2-2p^3q^2\alpha d,$$

$$=pq\alpha^2(q^2+2pq+p^2),\text{ and since}$$

$$(p^2+2pq+q^2)\text{ equals unity,}$$

$$=pq\alpha^2.$$

Table 4.10: Genotypic values, frequencies of parents and mean genotypic values of progeny

Parents			Mean genotypic values of progeny
Genotypes	Frequencies	Genotypic values	
A_1A_1	p^2	$2q(\alpha-qd)$	$q\alpha$
A_1A_2	$2pq$	$(q-p)\alpha+2pqd$	$\frac{1}{2}q\alpha-\frac{1}{2}p\alpha$
A_2A_2	q^2	$-2p(\alpha+pd)$	$-p\alpha$

It was shown in section 2.5, that $2pq\alpha^2$ is additive genetic variance. When several loci are taken into consideration this covariance will be $\frac{1}{2}\sigma^2_A$.

(*ii*) *Covariance of Half-sibs:* Half-sibs are the individuals having one parent in common. For example, *n* progeny families produced by crossing *n* lines with one tester are half-sib families. The covariance of half-sibs is got as variance of means of half-sib progeny families (Table 4.10). Since the mean genotypic values of progeny families have been expressed as deviation from population mean, variance is got as sum of (frequency × square of mean) over three kinds of half-sib families. Thus, covariance of half-sibs (Cov_{HS}) is:

$$p^2(q\alpha)^2+2pq\left(\frac{1}{2}q\alpha-\frac{1}{2}p\alpha\right)^2+q^2(-p\alpha)^2$$

$$=p^2q^2\alpha^2+2pq\left(\frac{1}{4}q^2\alpha^2-\frac{1}{2}pq\alpha^2+\frac{1}{4}p^2\alpha^2\right)+p^2q^2\alpha^2$$

$$=2p^2q^2\alpha^2+\frac{1}{2}pq^3\alpha^2-p^2q^2\alpha^2+\frac{1}{2}p^3q\alpha^2$$

$$=p^2q^2\alpha^2+\frac{1}{2}pq^3\alpha^2+\frac{1}{2}p^3q\alpha^2$$

$$=\frac{1}{2}pq\alpha^2(2pq+q^2+p^2)\text{, and since } p^2+2pq+q^2=1,$$

$$= \frac{1}{2} pq\alpha^2$$, which is quarter of additive genetic variance.

The expression shows that when several loci are considered, covariance of half-sib progeny families is equal to quarter of an additive genetic variance $\left(\frac{1}{4}\sigma_A^2\right)$.

During the course of experimentation, geneticists develop inbred lines from open pollinated populations. The inbreds are then used to produce half-sib and full-sib progeny families. Before the genetic expectations of covariances of such families are given, it should be pointed out that the coefficient of inbreeding of individuals may range from zero (no inbreeding) to 1 (completely inbred). While deducing the covariance of half-sibs or full-sibs, therefore, one should take into consideration the extent of coefficient of inbreeding. Coefficient of inbreeding is the probability that two genes at any locus in an individual are indentical by descent. If two genes originated by replication of one gene in the previous generation, they are said to be identical by descent. An individual may be called as an identical homozygote if it carries two genes at a locus which are identical by descent. However, if the individuals are homozygous, but the two genes (although of the same kind) have different origin (not identical), homozygotes are said to be 'Independent homozygotes'. The coefficient of inbreeding is denoted by *F*. Thus, covariance of half-sibs produced from lines with any degree of coefficient of inbreeding could be obtained as

$$\left(\frac{1+F}{4}\right)^i \sigma_A^2 + \sigma_{AA}^2 \;\ldots\ldots$$

where i is the number of times A appears in the variance. σ^2_A is the additive genetic variance and σ^2_{AA} is the variance due to non-alielic interaction of additive × additive kind. Here we will consider only digenic non-allelic interaction. For example, if we assume that parental population is completely inbred ($F = 1$), covariance of half-sib (Cov_{HS})

will be

$$\left(\frac{1+1}{4}\right)^{i} \sigma_{A}^{2} + \sigma_{AA}^{2} \qquad \ldots\ldots\ldots$$

$$= \left(\frac{2}{4}\right)^{1} \sigma_{A}^{2} + \left(\frac{2}{4}\right)^{2} \sigma_{AA}^{2} \qquad \ldots\ldots\ldots$$

$$= \frac{1}{2}\sigma_{A}^{2} + \frac{1}{4}\sigma_{AA}^{2} \qquad \ldots\ldots\ldots$$

On the other hand, if half-sib progenies are produced from individuals of an open pollinated population ($F = 0$), covariance half-sibs will be:

$$\left(\frac{1+0}{4}\right)^{i} \sigma_{A}^{2} + \sigma_{AA}^{2} \qquad \ldots\ldots\ldots$$

$$= \left(\frac{1}{4}\right)^{1} \sigma_{A}^{2} + \left(\frac{1}{4}\right)^{2} \sigma_{AA}^{2} \qquad \ldots\ldots\ldots$$

$$= \frac{1}{4}\sigma_{A}^{2} + \frac{1}{16}\sigma_{AA}^{2} \qquad \ldots\ldots\ldots$$

(iii) Covariance of Full-sib progeny Families: Full-sibs are individuals having both parents in common. Covariance of full-sibs is obtained as variance of means of full-sib progeny families. With respect to a single locus with two alleles, there will be three kinds of genotypes, *viz.* A_1A_1, A_1A_2 and A_2A_2. As shown in section 2.3, there will be six kinds of matings among these genotypes. Individuals within families resulting from the six kinds of matings are full-sibs. Variation of means of these progenies will yield covariance of full-sibs. Information needed to deduce covariance is presented in Table 4.11.

Table 4.11: Mating types, frequencies of matings and mean genotypic values of progenies and parents

Mating types	Mating frequencies	Genotypic values of progeny			Mean genotypic values of	
		A_1A_1	A_1A_2	A_2A_2	Progeny	Parents
$A_1A_1 \times A_1A_1$	p^4	a	–	–	a	a
$A_1A_1 \times A_1A_2$	$4p^3q$	$\frac{1}{2}a$	$\frac{1}{2}d$	–	$\frac{1}{2}(d+a)$	$\frac{1}{2}(a+d)$
$A_1A_1 \times A_2A_2$	$2p^2q^2$	–	d	–	d	0
$A_1A_2 \times A_1A_2$	$4p^2q^2$	$\frac{1}{4}a$	$\frac{1}{2}d$	$\frac{1}{4}-a$	$\frac{1}{2}d$	d
$A_1A_2 \times A_2A_2$	$4pq^3$	–	$\frac{1}{2}d$	$\frac{1}{2}-a$	$\frac{1}{2}(d-a)$	$\frac{1}{2}(d-a)$
$A_2A_2 \times A_2A_2$	q^4	–	–	$-a$	$-a$	$-a$

Contribution of this locus to the sum of squares is got as:

$$p^4(a)^2 + 4p^3q\left(\frac{1}{2}a+\frac{1}{2}d\right)^2 + 2p^2q^2(d)^2 +$$

$$4p^2q^2\left(\frac{1}{2}d\right)^2 + 4pq^3\left(\frac{1}{2}d-\frac{1}{2}a\right)^2 + q^4(-a)^2,$$

$$= p^4a^2 + P^3qa^2 + 2p^3qad + p^3qd^2 + 2p^2q^2d^2 +$$
$$p^2q^2d^2 + pq^3d^2 - 2pq^3ad + pq^3a^2 + q^4a^2.$$

Subtraction of correction factor from this sum of square gives covariance of full-sibs. Correction factor is square of population mean, *i.e.* $[a(p-q) + 2pqd]^2$. Covariance of full-sibs (Cov_{FS}) is thus:

$$pq\alpha^2 + p^2q^2d^2.$$

This covariance is equal to $\frac{1}{2}\sigma_A^2 + \frac{1}{4}\sigma_D^2$ when several loci are taken into consideration. Covariance of full-sibs includes not only additive variance but also dominance variance.

If the coefficient of inbreeding is taken into consideration, covariance of full-sibs (Cov_{FS}) is got as:

$$\left(\frac{1+F}{2}\right)^{i+2j} \sigma^2_A + \sigma^2_D + \sigma^2_{AA} + \sigma^2_{AD} + \sigma^2_{DD} \cdots\cdots$$

where i is the number of times A appears in variance and j is the number of times D appears in variance. σ^2_{AD}, and σ^2_{DD} are the interaction components of additive × dominance and dominance × dominance kinds, respectively. For example, covariance of full-sib families for an open pollinated crop species, such as maize ($F = 0$), will be

$$\left(\frac{1}{2}\right)^1 \sigma^2_A + \left(\frac{1}{2}\right)^2 \sigma^2_{AA} + \left(\frac{1}{2}\right)^2 \sigma^2_D + \left(\frac{1}{2}\right)^3 \sigma^2_{AD} + \left(\frac{1}{2}\right)^4 \sigma^2_{DD}$$

$$= \frac{1}{2}\sigma^2_A + \frac{1}{4}\sigma^2_{AA} + \frac{1}{4}\sigma^2_D + \frac{1}{8}\sigma^2_{AD} + \frac{1}{16}\sigma^2_{DD}.$$

However, if the coefficient of inbreeding is 0.50, this covariance will be:

$$\left(\frac{1+0.5}{2}\right)\sigma^2_A + \left(\frac{1+0.5}{2}\right)^2 \sigma^2_{AA} + \left(\frac{1+0.5}{2}\right)^2 \sigma^2_D +$$

$$\left(\frac{1+0.5}{2}\right)^3 \sigma^2_{AD} + \left(\frac{1+0.5}{2}\right)^4 \sigma^2_{DD}$$

$$= \left(\frac{1.50}{2}\right)\sigma^2_A + \left(\frac{1.50}{2}\right)^2 \sigma^2_{AA} + \left(\frac{1.50}{2}\right)^2 \sigma^2_D +$$

$$\left(\frac{1.50}{2}\right)^3 \sigma^2_{AD} + \left(\frac{1.50}{2}\right)^4 \sigma^2_{DD}$$

$$= 0.7500\,\sigma^2_A + 0.5625\sigma^2_{AA} + 0.5625\sigma^2_D +$$

$$0.4218\sigma^2_{AD} + 0.3164\sigma^2_{DD}.$$

(iv) Covariance of Mean of Offspring and Mean of Two Parents: Suppose two parental lines P_1 and P_2 are crossed to produce offspring (denoted by O). We have to find the covariance of genotypic values of

$\frac{1}{2}(P_1 + P_2)$ and $\overline{O}$. From the information provided in Table 4.11, sum of the products of (frequency of mating × mean of progeny × mid-parental value) over six matings is obtained. Sum of cross products is, therefore,

$$p^4 (a)^2 + 4p^3 q\left(\frac{1}{2}a + \frac{1}{2}d\right)^2 + 2p^2 q^2 (d \times 0) +$$

$$4p^2 q^2\left(\frac{1}{2}d \times d\right) + 4pq^3\left(\frac{1}{2}d - \frac{1}{2}a\right)^2 + q^4 (-a)^2.$$

$$= p^4a^2 + p^3qa^2 + 2p^3qad + p^3qd^2 + 2p^2q^2d^2 +$$
$$pq^3d^2 - 2pq^3ad + pq^3a^2 + q^4a^2$$
$$= p^3a^2 + q^3a^2 + 2p^2qad - 2pq^2ad + pqd^2.$$

Covariance is obtained following deduction of correction factor from this sum of cross products. Correction factor is square of the population mean because means of both parental and offspring generation are identical for a population in Hardy-Weinberg equilibrium. Covariance derived in this way is $pq\alpha^2$. Covariance of offspring with mid-parent is thus equal to half the additive variance, when several loci are considered. Covariance of offspring with one parent and covariance of offspring with mean of two parents are thus identical.

In the preceding paragraphs of this section we assumed absence of non-allelic interaction. Now we must make room for interaction variance in genotypic covariances of various kinds of relatives. A generalisation can be made in this regard, as suggested by Falconer (1960). For example, if the coefficient of σ^2_A in covariance is x, the interaction component σ^2_{AA} will be present with coefficient x^2. Covariance will comprise of σ^2_{AD} and σ^2_{DD} with the coefficients xy and y^2, respectively, if coefficients of σ^2_A and σ^2_D are x and y, respectively. Thus, in the presence of non-allelic interaction, covariance of full-sibs (Cov_{FS}) will be:

$$\frac{1}{2}\sigma^2_A + \frac{1}{4}\sigma^2_{AA} + \frac{1}{4}\sigma^2_D + \frac{1}{8}\sigma^2_{AD} + \frac{1}{16}\sigma^2_{DD}.$$

4.6.2 *Covariance of Relatives in Populations Produced by Controlled Crossing*

Geneticists usually employ inbred lines to develop experimental material. Two inbred lines can be crossed to develop a selfing series, such as F_2, F_3, F_4, *etc.*Covariance of two such families could be used to estimate the magnitude of additive and dominance variance. Fisher, Immer and Tedin (1932) published genetic expectations of covariances of some relatives. However, Mather and Jinks (1971, 1977 and 1982) further developed this aspect.

Breeders cross two diverse inbred lines in a bid to generate variability for a character which they intend to improve. From the F_2 generation they select plants on the basis of their phenotype. F_3 progeny rows are grown from seeds collected on selected plants. It would be of interest to measure regression of F_3 progeny family means on means of their F_2 parents. Let us deduce the covariance of means of F_2 parents and means of their F_3 progeny families. As a simple case we assume that the inbred lines which produced F_2 generation differed for a single locus with two alleles, viz. A_1 and A_2. Information required to derive covariance is presented in Table 4.12 (we will follow the symbols of Fisher *et al.*, 1932 in what follows).

TABLE 4.12: Showing genotypes of F_2 and F_3 generations and their mean genotypic values

Genotype in F_2	Frequency of genotype in F_2	Genotypic value in F_3			Mean genotypic value	
		A_1A_1	A_1A_2	A_2A_2	F_3 progeny	F_2 parent
A_1A_1	$\frac{1}{4}$	d	–	–	d	d
A_1A_2	$\frac{1}{2}$	$\frac{1}{4}d$	$\frac{1}{2}h$	$\frac{1}{4}-d$	$\frac{1}{2}h$	h
A_2A_2	$\frac{1}{4}$	–	–	$-d$	$-d$	$-d$

From this table sum of cross products is got as:

$$\frac{1}{4}(d \times d)+\frac{1}{2}\left(\frac{1}{2}h \times h\right)+\frac{1}{4}(-d \times -d)$$

$$=\frac{1}{4}d^2+\frac{1}{4}h^2+\frac{1}{4}d^2$$

$$=\frac{1}{2}d^2+\frac{1}{4}h^2.$$

Correction factor is simply a product of $\bar{F}_2$ and $\bar{F}_3$ (because sum of the frequencies in F_2 as well as in F_3 generation is unity, and total of genotypic values is also the mean). Mean genotypic values of F_2 and F_3 families are $\frac{1}{2}h$ and $\frac{1}{4}h$, respectively, (section 3.2). Correction factor is, therefore, $\frac{1}{2}h \times \frac{1}{4}h = \frac{1}{8}h^2$. Genotypic covariance of F_2 and F_3 (C_{ovF2F3}) is, thus:

$$\frac{1}{2}d^2+\frac{1}{4}h^2-\frac{1}{8}h^2$$

$$=\frac{1}{2}d^2+\frac{1}{8}h^2$$

When several loci the governing the inheritance of a metrical trait are taken into consideration covariance of F_2 means with means of their F_3 progeny families would be $\frac{1}{2}S(d^2)+\frac{1}{8}S(h^2)$. If we denote $S(d^2)$ and $S(h^2)$ by D and H, respectively then Cov_{F2F3} could be expressed as:

$$\frac{1}{2}D+\frac{1}{8}H.$$

In genetic studies several kinds of generations are developed by selfing. It will be useful to give a generalised expression for genotypic covariance of two generations. Expected value for heritable component of covariance of means of two generations, *viz.* $(n-1)$ and n, is given by:

$$\left(\frac{1}{2}\right)^{j} D+\left(\frac{1}{2}\right)^{2n-j-2} H.$$

For example, we may like to find the value of genetic covariance of means of F_3 progeny families with means of groups of F_4 generation. Families within a group of F_4 generation descend from same family in F_3.

Here $n = 4$, hence $Cov_{F3,\ F4}$ is:

$$\frac{1}{2}D+\left(\frac{1}{2}\right)^{2\times4-2-1}H$$

$$=\frac{1}{2}D+\frac{1}{32}H.$$

In addition to the genotypic covariance, environmental covariance also contributes to phenotypic covariance. But if environmental variances of two relatives are not correlated, environmental covariance does not contribute to the phenotypic covariance. Proper randomisation of individuals belonging to different generations will enable to achieve this.

We have assumed in preceding paragraphs absence of non-allelic interaction. Since the mean expressions of different generations are influenced by non-allelic interactions of various kinds, their variances and covariances are also influenced by non-allelic interaction. In the absence of digenic non-allelic interaction, heritable variance of F_2 and variance of means of F_3 families with respect to two loci, each with two alleles, *i.e.*, A_1, A_2 and B_1, B_2, would be:

$$V_{1F_3}=\frac{1}{2}d_a^2+\frac{1}{2}d_b^2+\frac{1}{4}h_a^2+\frac{1}{4}h_b^2$$

and $$V_{1F_3}=\frac{1}{2}d_a^2+\frac{1}{2}d_b^2+\frac{1}{16}h_a^2+\frac{1}{16}h_b^2$$

With digenic non-allelic interaction genotypic variances of F_2 and means of F_3 progeny families appear as:

$$V_{1F_2}=\frac{1}{2}\left(d_a+\frac{1}{2}j_{ab}\right)^2+\frac{1}{2}\left(d_b+\frac{1}{2}j_{ba}\right)^2+\frac{1}{4}\left(h_a+\frac{1}{2}l_{ab}\right)^2$$

$$+\frac{1}{4}\left(h_b+\frac{1}{2}l_{ab}\right)^2+\frac{1}{4}(i_{ab})^2+\frac{1}{8}(j_{ab})^2+\frac{1}{8}(j_{ba})^2+\frac{1}{16}(l_{ab})^2, \text{and}$$

$$V_{1F_3}=\frac{1}{2}\left(d_a+\frac{1}{4}j_{ab}\right)^2+\frac{1}{2}\left(d_b+\frac{1}{4}j_{ba}\right)^2+\frac{1}{16}\left(h_a+\frac{1}{4}l_{ab}\right)^2$$

$$+\frac{1}{16}\left(h_b+\frac{1}{4}l_{ab}\right)^2+\frac{1}{4}(i_{ab})^2+\frac{1}{32}(j_{ab})^2+\frac{1}{32}(j_{ba})^2+\frac{1}{256}(l_{ab})^2.$$

Genotypic covariance of F_2 and F_3 with respect to these loci, in the absence of digenic non-allelic interaction, would be:

$$\frac{1}{2}d_a^2+\frac{1}{2}d_b^2+\frac{1}{8}h_a^2+\frac{1}{8}h_b^2.$$

When digenic non-allelic interaction is present, covariance is the geometric mean of variances of two generations being considered. Thus Cov_{F2F3} could be expressed as:

$$\frac{1}{2}\left(d_a+\frac{1}{2}j_{ab}\right)\left(d_a+\frac{1}{4}j_{ab}\right)+\frac{1}{2}\left(d_b+\frac{1}{2}j_{ba}\right)\left(d_b+\frac{1}{4}j_{ba}\right)+$$

$$\frac{1}{8}\left(h_a+\frac{1}{2}l_{ab}\right)\left(h_a+\frac{1}{4}l_{ab}\right)+\frac{1}{8}\left(h_b+\frac{1}{2}l_{ab}\right)\left(h_b+\frac{1}{4}l_{ab}\right)+$$

$$\frac{1}{4}(i_{ab})^2+\frac{1}{16}(j_{ab})^2+\frac{1}{16}(j_{ba})^2+\frac{1}{64}(l_{ab})^2.$$

Coefficients of pure forms of digenic non-allelic interaction parameters are products of their main effects as they have been observed for other rank one variances. Additive and dominance components of covariance could be biased upwards or downwards depending upon the signs and magnitudes of non-allelic interaction parameters, especially the additive × dominance and dominance × dominance kinds. Magnitude of total covariance can also increase or decrease depending upon the signs and magnitudes of pure forms of digenic non-allelic interaction parameters.

Contribution of linked gene pairs to the heritable variances of various ranks in different generations was described in section 4.5.2. Linkage also influences genotypic covariance. Since we are considering only rank 1 covariances, the constitution of additive and dominance components of covariances is similar to V_{1F2}, V_{1F3}, V_{1S3} *etc.* in the absence of non-allelic interaction. Thus Cov_{F2F3} would be:

$$\frac{1}{2}[d_a^2 + d_b^2 \pm 2(1-2p)d_a d_b] + \frac{1}{8}[h_a^2 + h_b^2 + 2(1-2p)^2 h_a h_b].$$

Constitution of additive and dominance components of covariances of rank 1 between other generations is similar to V_{1F2}, *etc.* Like the variances, therefore, magnitude of covariances depends upon the signs of interaction parameters and the frequency of recombination.

4.7 Heritability

Essential features of most, if not all, breeding programmes are:

(i) Selection of plants with desirable phenotypes from genetically variable population, and

(ii) Utilisation of these selected plants for creation of new population to be used as potential new commercial varieties or as a base for new cycle of selection.

Genetic advance, *i.e.* improvement in genotypic value of new population compared with base population, depends among other things upon the magnitude of differences among the genotypic values of individuals in the base population. If all or most of the variability among the individuals in base population is attributable to non-heritable agencies, selection of phenotypically superior individuals from the population will not lead to improvement. What a geneticist can directly measure is the phenotypic value of an individual. Success of a breeder in changing the characteristics of a population, therefore, depends upon the degree of correspondence between the phenotypic values and the genotypic values. A quantitative measure which provides information about the correspondence between genotypic variance and phenotypic variance is heritability. This term was originally proposed by Lush (1943) to describe the ratio of variance due to hereditary differences (σ^2_g) to the total phenotypic variance (σ^2_p). This ratio is expressed in per cent. If the precentage is large, character is regarded as highly heritable. On the other hand, if it is smaller, environmental agency is considered as mostly responsible for phenotypic mainfestation of the character. This ratio is now known as "broad sense heritability". The concept of broad sense heritability is useful if interest is in relative importance of genotype and environment in the determination of phenotypic values. But it does not indicate the progress which might be made through selection within a particular population.

It was pointed out in section 2.5 that the mean genotypic value of a progeny is determined by the average effects of genes transmitted by parents in question. In other words, it is the breeding value of parents which determines the genetic properties of progeny. The degree of resemblance between parents and offspring generation is determined by the breeding value. Hence it is the proportion of phenotypic variation that is made up of the variation attributable to breeding values (known as additive genetic variance) which is of interest to the breeder. The ratio of additive genetic variance (σ^2_A) to the phenotypic variance (σ^2_p) is known as "narrow sense heritability" (h^2). Thus

$$\hat{h}^2 = \frac{\sigma^2_A}{\sigma^2_p} \times 100.$$

Narrow sense heritability measures the extent of correspondence between breeding values and phenotypic values. Since the phenotypic variance is made up of genotypic variance (σ^2_g) and non-heritable variance (σ^2_e), narrow sense heritability can also be expressed as:

$$\hat{h}^2 = \frac{\sigma^2_A}{\sigma^2_g + \sigma^2_e}, \text{ and since,}$$

$$\sigma^2_g = \sigma^2_A + \sigma^2_D + \sigma^2_I,$$

$$\hat{h}^2 = \frac{\sigma^2_A}{\sigma^2_A + \sigma^2_D + \sigma^2_I + \sigma^2_e}$$

Narrow sense heritability expresses the magnitude of genotypic variance in the population, which is mainly responsible for changing the genetic composition of population through selection. It also provides a basis to predict accuracy with which selection for genotypes could be made based on phenotypic values of individuals or groups of individuals.

Heritability can be expressed also as regression of breeding values (BV) on phenotypic values (P). Thus heritability (h^2) = $b_{BV.P}$ Derivation of this relationship is simple. Let us split the phenotypic value into breeding value (BV) and the rest (R) which comprises of dominance deviation, interaction deviation and environmental deviation. Thus $P = BV + R$. Covariance of breeding values and phenotypic values is, therefore:

$$BV.(BV + R)$$
$$= BV^2 + BV.R.$$

Since breeding values are not correlated with dominance deviations, interaction deviations, etc. $Cov_{BV.R}$ is BV^2. Here we should note two things. The breeding values and dominance deviations are usually expressed as deviation from the population mean. And secondly the sum of frequencies of 3 genotypes with respect to a single locus with two alleles (A_1,A_2), is unity. Therefore, BV^2 is also the variance of breeding values, *i.e.* σ^2_A. Thus $b_{BV.P}$ is

$$\frac{\sigma^2_A}{\sigma^2_P} = h^2$$

It is important to note that heritability is a property not only of the character being studied, but also the population being sampled and the environmental circumstances to which individuals have been subjected. Since the value of heritability depends upon the magnitude of all components of phenotypic variance, change in the amount of any one of these components will alter it. It was shown is section 4.3 that genotypic variance and its components are influenced by the gene frequencies. Because the frequencies of genes differ from one population to another, estimate of heritability also varies from one population to another for a given character. Magnitude of heritability can be influenced by developments that have occurred in the origin of material. A character in a population which has been under intense selection should be expected to have lower heritability than the same trait in a population where additive genetic variance has not been reduced by selection pressure, when both populations are evaluated under identical environmental conditions. Also, the heritability of a character, such as yield, may be relatively high when measured in early segregating generations of a population produced by crossing widely divergent material, such as race and species.

Heritability also depends upon the type of gene action involved for the expression of a character. In general, characters which are controlled largely by genes acting in an additive fashion have higher values of heritability than the characters governed by genes with large non-additive effects. Populations which are genetically more uniform are expected to show lower heritability than the genetically variable populations. In particular, small populations maintained long enough for an appreciable amount of fixation of genes to have taken place are expected to show lower heritability than the large populations.

Environmental variance is also a component of phenotypic variance. Environmental variance depends upon the conditions of management. More variable environmental conditions reduce the magnitude of heritability and more uniform conditions increase it. Therefore, whenever a value is stated for heritability of a character, it refers to a particular population under particular environmental conditions.

In plants, less use and importance has been attached to the heritability *per se* than in domestic animals. This is partly due to the field designs and experimental procedures with plants which allow refinements resulting in reduction of environmental variance. Thus, without changing the magnitude of additive genetic variance, heritability increases and makes the comparison of heritability values derived from different experiments rather meaningless. Moreover, the original concept of heritability was for cross-fertilising species and many crop plants are self-fertilised. The definition of heritability changes according to the nature of usable genetic variability, the experimental unit being considered and the inference population assumed. The portion of total genetic variability that is usable differs depending upon whether the crop is cross-pollinated, self-pollinated or asexually propagated. In the asexually propagated crops, for example, broad sense heritability would be relevant because the entire genotypic variability is usable. The reference unit in plants may be a plant, a field plot, replicated plot in one environment, replicated plots in two or more environments. The plots may consist of progeny from open-pollinated individual, bulked progeny in advanced generation of selfing or other type of plant material. These will influence the definition of heritability.

According to Robinson (1966) heritability estimates in cultivated plants can be placed in following categories:

(1) Low heritability (5 to 10 per cent)
e.g. grain yield
(2) Medium heritability (10 to 30 per cent)
e.g. components of yield, components of plant height.
(3) High heritability (30 to 60 per cent)
e.g. Maturity characters, chemical composition of characters.

This classification is approximate and represents averages of heritability estimates over various crop plants, procedures of determination and several environments comprising of locations and years.

4.8. Estimation of Heritability

Warner (1952) classified procedures employed to estimate heritability into three main categories:

(i) Parent-progeny regression
(ii) Estimation of variance components from an analysis of variance, and
(iii) Approximation of non-heritable variance from genetically uniform population to estimate total genetic variance.

First two procedures will be described in this section. The third procedure is not precise and currently used in plants and hence will not be described.

4.8.1 *Parent-progeny Regression*

One of the common methods of determining heritability of attributes in plants is by progeny-parent regression, proposed by Lush (1940). This procedure involves regressing of the mean value of a characteristic in the progeny upon the value for same characteristic in the parent. In section 4.6.1, covariance of parent and progeny was shown to be equal to $\frac{1}{2}\sigma^2_A$. Regression of offspring on one parent (b_{OP}), therefore, provides an estimate of heritability $\left(\frac{1}{2}h^2\right)$. Thus

$$b_{OP} = \frac{\frac{1}{2}\sigma^2_A}{\sigma^2_P} = \frac{1}{2}h^2$$

where σ^2_P is the phenotypic variance of the parents. In random mating population, therefore, it is necessary to double the regression value to obtain heritability value.

Covariance of mid-parental values and mean genotypic values of the progeny was shown to be equal to $\frac{1}{2}\sigma^2_A$ in section 4.6.1. Regression of offspring on mid-parents also provides an estimate of heritability (h^2). Thus $b_{O\overline{P}} = \frac{1}{2}\sigma^2_A / \frac{1}{2}\sigma^2_P$. Total phenotypic variance of mid–parents is $\frac{1}{2}\sigma^2_P$. Why? Let us see. We require variance of $\left(\frac{1}{2}P_1 + \frac{1}{2}P_2\right)$. Since $\frac{1}{2}$ is a constant, var $\frac{1}{2}(P_1 + P_2)$ is $\frac{1}{4}V_{P1} + \frac{1}{4}V_{P2}$. If the phenotypic variances of P_1 and P_2 are equal, $\frac{1}{4}V_{P1} + \frac{1}{4}V_{P2} = \frac{1}{2}V_P$. A complication in the use of regression of offspring on mid-parent arises if the variances of two parents are not equal. Heritability should be estimated separately for each parent, *i.e.*, regression of offspring on P_1 and P_2, when the variances of two parents are not equal.

In practice, parent-progeny regression for characteristics in plants often involve regressing the data obtained from progeny grown in one year upon the parental data recorded in previous year. For example, F_2 generation is raised in one year, and the F_3 progenies of plants selected in F_2 generation in the subsequent year. Obviously, any environmental factor which tends to inflate or reduce the range of phenotypic variation of progenies could affect the heritability percentage obtained, although the ratio of components of variances remains similar to that of the parents. For instance, if the grain yield of parental strains ranged from 60-80 quintals/ha when grown in one year and range among the progenies was reduced by effect of environment to 20-30 quintals/ha, the ceiling of heritability percentage would be approximately 50 per cent. This assumes that the ratio of population ranges is related to regression coefficients. If the years are interchanged, the approximate ceiling would be 200 per cent. Thus it is difficult to determine whether heritability of given magnitude is low, intermediate or high unless ceiling is known for each set of data. Frey and Horner (1957) suggested a modification of parent-progeny regression procedure to determine heritability percentage, which has a ceiling of 100 per cent in all the situations, irrespective of the postulated environmental scaling effects. This method is known as "heritability in standard units". Standard unit heritability is obtained by using standardised values of progeny and parents for calculation of regression of progeny on parents. Thus, each observation recorded on progeny is divided by its standard deviation. Similarly standardised values are obtained for parents. Such a regression coefficient is equal to correlation coefficient on original units. Standard unit heritability corrects only for a particular type of genotype-environment interaction, which tends to cause an expansion or contraction of the scale. This method has an advantage over conventional method. The most important advantage is that the ceiling for heritability values is 100 per cent. With conventional methods,on the other hand, the ceilings of heritability percentages change with each set of data. Frey and Horner (1957) found that in case of heading date in oats, the predicted gain based on standard heritability came closer to the actual gain obtained from selection. The standard unit method for calculating heritability percentage is useful only when a certain type of scaling effect is operating. If environment does not cause an expansion or contraction of phenotypic variability present in the population, then standard unit heritability will in all probability be similar to that obtained by conventional method.

4.8.2 *Estimation of Variance Components from Analysis of Variance*

In the initial stages of a breeding programme, breeder looks for genetic variability for attributes which need improvement. The extent of genetic variability could be detected by means of a relatively simple experiment. Available genotypes are grown in randomised block design with r replications (Table 4.13). Analysis of variance provides an appropriate basis to detect existence of genetic variability. Linear mathematical model for observation recorded on *i*th genotype growing in *j*th replication is:

$$Y_{ij} = \mu + g_i + e_{ij}$$

where μ is the general mean, g_i the effect of *i*th genotype and e_{ij} the error associated with particular measurement. The genotypes are assumed to be distributed with mean μ_g and variance σ^2_g.

TABLE 4.13: Analysis of variance when *g* genotypes are raised in R.B.D. with *r* replications

source	*df*	S.S.	MS	Expectation mean square
Replications	$(r-1)$			
Among genotypes	$(g-1)$	$r\sum_i (y_{i.} - Y_{..})^2$	M_1	$\sigma_e^2 + r\sigma_g^2$
Within genotypes	$(r-1)(g-1)$	$\sum_{ij}(y_{ij} - Y_{i.})^2$	M_2	σ_e^2
Total	$(rg-1)$	$\sum_{ji}(y_{ij} - Y_{..})^2$		

From the mean squares, estimate of genotypic variance (σ^2_g) is got as:

$$\hat{\sigma}_g^2 = \frac{M_1 - M_2}{r}$$

$$= \frac{\sigma_e^2 + r\sigma_g^2 - \sigma_e^2}{r}$$

$$= \sigma_g^2$$

And estimate of σ^2_e, the environmental variance, is provided by M_2. Hence the estimate of phenotypic variance (σ^2_P) is:

$$\sigma_g^2 + \sigma_e^2.$$

Broad sense heritability (h^2) is then calculated as:

$$\frac{\sigma_g^2}{\sigma_P^2} \times 100.$$

Worked Example

Twentyeight genotypes of sorghum were raised in randomised block design with two replications. Data were recorded on 1000-grain weight. Result of analysis of variance is presented below:

Source	*df*	Mean square
Replications	1	4.352
Genotypes	27	18.6301**
Error	27	2.4984

** Significant at one per cent level.

Estimate of genotypic variance is obtained as:

$$\sigma^2_g = \frac{18.6301 - 2.4984}{2}$$

$$= 8.0658$$

Estimate of environmental variance is:

$\sigma^2_e = 2.4984$

Estimate of phenotypic variance (σ^2_P) will be, therefore,

$8.0658 + 2.4984 = 10.5642$

Broad sense heritability is then:

$$\frac{8.0658}{10.5642} \times 100 = 76.35 \textit{ per cent}$$

Experiments designed to obtain the estimates of genotypic variance should be conducted in adequate number of environments. Genotypic variance calculated from genotypes grown at one location for one year will be biased. If the genotypes are grown at one location for several years or for one year at several locations, certain interaction components such as σ^2_{gl} or σ^2_{gy} remain associated with σ^2_{g}, consequently the estimate of genotypic variance is biased. For example, from the Tables 4.14, 4.15, and 4.16 it will be clear that only when genotypes are raised at several locations (where the variety is to be ultimately grown) for several years, the estimate of genotypic variance

(σ^2_g) will be free from such interaction components such as σ^2_{gly}, σ^2_{gy} and σ^2_{gl}. Expected progress based on biased estimate of σ^2_g will not be in agreement with observed gains. Complications arising from such issues will be discussed in a separate chapter.

TABLE 4.14: Format for ANOVA when genotypes are raised at several locations for one year

Source	*df*	MS	Expectation MS
Replications within locations	$l\,(r-1)$	–	–
Locations	$(l-1)$	–	–
Genotypes	$(g-1)$	M_1	$\sigma^2_e + r\sigma^2_{gl} + rl\sigma^2_g$
Genotypes × locations	$(g-1)\,(l-1)$	M_2	$\sigma^2_e + r\sigma^2_{gl}$
Pooled Error	$l(r-1)\,(g-1)$	M_3	σ^2_e

where r = No. of replications

l = No. of locations

σ^2_{gl} = Genotype-location interaction variance.

TABLE 4.15 : Structure for ANOVA when genotypes are raised for several years at several locations.

Source	*df*	MS	Expectation MS
Replications within locations in years	$yl\,(r-1)$	–	–
Years	$(y-1)$	–	–
Locations	$(l-1)$	–	–
Years × locations	$(y-1)\,(l-1)$	–	–
Genotypes	$(g-1)$	M_1	$\sigma^2_e + r\sigma^2_{gly} + ry\sigma 2_{gl} + rl\sigma^2_{gy} + rly\sigma^2_g$
Genotypes × years	$(g-1)\,(y-1)$	M_2	$\sigma^2_e + r\sigma^2 gly + rl\sigma^2 gy$
Genotypes × locations	$(g-1)\,(l-1)$	M_3	$\sigma^2_e + r\sigma^2 gly + ry\sigma^2 gl$
Genotypes × years × locations	$(g-1)\,(y-1)\,(l-1)$	M_4	$\sigma^2_e + r\sigma^2_{gly}$
Pooled Error	$yl(r-1)\,(g-1)$	M_5	σ^2_e

Where σ^2_{gly} = genotypes × years × locations interations variance,

σ^2_{gy} = genotypes × years interaction variance.

TABLE 4.16. Showing various interaction variance components clubbed with σ^2_g

Genotypes raised at/in	Components actually obtained instead of	
	σ^2_{ge*}	σ^2_g
One year in one location	–	$\sigma^2_{gly} + \sigma^2_{gy} + \sigma^2_{gl} + \sigma^2_g$
One year at several locations	$\sigma^2_{gly} + \sigma^2_{gl}$	$\sigma^2_{gy} + \sigma^2_g$
One location for several years	$\sigma^2_{gly} + \sigma^2_{gy}$	$\sigma^2_{gl} + \sigma^2_g$
Several years at several locations	$\sigma^2_{gly} + \sigma^2_{gy} + \sigma^2_{gl}$	σ^2_g

* σ^2_{ge} = Genotypes × environment interaction variance.

Certain mating designs permit estimation of components of genotypic variance, (*i.e.*, σ^2_A and σ^2_D), which could be used to estimate narrow sense heritability. The results of analysis of variance of these mating designs also provide direct tests of significance of σ^2_A and σ^2_D (with some exceptions). Simple procedures have been developed by Warner (1952) and Mather (1949) to estimate the magnitude of additive, dominance and environmental variance from segregating material. It will be useful to know these methods.

4.8.3 *Mather's* (1949) *D and H Components*

The concept of partitioning heritable variation of generations developed by selfing series was given by Fisher, Immer and Tedin (1932), which was elaborated further by Mather (1949).

It was shown in section 4.5 that heritable variation of F_2 generation, in the absence of non-allelic interaction, comprises of·

$$\frac{1}{2}S(d^2) + \frac{1}{4}S(h^2).$$

And since we preferred to denote $S(d^2)$ and $S(h^2)$ by new symbols D and H respectively, heritable variance of F_2 was described as:

$$\frac{1}{2}D+\frac{1}{4}H.$$

Sum of heritable variances of Bc_1 and Bc_2 generations was also derived in this section. It was shown to be : ½ D + ½H.

Phenotypic variances of F_2, Bc_1 and Bc_2 generations include environmental variance (E) and, therefore, V_{1F2} and $V_{Bc\,1}$ + $V_{Bc\,2}$ could be expressed as:

$$V_{1F_2}=\frac{1}{2}D+\frac{1}{4}H+E$$

$$V_{Bc_1}+V_{Bc_2}=\frac{1}{2}D+\frac{1}{2}H+2E.$$

Narrow sense heritability for a character could be obtained following Warner (1952). He proposed a method to estimate narrow sense heritability based on phenotypic variation of F_2, B_{C1} and B_{C2} generations. Following assumptions are involved in the estimation of narrow sense heritability (Warner, 1952):

(i) Contributions made by heritable and non-heritable agencies to the variances of various generations are independent,

(ii) Effects of genes at various loci, influencing the expression of a given character are additive on an average, and

(iii) The non-heritable components of V_{F_2}, V_{BC_1} and V_{BC_2} are of comparable magnitudes.

Randomisation of experimental meterial will take care of correlation between heritable and non-heritable agencies. Adequacy of the additive-dominance model (*i.e.*, absence of non-allelic interaction) can be detected by means of scaling tests (Mather, 1949). Transformation of data could be helpful to induce additivity of gene effects at different loci. Warner (1952) advocated raising several hundred individuals of F_2, B_{C1} and B_{C2} generations to minimise sampling variance.

Following Warner (1952), estimate of additive variance is obtained as:

$$2V_{1F_2}=D+\frac{1}{2}H+2E$$

$$-(V_{Bc1}+V_{Bc2})=\frac{\frac{1}{2}D+\frac{1}{2}H+2E}{\frac{1}{2}D}$$

Ratio of $\frac{1}{2}D$ to V_{1F2} gives narrow sense heritability because V_{1F2} is $\frac{1}{2}D+\frac{1}{4}H+\text{E}$. Thus, narrow sense heritability is:

$$\frac{\frac{1}{2}D}{\frac{1}{2}D+\frac{1}{4}H+E}\times 100.$$

Estimate of E, the environmental variance, can be got as an average of the variances of three non-segregating generations, namely P_1, P_2 and F_1. By virtue of better buffering, F_1 generation usually tends to manifest lower non-heritable variation than the true breeding parental lines. This is especially true for heterozygous individuals of most cross-fertilised crops. Hence the estimate of E is obtained as a weighted average of variations of P_1, P_2 and F_1 generations. Proportions of genotypes similar to P_1, P_2, and F_1 are expected to be $\frac{1}{4}$, $\frac{1}{4}$ and $\frac{1}{2}$, respectively in F_2 generation. Hence estimate of E will be:

$$\frac{1}{4}V_{P_1}+\frac{1}{4}V_{P_2}+\frac{1}{2}V_{F_1}$$

Worked Example

Six generations of sorghum, *viz*, P_1, P_2, F_1, F_2, B_{C_1} and B_{C_2} were raised in a randomised block design with two replications. Observations were recorded on plant height (cm). Variances of three generations, *viz*, F_2, B_{C1} and B_{C2} are given below:

Statistics	Expected components	Observed values
V_{1F_2}	$\frac{1}{2}D+\frac{1}{4}H+E$	80.2036
V_{Bc_1}	$\frac{1}{4}D+\frac{1}{4}H-\frac{1}{2}F+E$	33.6440
V_{Bc_2}	$\frac{1}{4}D+\frac{1}{4}H+\frac{1}{2}F+E$	93.3680

Estimate of ½ D is calculated as:

$$2V_{1F_2}-(V_{Bc_1}+V_{Bc_2})$$
$$=2(80.2036)-(33.6440+93.3680)$$
$$=160.4072-127.0120$$
$$=33.3952$$

Narrow sense heritability is:

$$\frac{33.3952}{80.2036}\times 100$$
$$=41.63\%$$

In this experiment, variances of non-segregating generations were also measured. These are:

Generations	Variances
P_1	36.8333
P_2	43.4160
F_1	40.5000

Thus estimate of E would be

$$\frac{1}{4}(36.8333)+\frac{1}{4}(43.4160)+\frac{1}{2}(40.5000)$$
$$=40.3123$$

Substituting the values of ½ D and E in V_{1F_2} we get ¼ H as shown below:

$$V_{1F_2}=\frac{1}{2}D+\frac{1}{4}\mathrm{H}+\mathrm{E}=80.2036$$
$$=33.3952+\tfrac{1}{4}\mathrm{H}+40.3123=80.2036$$
$$\therefore\quad \tfrac{1}{4}H=80.2036-33.3952-40.3123$$
$$=6.4959.$$

Estimates of *D*, *H* and *E* for plant height of sorghum are thus:

$$D = 2\left(\frac{1}{2}D\right) = 66.7904$$

$$H = 4\left(\frac{1}{4}H\right) = 25.9836$$

$$E = 40.3123.$$

Relative magnitudes of these components of variations suggest that additive genetic variance is the predominant determinant of variation for plant height. Improvement for this character, is therefore, possible through simple selection procedures.

It is possible to estimate four components of variation. *viz*, *D*, *H*, *F* and *E*, through perfect fit solutions (Mather and Jinks, 1977). *D* depends on difference between individuals distinguished by being homozygous for two allelomorphs of various genes. *H* depends on departure of hetrozygote from the mean of the two comparable homozygotes. *F* is the linear function of dominance and is in fact a weighted sum of *h*'s over all the loci. The sign of F [= S (*dh*)] provides information regarding dominance of genes with increasing or decreasing effects. If genes with positive effects are on the whole dominant, *i.e.*, sign of *h* is positive, sign of *F* will be positive. If genes with negative effects on the character are dominant, sign of *h* and consequently the sign of *F* will be negative. Thus positive sign of *F* implies that the genes with increasing effects are on the whole dominant and *vice versa*. When there is no dominance, i.e., $h = 0$, *F* will be zero. If $d = 0$, *i.e.*, the mean measurements of two parents are equal, *F* will be zero.

Estimate of *D* is obtained as $4V_{F_2} - 2(V_{Bc_1} + V_{Bc_2})$. Why? The variation observed for F_2 is composed of $\frac{1}{2}D + \frac{1}{4}H + E$. Summed variances of B_{c_1} and B_{c_2} generations comprise of $\frac{1}{2}D + \frac{1}{2}H + 2E$. Substituting these values in $4V_{F_2} - 2(V_{Bc_1} + V_{Bc_2})$ we get:

$$4\left(\frac{1}{2}D + \frac{1}{4}H + E\right) - 2\left(\frac{1}{2}D + \frac{1}{2}H + 2E\right)$$

$$= 2D + H + 4E - D - H - 4E$$

$$= D.$$

Estimate of *H* is got as:

$$4\left[\left(V_{Bc_1}+V_{Bc_2}\right)-V_{F_2}-E\right].$$

F is estimated as difference between variances of two backcross generations, namely, V_{Bc_1} and V_{Bc_2}. Thus,

$$F = V_{Bc_2} - V_{Bc_1}.$$

Worked Example

Information provided for previous worked example (Plant height in sorghum) will be used to illustrate estimation of D, H, F and E. Thus,

$$\begin{aligned}
D &= 4(80.2036) - 2(33.6640 + 93.3680] \\
&= 320.8144 - 254.064 \\
&= 66.7504 \\
H &= 4[(33.6640 + 93.3680) - 80.2036 - 40.3123] \\
&= 4(127.032 - 80.2036 - 40.3123) \\
&= 26.0644 \\
F &= 93.3680 - 33.6640 \\
&= 59.7240 \\
E &= \frac{1}{4}(36.8333) + \frac{1}{4}(43.4160) + \frac{1}{2}(40.5000) \\
&= 40.3123
\end{aligned}$$

Three statistics provided estimates of three parameters, *viz.* D, H and F, hence a chi-square test cannot be applied to test the significance of these parameters.

4.8.4 *Mather's (1949) Least Square Analysis*

Based on the principles of least squares, Mather (1949) proposed a technique which could be adopted for estimation of components of variation, provided the number of statistics available exceeds the number of parameters desired. It was further developed by Mather and Vines (1952). Several mating designs (Chapters, 5, 6, and 7) have been developed which permit not only testing of the significance of components of heritable variation but also their estimation. Least square analysis of Mather (1949), which is a form of multivariate analysis, has two advantages over the analysis of variance of mating designs. Analysis of variance of mating designs is based on information collected on certain kinds of families, *e.g.* half-sibs and/or full-sibs. Although analyses of variance of mating designs provide a test of significance of additive and dominance components of genotypic variance, number of mean squares are so restricted that little can be done to test the validity of assumption regarding independence of genes in inheritance and action. Moreover, the technique of analysis of variance of mating designs does not allow combining any number of statistics from any number of generations in a single analysis. Mather's (1949) least square analysis can accommodate information available from any kind and number of generations. Because the estimates of components of variation are based on statistics recorded on a number of generations, Mather's (1949) analysis appears more reliable and useful.

This analysis assumes adequacy of additive-dominance model. Scaling tests provide information to this effect. Let us examine the technique. We assume that the statistics available are V_{1F_2}, V_{1F_3}, $W_{1F_{23}}$, V_{2F_3}, E_1 and E_2. Using information provided by these statistics, components D, H, E_1 and E_2 have to be estimated. E_1 is measured as variation of individuals within true breeding families and E_2 as variation of means of true breeding families. Since estimates of four parameters are desired we need four normal equations which are obtained as described in section 3.3.2. For this purpose a table is set up as shown below:

Statistics	Coefficients of components					Observed
	D	H	E_1	E_2		values
V_{1F_2}	$\frac{1}{2}$	$\frac{1}{4}$	1	–	=	X_1
V_{1F_3}	$\frac{1}{2}$	$\frac{1}{16}$	–	1	=	X_2
$W_{1F_{23}}$	$\frac{1}{2}$	$\frac{1}{8}$	–	–	=	X_3
V_{2F_3}	$\frac{1}{4}$	$\frac{1}{8}$	1	–	=	X_4
E_1	–	–	1	–	=	X_5
E_2	–	–	–	1	=	X_6

First step to obtain first normal equation is to multiply each item in the row with the coefficient of parameter D, including the coefficient of D itself. For example, multiplication of first row with ½ will give.

$$\left(\frac{1}{2}\times\frac{1}{2}\right)D+\left(\frac{1}{2}\times\frac{1}{4}\right)H+\left(1\times\frac{1}{2}\right)E_1+\left(0\times\frac{1}{2}\right)E_2 = X_1\times\frac{1}{2}$$

$$\frac{1}{4}D+\frac{1}{8}H+\frac{1}{2}E_1=\frac{1}{2}X_1$$

Arrange the products so obtained from six multiplications as:

$$\frac{1}{4}D+\frac{1}{8}H+\frac{1}{2}E_1 = \frac{1}{2}X_1$$

$$\frac{1}{4}D+\frac{1}{32}H+\frac{1}{2}E_2 = \frac{1}{2}X_2$$

$$\frac{1}{4}D+\frac{1}{16}H = \frac{1}{2}X_3$$

$$\frac{1}{16}D+\frac{1}{32}H+\frac{1}{4}E_1 = \frac{1}{4}X_4$$

Total $$\frac{13}{16}D+\frac{1}{4}H+\frac{3}{4}E_1+\frac{1}{2}E_2 = \frac{1}{2}X_1+\frac{1}{2}X_2+\frac{1}{2}X_3+\frac{1}{4}X_4$$

Total at the bottom gives first normal equation. Calculate the 2nd, 3rd and 4th normal equations in similar fashion, employing the coefficients of H, E_1, and E_2 in turn. The elements of four normal equations are then arranged as:

$$\begin{bmatrix} a_{11} & a_{12} & a_{13} & a_{14} \\ a_{21} & a_{22} & a_{23} & a_{24} \\ a_{31} & a_{32} & a_{33} & a_{34} \\ a_{41} & a_{42} & a_{43} & a_{44} \end{bmatrix} \begin{bmatrix} \hat{D} \\ \hat{H} \\ \hat{E}_1 \\ \hat{E}_2 \end{bmatrix} = \begin{bmatrix} \frac{1}{2}X_1+\frac{1}{2}X_2+\frac{1}{2}X_3+\frac{1}{4}X_4 \\ \frac{1}{4}X_2+\frac{1}{16}X_2+\frac{1}{8}X_3+\frac{1}{8}X_4 \\ X_1 \quad +X_4 \quad +X_5 \\ X_2 \quad +X_6 \end{bmatrix}$$

J $\qquad M \qquad S$

Matrix J is information matrix. M is the matrix of parameters to be estimated and S the matrix of scores. Estimates of D, H, E_1 and E_2 could be obtained as:

$$M = SJ^{-1}$$

J^{-1} is the inverse of matrix J. The inverse could be obtained as described in Appendix I.

Although this method is simple to use, it has some disadvantages

(Mather and Jinks, 1971). It was shown in section 4.5 that the variance of F_3 generation, for example, has two components, *viz*, V_{1F_3} and V_{2F_3}.

Rank 1 variance was described as

$$\frac{1}{2}D+\frac{1}{16}H+E_b+\frac{1}{n}V_{2F_3}$$

and rank two variance as:

$$\frac{1}{4}D+\frac{1}{8}H+E_w.$$

Likewise V_{S_3} has two components, *viz.*, V_{1S_3} and V_{2S_3}. Each rank 1 variance comprises of a sampling variance attributable to the rank 2 variance. Hence, rank 1 variance tends to be inflated due to the higher rank variances. This inflation is ignored in the simple method proposed by Mather (1949).

It is assumed in Mather's (1949) least square analysis that all the statistics employed for calculation of components of variance are known with equal precision. Nevertheless, this may not be always true. Hence, statistics known with more precision should be given more weight.

An assumption implicit in Mather's (1949) least square analysis is that the various statistics, employed for estimation purpose, are not correlated. At times this may not be correct. In plants we grow F_2 in one season and select individuals to be advanced to F_3. Usually it is not possible to grow same F_2 individuals, which were chosen as parents of F_3, along with F_3 progenies. Instead, we grow remnant seed harvested from F_1 plant (F_2 seed) in the experiment comprising of P_1, P_2, F_1, F_2 and F_3. Hence, measurements made on individuals of F_2 and F_3 generation may not be correlated. Nelder (1960) and Hayman (1960) developed method for estimation of components of variances which take care of the precision of individual statistics as well as the correlations among them.

Calculated values of D, H, E_1 and E_2 could be used to find the expected values of various statistics employed for analysis. Sum of squares, *i.e.*, (observed value—expected value)^2, over all the statistics is then obtained. Division of sum of squares by appropriate number of degrees of freedom gives mean square deviation (S^2). What is the appropriate degree of freedom? If n statistics are employed to estimates components of variation the degree of freedom will be $(n-s)$. Diagonal elements of J^{-1} matrix are variances of the components being estimated. The standard errors for estimates of D, H, E_1 and E_2 are then calculated as square root of the product of S^2 and the diagonal element of J^{-1} corresponding to each component. Let us take up a worked example for clarity.

Worked Example

Two varieties of sorghum, viz. CSV 4 and E 35-1, were crossed and F_2 generation of this cross was raised. Plants were selected in F_2 generation and advanced to F_3. An experiment was planted comprising of P_1, P_2, F_1, F_3 progenies (each descending from different F_2 plants) and F_2 (from remnant F_2 seed). Observations were recorded on height of 10 plants/ generation.

Variation for plant height within each of the parental lines, and F_1 generation and variation of means of parental lines and F_1 were obtained, which represent E_1 and E_2, respectively. Information required for least square analysis is provided in the Table 4.17. Thus, six statistics are available to estimate four components of variation.

TABLE 4.17: Variances and covariances for plant height in sorghum

Statistics	Coefficients of components				Observed value
	D	H	E_1	E_2	
V_{1F_2}	$\frac{1}{2}$	$\frac{1}{4}$	1	–	925.5454
V_{1F_3}	$\frac{1}{2}$	$\frac{1}{16}$	–	1	611.6400
$W_{F_{23}}$	$\frac{1}{2}$	$\frac{1}{8}$	–	–	535.9090
V_{2F_3}	$\frac{1}{4}$	$\frac{1}{8}$	1	–	483.2475
E_1	–	–	1	–	76.6166
E_2	–	–	–	1	94.3266

To get the first normal equation, we multiply each element of row by the coefficient of D. Result of multiplication is presented in the following table. Sum at the bottom yields the first normal equation.

	D	H	E_1	E_2	Observed value
	$\frac{1}{4}$	$\frac{1}{8}$	$\frac{1}{2}$	0	464.7727
	$\frac{1}{4}$	$\frac{1}{32}$	0	$\frac{1}{2}$	305.8200
	$\frac{1}{4}$	$\frac{1}{16}$	0	0	267.9545
	$\frac{1}{16}$	$\frac{1}{32}$	$\frac{1}{4}$	0	120.8118
Total	$\frac{13}{16}D$	$\frac{1}{4}H$	$\frac{3}{4}E_1$	$\frac{1}{2}E_2$	1159.5390

Second normal equation is got in the same fashion, however, coefficients of H are used for multipliction. Thus second normal equation is shown at the end of following table:

	D	H	E_1	E_2	Observed value
	$\frac{1}{8}$	$\frac{1}{16}$	$\frac{1}{4}$	0	232.3863
	$\frac{1}{32}$	$\frac{1}{256}$	0	$\frac{1}{16}$	38.2275
	$\frac{1}{16}$	$\frac{1}{64}$	0	0	66.9886
	$\frac{1}{32}$	$\frac{1}{64}$	$\frac{1}{8}$	0	60.4059
Total	$\frac{1}{4}D$	$\frac{25}{256}H$	$\frac{3}{8}E_1$	$\frac{1}{16}E_2$	398.0083

Coefficients, of E_1 are used as a multiplier to get the third normal equation. Third normal equation is shown at the bottom of table presented below:

	D	H	E_1	E_2	Observed value
	$\frac{1}{2}$	$\frac{1}{4}$	1	0	929.5454
	$\frac{1}{4}$	$\frac{1}{8}$	1	0	483.2475
	0	0	1	0	76.6166
Total	$\frac{3}{4}D$	$\frac{3}{8}H$	$3E_1$	$0E_2$	1489.4095

Fourth normal equation is found in similar manner using coefficients of E_2 as a multiplier. Result of such a multiplication is shown in the following table.

	D	H	E_1	E_2	Observed value
	$\frac{1}{2}$	$\frac{1}{16}$	0	1	611.6400
	0	0	0	1	94.3266
Total	$\frac{1}{2}D$	$\frac{1}{16}H$	$0E_1$	$2E_2$	705.9666

Four normal equations so obtained are arranged in matrix form as:

$$\begin{bmatrix} \frac{13}{16}D & \frac{1}{4}H & \frac{3}{4}E_1 & \frac{1}{2}E_2 \\ \frac{1}{4}D & \frac{25}{256}H & \frac{3}{8}E_1 & \frac{1}{16}E_2 \\ \frac{3}{4}D & \frac{3}{8}H & 3E_1 & 0E_2 \\ \frac{1}{2}D & \frac{1}{16}H & 0E_1 & 2E_2 \end{bmatrix} \begin{bmatrix} \hat{D} \\ \hat{H} \\ \hat{E}_1 \\ \hat{E}_2 \end{bmatrix} = \begin{bmatrix} 1159.3590 \\ 398.0083 \\ 1489.4095 \\ 705.9666 \end{bmatrix}$$

$$J \qquad\qquad M \quad S$$

Values in the J matrix are converted to decimals, for convenience, as shown below:

$$\begin{bmatrix} 0.8125 & 0.2500 & 0.7500 & 0.5000 \\ 0.2500 & 0.0976 & 0.3750 & 0.0625 \\ 0.7500 & 0.3750 & 3.0000 & 0.0000 \\ 0.5000 & 0.0625 & 0.0000 & 2.0000 \end{bmatrix} \begin{bmatrix} \hat{D} \\ \hat{H} \\ \hat{E}_1 \\ \hat{E}_2 \end{bmatrix} = \begin{bmatrix} 1159.3590 \\ 398.0083 \\ 1489.4095 \\ 705.9666 \end{bmatrix}$$

$$J \qquad M \qquad S$$

After getting J^{-1}, these matrices can be arranged as under:

$$\begin{bmatrix} D \\ H \\ E_1 \\ E_2 \end{bmatrix} = \begin{bmatrix} 10.5496 & -30.4168 & 1.1644 & -1.6865 \\ -30.4168 & 108.2088 & -5.9211 & 4.2218 \\ 1.1644 & -5.9211 & 0.7823 & -0.1060 \\ -1.6865 & 4.2218 & -0.1060 & 0.7896 \end{bmatrix} \begin{bmatrix} 1159.3590 \\ 398.0083 \\ 1489.4095 \\ 705.9666 \end{bmatrix}$$

$$M \qquad J^{-1} \qquad S$$

Estimates of four components are got as:

$$\begin{aligned} \hat{D} &= (10.5496 \times 1159.3590) + (-30.4168 \times 398.0083) + \\ &\quad (1.1644 \times 1489.4095) + (-1.6865 \times 705.9666) \\ &= 668.2905 \\ \hat{H} &= (-30.4168 \times 1159.3590) + (108.2088 \times 398.0083) + \\ &\quad (-5.9211 \times 1489.4095) + (4.2218 \times 705.9666) \\ &= 1965.5169 \\ \hat{E}_1 &= (1.1644 \times 1159.3590) + (-5.9211 \times 398.0083) + \\ &\quad (0.7823 \times 1489.4095) + (-0.1060 \times 705.9666) \\ &= 83.6432 \\ \hat{E}_2 &= (-1.6865 \times 1159.3590) + (4.2218 \times 398.0083) + \\ &\quad (-0.1060 \times 1489.4095) + (0.7896 \times 705.9666) \\ &= 124.6063 \end{aligned}$$

The expected values of various statistics are now constructed from estimates of D, H, E_1 and E_2. For example, we know that V_{1F_2} is made up of $\frac{1}{2}D + \frac{1}{4}H + E_1$. Substituting the values of these components, we get the expected value of V_{1F_2}. Thus,

$$\frac{1}{2}(668.2905)+\frac{1}{4}(1965.5169)+83.6432$$
$$=909.1676$$

Expected values of other statistics are presented in Table 4.18.

TABLE 4.18. Observed and expected values of statistics for plant height in sorghum

Statistics	Observed (*O*)	Expected (*E*)	Deviation (*O–E*)
V_{1F_2}	929.5454	909.1676	20.3778
V_{1F_3}	611.6400	581.5963	30.0437
$W_{1F_{23}}$	535.9090	579.8348	–43.9253
V_{2F_3}	483.2475	496.4054	–13.1579
E_1	76.6166	83.6432	–7.0266
E_2	94.3266	124.6063	–30.2797

Deviations in Table 4.18 are squared and added over six statistics. This sum of squared deviations is found to be 4386.6742. Since six statistics were used to find the estimates of four components, two degrees of freedom are available to find mean squared deviations (S^2). Thus,

$$S^2=\frac{4386.6742}{2}=2193.3371.$$

Standard errors of $\hat{D}$, $\hat{H}$, $\hat{E}_1$, and $\hat{E}_2$ are calculated as:

$$S.E._D=(10.5496^2 2193.3371)^{\frac{1}{2}}$$
$$=152.1145$$

$$S.E._H=(108.2088^2\ 2193.3371)^{\frac{1}{2}}$$
$$=487.1738$$

$$S.E._{E_1}=(0.7823^2\ 2193.3371)^{\frac{1}{2}}$$
$$=41.4227$$

and finally

$$S.E._{E_2}=(0.7896^2\ 2193.3371)^{\frac{1}{2}}$$
$$=41.6156.$$

Test of significance revealed that these components of variances were significantly different from zero (Table 4.19). Estimate of dominance component is relatively larger in magnitude. Thus large part of observed variability is not fixable in nature. Because additive component is also significant, some variation is fixable.

TABLE 4.19: Estimates of components of variation for plant height in sorghum

Components	Estimates		
$\hat{D}$	668.2905**	±	152.1145
$\hat{H}$	1965.5169**	±	487.1738
$\hat{E}_1$	83.6432*	±	41.4227
$\hat{E}_2$	124.6063**	±	41.6156

It should be pointed out that estimates of components of variation based on so small number of degrees of freedom are not reliable. To be reliable, estimates should be based on adequate number of statistics grown in an experimental design which is replicated at least four times.

Standard errors of the estimates of components can be obtained in two ways when the experimental material is replicated, *viz.* from the error variance of heterogeneity test and in empirical manner.

When the experimental material is replicated, estimates of components are obtained for each replication separately using values of various statistics. Estimated values of these components are then employed to find the expected values of statistics in each replication. From the observed and expected values of statistics, sum of squares of deviations are obtained for each replication.

If n statistics are used to calculate s components, each sum of square will be based on $(n-s)$ degrees of freedom. A chi-square test will indicate whether the s components are adequate to explain the observed variation. A test of heterogeneity will indicate whether the s components are adequate for each part of the experiment and also for the entire experiment. Using the mean value of each statistic over the r replications, in which the material is grown, "overall" estimate of s components are calculated. These "overall" estimates are used to calculate expected values and subsequently an "overall" sum of square. This "overall" sum of square is also based on ($n - s$) degrees of freedom. Since the mean values of statistics are used to calculate overall sum of squares, overall sum of square should be multiplied with r (number of replications) in order to make it comparable with total sum of squares. An analysis of variance table is set up as shown in Table 4.20. Test the significance of overall mean square against heterogeneity mean square. Non-significance implies that the s components of variance are adequate to account for variation observed in the entire experiment as well as in r parts of the experiment considered separately.

TABLE 4.20: ANOVA for heterogeneity of components of variation

Source	*df*	*SS*	*MS*
"Overall"	$(n - s)$		
Heterogeneity	By difference		
Total	$r\ (n - s)$		

When the overall and heterogeneity mean squares do not differ significantly they are combined to provide an estimate of error variance. Standard errors of the s components are given by square root of product of the diagonal element of J^{-1} matrix and error variance. This assumes that error variance is common to all the statistics.

Since the overall estimate is got over replications, standard errors of components of variances will be $\left(\frac{1}{r}\right)^{\frac{1}{2}}$ times the standard error of individual estimates.

Standard error could be calculated in an empirical manner. Since r estimates of each component are available, variance of each component is got as a variation of r estimates. For example, if experimental material is replicated six times, 6 estimates of D would be available. Variance of six estimates will give variance of D. However, estimates of standard errors obtained from analysis of variance are more precise because they depend upon larger degrees of freedom, *viz.* $r\ (n - s)$, as compared with empirical estimates which are based on $(r - 1)$ degrees of freedom only. However, empirical estimate would be more desirable if based on larger number of replications, *e.g.*, four and more. (Mather, personal communication).

5

NORTH CAROLINA MATING DESIGNS

5.1 Mating Designs and Assumptions

In the last chapter methods were described which enable estimation of the additive and dominance components of heritable variation of quantitative attributes. These methods do not offer a direct test of significance of either additive or dominance components. However, certain mating designs permit not only a test of significance of additive and dominance components of variation but also enable estimation of their magnitudes. Relatives are developed by some system of matings — the mating designs — which are grown in a set of environmental conditions — the environmental designs. A quadratic analysis of observations leads to the estimates of components of variances and covariances of the design which are then interpreted genetically. The term 'mating design' refers to a system of mating employed to develop progenies of certain kinds. The manner in which progenies so developed are subjected to environment is the "environmental design". For each mating design an environmental design must be superimposed.

Cockerham (1963) classified mating designs as one, two, three and four factors designs, depending upon the number of ancestors per progeny over which control is exercised. Common mating designs such as diallel cross, North Carolina designs (I, II, and III), line × tester and partial diallel are two factor designs.The triallel and quadriallel crosses are three and four factor mating designs, respectively. A set of half-sib families or polycross progenies constitute one factor design.

Choice of mating design depends primarily on two things, *viz.*

simplicity of the design and information provided by the design. One factor design is suitable for detecting presence of genetic variability. In the absence of non-allelic interaction, two factor mating design is convenient for the estimation of additive and dominance components of variance. However, complex mating designs are required for the estimation of additive, dominance and epistatic components of genotypic variance. All these mating designs were developed to suit cross-pollinated species and those self-pollinated crop species which could be crossed easily. It is natural that mating designs most often employed are those which can be readily analysed by standard statistical procedures and interpreted into the components of variance of the design. To interpret genetically, components of variance of a design are translated into covariances of relatives. It is the covariances of relatives which are often readily interpretable into components of genotypic variance (section 4.6). In most of the cases estimates of variance components, obtained through translation of covariances of relatives, refer to the population from which individuals for mating have been sampled. This is the reference population, both for genotypes and environments, and it is in terms of variances of the reference population that various procedures and designs are interpreted. In few circumstances only, variances can be translated from one population to another. The reference population may be a variety or a racial mixture of varieties or a genetic mixture of many homozygous lines or segregating material arising from a cross between two homozygous lines.

Comstock and Robinson (1948, 1952) proposed three mating designs. A few assumptions have to be satisfied for valid inferences. Comstock and Robinson (1952) made following assumptions while deriving the expectations of mean squares. (By expectations of mean squares we mean a value that we would approach as a limit if the amount of data is infinitely large):

1. Random choice of those individuals which are mated to produce experimental progeny.
2. Random distribution of genotypes relative to variations in the

environment. The experimental errors are assumed to be independent, and

3. That there are no non-genetic maternal effects.

Interpretation of the variance components of the design also involve some assumptions (Comstock and Robinson, 1952). These are:

(i) Regular diploid behaviour of chromosomes at meiosis.

(ii) Gene frequency in the population should be one-half at all the loci which govern the inheritance of character being studied. In other words, it is assumed that $p = q = 0.50$ at all the loci.

(iii) There are no multiple alleles.

(iv) There is no linkage among the genes. If there is linkage, then the repulsion and coupling phase linkages are in equilibrium, and lastly

(v) There is no non-allelic interaction.

Assumption of the diploid inheritance includes regular amphidiploids and can be modified to include autopolyploidy, so long as the parameter alpha (coefficient of double reduction) equals zero (Dudley and Moll, 1969), and meiosis is regular.

The experimental material of North Carolina Experimental designs I, II and III is developed from F_2 generation as a base material. If the F_2 generation is developed from two true breeding homozygous lines, assumption regarding gene frequencies is satisfied. Natural selection might, however, influence the gene frequencies to some extent. A good stand of usable plants constitutes an insurance in favour of this assumption (Comstock and Robinson, 1952). This assumption is not necessary for North Carolina design III.

Alternative alleles arise as a result of mutation. Multiple alleles arise likewise at a locus. If individuals chosen to be the parents of F_2 generation do not exhibit multiple allelism, there is a remote possibility that multiple alleles will bias the estimates of components of genotypic variance.

Inheritance of quantitative characters is governed by several gene pairs. Hence, assumption that coupling and repulsion phase linkages are in equilibrium is not valid in studies of populations which are only a few generations removed from pure line crosses. This is particularly true if recombination frequency is low. True breeding parental lines which are crossed to produce an F_1 and subsequently the F_2 population, are expected to bear on each of the chromosomes several genes which influence not only a given character but also other metric characters. One generation of random mating is, therefore, not likely to lead the population to Hardy-Weinberg equilibrium (section 2.3.3). Hence, linkage equilibrium may not be reached in F_2 generation. Effect of linkage is to cause an upward bias in the estimate of average degree of dominance (Comstock and Robinson, 1948). Values of '*a*' (average degree of dominance — a symbol used by Comstock and Robinson, 1948, 1952), greater than unity may result either from true overdominance or from genes linked in repulsion. Interpretation of the genetic components of variance should, therefore, be made with caution.

It is also not realistic to assume that non-allelic interaction is not operative. Comstock and Robinson (1948) are of the view that epistasis may cause an upward bias in the estimate of average degree of dominance. In section 4.5.1, contribution of non-allelic interaction of genes to the heritable variances of various generations was explained.

Several matings designs have been proposed. In this chapter we will consider the three North Carolina experimental designs (Comstock and Robinson, 1952), and the line × tester design (Kempthorne, 1957).

North Carolina mating designs were developed to measure average degree of dominance involved in the action of genes governing the inheritance of quantitative characters.

The line × tester design permits evaluation of general combining abilities of lines crossed to a set of testers as well as the general combining abilities of the latter. Estimates of specific combining ability effects of crosses are also provided by the this mating design.

The mating designs proposed by Comstock and Robinson (1952)

have two aspects, *viz.*

(i) The first aspect deals with development of experimental material. Base population is F_2 generation for all the designs. In designs I and II, plants are randomly chosen to be used as pollen and seed parents and mated in certain ways. On the other hand, plants selected in F_2 generation are mated to both the inbred parents in design III.

(ii) Field arrangement of the experimental material is second aspect. Since large number of progenies are raised with the object of getting reliable estimates of components of genotypic variances, appropriate experimental designs are essential. Major difference between choice of the designs for experiments of this kind and other agronomic experiments is that the quantities of interest are variances rather than means. Experimental designs such as lattice, which confound genetic and environmental differences among the means, are not satisfactory. Replications-in-blocks design proposed by Comstock and Robinson (1952) is satisfactory when blocking of genetic material is necessary in order to control the environmental variability. However, the mating design must be such that it permits the set of progenies to be randomly assigned to the blocks in a way that will allow an independent estimate of variances of interest from analysis of each block.

5.2. North Carolina Design I

The base population employed to produce experimental material of this design is F_2 generation of a cross between two inbred lines. From this base population, randomly chosen *sm* plants are used as pollen parents (males). Each pollen parent is mated to randomly chosen *f* plants used as seed parent (female). A female plant crossed with a given male plant (pollen parent) shall not be involved in matings with other pollen parents (Fig.5.1). Consequently there will be *smf* matings and *smf* progeny families. For example, if 16 plants are selected as male parents, and each male is mated to 3 different female plants, there will be in all 48 (*smf*) female plants and fortyeight progeny families. A group of progenies having one common male parent is called a male group.

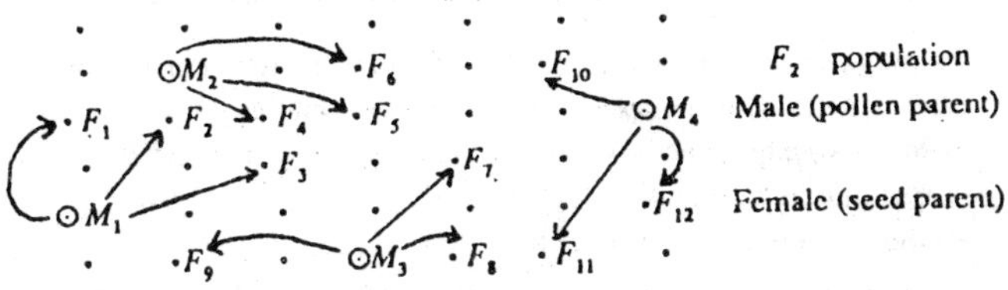

FIG. 5.1 : *Biparental mating*

For field arrangement *sm* male groups, each comprising of *f* progeny families, are divided into *s* sets. Each set of progenies is the experimental material for a separate unit of experiment. In mating designs a 'set' is a replicated experiment comprising of a group of genotypes. Different sets are made up of different male groups. Thus, 16 male groups in the example under consideration may be divided into 4 sets, each comprising of 4 male groups. Each male group consists of three half-sib progeny families and hence one set will comprise of 12 half-sib progeny families. Each set is planted in a randomised block design with *r* replications. Observations are recorded on *k* plants per plot. Format for the analysis of variance is given in Table 5.1.

TABLE 5.1: ANOVA for NC design I (on plants basis)

Source	*df*	MS	Expectation of MS.*
Sets	$(s-1)$		
Replications in sets	$s(r-1)$		
Males in sets	$s(m-1)$	M_1	$\sigma^2_e + k\sigma^2_p + rk\sigma^2_f + rkf\sigma^2 m$
Females in males in sets	$sm(f-1)$	M_2	$\sigma^2_e + k\sigma^2 p + rk\sigma^2 f$
Plots in females in males	$smf(r-1)$	M_3	$\sigma^2_e + k\sigma^2_p$
Remainder	$smfr(k-1)$	M_4	σ^2_e

* σ^2_e is the error variance and comprises of 'intra' plot environmental variance and genetic variance among individuals of same progeny. (There will be within progeny genetic variance because progeny results from a cross of two random F_2 plants).

σ^2_p is the variance of plot effects.

σ^2_m is the variance of progeny of different males mated to different females.

σ^2_f is the variance of progeny families of different females.

Classification of the *smf* progeny families so developed is made in an hierarchical fashion. In the hierarchical population members are in groups of families, subfamilies, sub-subfamilies and so on. This is also known as the 'nested' classification. Inferences drawn from this experiment refer to the population from which individuals have been chosen for mating and not to the individuals themselves. Thus it is a random effects model. It is assumed in this model that the sets, replications in sets, male in sets and females in males in sets are randomly distributed with zero mean and variances σ^2_s, σ^2_r, σ^2_m and σ^2_f, respectively. Errors are also assumed to be distributed with zero mean but variance σ^2_e.

5.2.1 *Estimation of Variance Components*

After analysing the data, significance of variance components is tested by means of *F* test. An appropriate denominator should be chosen for *F* test. For example, if the observations are recorded on plot basis (Table 5.2), an appropriate denominator for testing the significance of mean square of females in males in sets would be the remainder mean square.

The reason being that the null hypothesis (H_0) is $\sigma^2_f = 0$. If we choose M_{13} as a denominator for *F* test and σ^2_f is really zero, then *F* would be unity within the limits of sampling variation. This is an appropriate F test. Thus,

$$F_{(\text{females})} = \frac{M_{12}}{M_{13}} = \frac{\sigma_e^2 + r\sigma_f^2}{\sigma_e^2} = 1.$$

TABLE 5.2: Analysis of variance of NCI (plot basis)

Source	*df*	MS	Expectation of MS
Sets	$(s-1)$		
Replications in sets	$s(r-1)$		
Males in sets	$s(m-1)$	M_{11}	$\sigma^2_e + r\sigma^2_f + rf\sigma^2_m$
Females in males in sets	$sm(f-1)$	M_{12}	$\sigma^2_e + r\sigma^2_f$
Remainder	$s(r-1)$ $(mf-1)$	M_{13}	σ^2_e

What should be an appropriate denominator for males? If the null hypothesis (H_0) is $\sigma^2_m = 0$, following F test will wrongly infer about significance of genetic differences among the males, provided $\sigma^2_f \neq 0$. Thus,

$$F_{(males)} = \frac{M_{11}}{M_{13}} = \frac{\sigma_e^2 + r\sigma_f^2 + rf\sigma_m^2}{\sigma_e^2} \neq 1.$$

This shows that if $\sigma^2_f \neq 0$, the ratio $\frac{M_{11}}{M_{13}}$ will be greater than unity leading to a wrong inference regarding genetic differences among the males. When $\sigma^2_f \neq 0$, an appropriate denominator for the males mean square would be M_{12}. This ratio will be unity, when null hypothesis is correct as shown below

$$F_{(males)} = \frac{M_{11}}{M_{12}} = \frac{\sigma_e^2 + r\sigma_f^2 + rf\sigma_m^2}{\sigma_e^2 + r\sigma_f^2} = 1.$$

Significance of mean square for males suggests significant differences among the progeny families of different males (because of the genetic differences among the males). In this mating design each male is crossed with f seed plants. Therefore, the progeny families of a given male are half-sibs. Mean square for males, therefore, measures variance of half-sib progeny families. This variance is also the covariance of half-sibs and as shown in section 4.6.1 equals $\frac{1}{4}\sigma^2_A$. Significance of mean square for males, therefore, provides a direct test of significance of additive genetic variance.

When mean square for females in males is significant, we infer that there are significant genetic differences among the plants randomly chosen as the seed parents. Since the experimental material produced by this mating design is a biparental progeny (S_3), total heritable variation of the experimental material is $\frac{1}{2}\sigma^2_A + \frac{1}{4}\sigma^2_D$ (section 4.5). The expectation of heritable variation of males equals $\frac{1}{4}\sigma^2_A$, therefore, the heritable variation of progenies of the females can be obtained as a difference. Thus,

$$\sigma^2_f = \left(\frac{1}{2}\sigma^2_A + \frac{1}{4}\sigma^2_D\right) - \frac{1}{4}\sigma^2_A$$

$$= \frac{1}{4}\sigma^2_A + \frac{1}{4}\sigma^2_D.$$

A difficulty encountered by the students of biometrical genetics is regarding use of notations. Different notations have been used for the same effect. For example, Falconer (1960) used symbol 'a' to denote deviation of either homozygote from mid-point and d for the extent of departure of heterozygote from mid-point. Fisher *et al.* (1932) used d and h instead of a and d, respectively. We have preferred to use symbols a and d for random mating populations and d and h for populations developed by controlled matings. Comstock and Robinson (1948, 1952) used symbols μ and $a\,\mu$ for a and d (of Falconer) respectively. μ_i is the deviation of either homozygote from mid-point at i th locus and similarly $a_i\mu_i$ the departure of heterozygote at ith locus. Comstock and Robinson (1948) derived expected values for additive genetic and dominance variance, which are $\frac{1}{2}\Sigma\mu_i^2$ and $\frac{1}{4}\Sigma a_i^2\,\mu_i^2$, respectively, provided $p = q = \frac{1}{2}$. Relationship between σ^2_m and σ^2_f, on one hand, and genetic expectations for additive variance and dominance variance on the other could be expressed as:

$$\sigma^2_m = \frac{1}{8}\Sigma\mu_i^2, \sigma^2_f = \frac{1}{8}\Sigma\mu_i^2 + \frac{1}{16}\Sigma a_i^2\mu_i^2$$

Hence, estimates of σ^2_A and σ^2_D could be got as:

$$\sigma^2_A = 4\sigma^2_m \text{ and } \sigma^2_D = 4(\sigma^2_f - \sigma^2_m).$$

5.2.2 *Estimation of Average Degree of Dominance*

With respect to a single locus with two alleles, the degree of dominance may be measured as $\frac{d^2}{a^2}$. For *i*th locus it is got as $\frac{d_i^2}{a_i^2}$. However, complication arises when several loci, which influence the inheritance of an attribute, are considered. We cannot measure the degree of dominance at each locus because the effect of individual gene cannot be measured. However, estimate of average degree of dominance can be obtained. Should we be satisfied with an unweighted estimate of average degree of dominance over all the loci? All the loci which govern the expression of a character may not be equally important and hence an unweighted estimate of average degree of dominance may not be meaningful. Comstock and Robinson (1952) proposed to take a weighted estimate of average degree of dominance (denoted by a symbol $\bar{a}$). How should the weighting be done? Comstock and Robinson (1952) suggested weighting of a^2s at individual loci by corresponding μ^2s. The estimate of average degree of dominance will be greater than unity when individual '*a*'s are greater than unity at several locii. If $\bar{a}$ is greater than unity, overdominance in the action of genes is suggested. When the average degree of dominance is in the overdominance range all the loci may not be overdominant. According to Comstock and Robinson (1948), the average degree of dominance ($\bar{a}$) is calculated as:

$$\bar{a} = \left(\frac{\Sigma a^2 \mu^2}{\Sigma \mu^2}\right)^{1/2}$$

Inference regarding the average degree of dominance involved in the action of genes can be made from the calculated value of this ratio as under

Value of $\bar{a}$	*Degree of dominance*
0	No dominance
Greater than 0, but less than 1	Partial dominance
Equal to 1	Complete dominance
Greater than 1	Overdominance.

According to Comstock and Robinson (1948) $\sigma_A^2 = \frac{1}{2}\Sigma\mu_i^2$ and $\sigma_D^2 = \frac{1}{4}\Sigma a_i^2\mu_i^2$. Average degree of dominance is therefore calculated as $\sqrt{\frac{2\sigma_D^2}{\sigma_A^2}}$. Estimation of $\bar{a}$, the average degree of dominance, for N.C.I. is obtained as:

$$\sqrt{\frac{2(M_{12}(f+1) - M_{11} - fM_{13})}{M_{11} - M_{12}}}$$

This formula may be derived as:

$$\bar{a}^2 = \frac{\Sigma a^2\mu^2}{\Sigma\mu^2} = \frac{2(\sigma_f^2 - \sigma_m^2)}{\sigma_m^2}$$

Since σ_f^2, in this experimental design is calculated as $\frac{M_{12} - M_{13}}{r}$ and σ_m^2 as $\frac{M_{11} - M_{12}}{rf}$, the numerator would be:

$$2\left[\frac{(M_{12} - M_{13})}{r} - \frac{(M_{11} - M_{12})}{rf}\right]$$

$$= 2\left[\frac{fM_{12} - fM_{13} - M_{11} + M_{12}}{rf}\right]$$

$$= 2\left[\frac{M_{12}(f+1) - M_{11} - fM_{13}}{rf}\right]$$

The denominator is σ_m^2 which is estimated as:

$$\frac{M_{11} - M_{12}}{rf}$$

Therefore, $\bar{a}$ would be:

$$\sqrt{2\left[\frac{M_{12}(f+1)-M_{11}-fM_{13}}{rf}\right]\times\frac{rf}{M_{11}-M_{12}}}$$

$$=\sqrt{\frac{2(M_{12}(f+1)-M_{11}-fM_{13})}{M_{11}-M_{12}}}$$

5.2.3. Worked Example

Six plants were randomly chosen from the F_2 generation of sorghum and used as pollen parents. From the F_2 population, eighteen plants were randomly tagged to be used as female parents. Each of the six pollen plants (males) were crossed to three different female plants. Resulting 18 progeny families were divided into two sets, each comprising of 3 male groups. Each set was planted in a randomised block design with three replications. Grain yield was recorded on 5 plants/plot (Table 5.3). Correction factor is calculated in usual manner from grand total

$$C.F.=\frac{(\text{Grand total})^2}{N}$$

Total number of observations (*N*), is got as a product of number of males in sets, number of females in males in sets, number of progeny on which the observations have been recorded, number of replications in sets and number of sets. Thus *N* is the present example is

$3 \times 3 \times 5 \times 3 \times 2 = 270$

$$\text{Correction factor} = \frac{(5079.5)^2}{270}$$

$$= \frac{25801320.25}{270}$$

$$= 95560.4453$$

Total sum of squares is calculated from Table 5.3 as:

$[(12.5)^2 + (8.5)^2 + (6.0)^2 + (10.5)^2 \ldots\ldots\ldots\ldots +$
$(28.5)^2 + (29.0)^2]$ –Correction factor
$= 117779.50 – 95560.4453$
$=22219.0547$

Sum of square for sets is obtained from set totals as:

$$\frac{\sum_{i=1}^{s}(\text{Set total})^2}{m\times f\times p\times r} - \text{correction factor}$$

TABLE 5.3: Grain yield of biparental progeny (NCI design)

Set	Male Parent	Progeny	Replication 1			Replication 2			Replication 3			Females			Set total
			F_1	F_2	F_3	F_1	F_2	F_3	F_1	F_2	F_3	F_1	F_2	F_3	
1	2	3	4	5	6	7	8	9	10	11	12	13	14	15	16
I	1	1	12.5	8.5	20.0	18.0	6.5	10.5	20.5	9.0	7.0				
		2	8.5	4.5	25.0	12.0	5.0	15.0	22.0	10.0	8.5				
		3	6.0	5.0	22.0	16.0	8.0	15.0	18.0	8.5	9.0				
		4	10.5	6.0	24.5	12.5	7.5	13.5	25.0	6.5	7.5				
		5	8.5	5.5	20.5	15.0	5.5	14.0	18.5	8.0	8.0				
Total			46.0	29.5	112.0	73.5	32.5	68.0	104.0	42.0	40.0	223.5	104.0	220.0	
Male total												547.5			
	2	1	20.0	18.0	5.5	15.0	15.0	6.5	25.0	22.0	8.0				
		2	15.5	12.5	8.0	12.0	18.0	7.5	20.5	18.0	8.5				
		3	12.0	14.0	7.5	10.5	12.5	8.0	15.0	15.5	7.5				
		4	18.0	15.0	8.5	18.0	20.5	5.5	18.5	15.0	6.5				
		5	15.0	10.0	6.0	15.5	18.0	7.0	18.0	20.0	7.0				
Total			80.5	69.0	35.5	71.0	84.0	34.5	97.0	90.5	37.5	248.5	243.5	107.5	
Male total												599.5			

(Contd.)

TABLE 5.3 (*Contd.*)

1	2	3	4	5	6	7	8	9	10	11	12	13	14	15	16
	3	1	10.0	15.0	22.0	15.5	20.0	20.0	18.0	25.0	20.0				
		2	10.0	18.0	25.0	12.0	25.0	21.5	12.0	30.5	21.5				
		3	15.5	25.0	30.0	12.5	22.0	24.0	15.0	28.0	20.5				
		4	12.5	20.0	25.0	10.0	18.0	23.5	18.5	28.5	23.5				
		5	12.0	15.0	28.0	15.0	20.0	22.0	16.5	28.0	20.5				
Total			60.0	93.0	130.0	65.0	105.0	111.0	80.0	140.0	106.0	205.0	338.0	347.0	
Male total														890.0	
Rep.total					655.5			644.5			737.0				
Set total															2037.0
II	4	1	40.0	25.0	20.0	35.5	24.0	15.5	35.5	20.5	20.0				
		2	35.5	22.5	18.5	38.0	25.0	17.5	35.0	28.0	18.5				
		3	30.5	24.5	16.0	38.5	20.0	18.0	34.5	27.5	19.0				
		4	32.5	24.0	15.5	37.0	25.5	18.5	38.5	26.5	19.5				
		5	35.5	25.0	15.5	37.5	23.5	17.5	37.5	26.5	17.5				
Total			174.0	121.0	85.5	186.5	118.0	87.0	181.0	129.0	94.5	541.5	368.0	267.0	
Male total												1176.5			

(Contd.)

TABLE 5.3 : (*Contd*).

1	2	3	4	5	6	7	8	9	10	11	12	13	14	15	16
	5	1	8.0	18.5	6.0	6.5	20.0	8.0	10.0	22.0	9.0				
		2	9.5	20.5	5.5	7.5	23.0	8.5	9.5	20.5	9.5				
		3	7.5	17.0	7.5	8.0	22.5	7.5	8.5	21.5	8.5				
		4	10.0	19.0	7.5	9.0	22.5	9.0	9.0	21.0	9.0				
		5	8.5	19.5	5.5	8.5	20.5	8.5	8.5	21.0	8.5				
Total			43.5	94.5	32.0	39.5	108.5	41.5	45.5	106.0	44.5	128.5	309.0	118.0	
Male total													555.5		
	6	1	30.0	20.5	30.0	28.5	25.0	35.0	25.0	27.0	30.5				
		2	32.5	25.0	35.0	27.5	24.0	38.5	25.5	29.0	28.5				
		3	32.0	23.5	38.5	30.5	20.5	37.0	28.0	25.0	29.0				
		4	35.5	24.0	35.0	30.0	21.0	36.5	27.5	28.0	28.5				
		5	33.5	24.0	35.0	29.0	21.0	37.0	28.0	27.0	29.0				
Total			163.5	117.0	173.5	145.5	115.5	184.0	134.0	136.0	145.5	443.0	364.5	503.0	
Male total														1310.5	
Rep. total					1004.5			1022.0			1016.0				
Set total															3042.5
Grand total															5079.5

where m, f, p and r represent the number of males in sets, number of females in males in sets, number of plants and number of replications per sets, respectively. The term

$$\sum_{i=1}^{s} \frac{(\text{Set total})^2}{mfpr}$$

is a crude sum of square for sets.

$$\text{Set } s.s. = \frac{(2037)^2 + (3042.5)^2}{135} - CF$$
$$= 99305.0018 - 95560.4453$$
$$= 3744.5565.$$

The crude $s.s.$ for sets is 99305.0018.

Since the experimental population is classified in an hierarchical fashion, correction factor for replications in sets and males in sets is crude s.s.for sets. Thus replication sum of squares is found as:

$$\frac{1}{m \times f \times p}[(655.5)^2 + (644.5)^2 + (737.0)^2 + (1004.5)^2 + (1022.0)^2 + (1016.0)^2] - \text{Crude s.s (sets)}$$

$$= \frac{4473989.75}{3 \times 3 \times 5 = 45} - 99305.0018$$

$$= 116.9926.$$

Sum of squares for males in sets is got from male totals. Thus,

$$\text{Males } s.s. = \frac{1}{r \times f \times p}[(547.5)^2 + (599.5)^2 + (890.0)^2 + (1176.5)^2 + (555.5)^2 + (1310.5)^2] - \text{Crude } s.s. \text{ sets.}$$

$$= \frac{4861399.25}{45} - 99305.0018$$

$$= 108031.0944 - 99305.0018$$

$$= 8726.0926$$

Since each male in a set has been mated to three different females, correction factor for females sum of squares is crude sum of squares for males. Hence females sum of squares is got as:

$$\frac{1}{r \times p}[(223.5)^2 + (104.0)^2 + (220.0)^2 + \ldots\ldots + (503.0)^2] - \text{Crude } s.s. \text{ males}$$

$$= \frac{1}{15} [1726417.75] - 108031.0944$$
$$= 115094.5166 - 108031.0944$$
$$= 7063.4222.$$

Remainder sum of squares is obtained as a difference. Thus,

Remainder *s.s.*= Total s.s –(Sets *s.s.* + Rep. *s.s.* + Male *s.s.* + Females *s.s.*)

= 22219.0547 – (3744.5565 + 116.9926 + 8726.0926 + 7063.4222)

= 2567.9908

The analysis of variance is set up as shown in Table 5.4

TABLE 5.4: ANOVA for grain yield (NCI)

Source	*df*	*S.S.*	M.S.	*F*
Sets	1	3744.5565	3744.5665 **	46.66
Replications in sets	4	116.9926	29.2481	0.36
Males in sets	4	8726.0926	2182.5231 *	3.70
Females in males in sets	12	7063.4222	588.6185 **	7.33
Remainder	32	2567.9908	80.2497	

The results reveal that mean square for sets is highly significant when tested against remainder mean square. Thus there were significant differences between the two sets. Replications mean square is, however, non-significant.

The mean square for females is found to be highly significant when remainder mean square is used as a denominator for *F* test. This significance indicates significant genetic differences among the plants employed as seed parents. Mean square for males is tested against females mean square. The *F* ratio is significant at 5 per cent level. Thus there were significant genetic differences among the plants chosen as pollen parents. Significance of mean square for males is also the significance of additive component of genotypic variance. Hence, additive genetic variance was important for variation observed for grain yield in the parental population (This is a random effects model).

Estimates of variance components are obtained from mean squares presented in Table 5.4. Thus,

$$\hat{\sigma}_m^2 = \frac{2181.5231 - 588.6185}{3 \times 3 = 9}$$

$$= \frac{1592.9046}{9}$$

$$= 176.9894.$$

The σ_m^2 measures $\frac{1}{4}\sigma_A^2$. Therefore, σ_A^2 will be 4 × 176.9894 =707.9576

$$\sigma_f^2 = \frac{588.6185 - 80.24}{3}$$

$$= \frac{508.3688}{3}$$

$$= 169.4562$$

Since $\hat{\sigma}_f^2$ is a measure of $\frac{1}{4}\sigma_A^2 + \frac{1}{4}\sigma_D^2$, estimate of $\frac{1}{4}\sigma_D^2$ is obtained as :

$$\sigma_f^2 - \sigma_m^2$$

$$= 169.4562 - 176.9894$$

$$= -7.5332$$

Estimate of $\frac{\sigma_D^2}{4}$ is negative. Since variances are quadratic functions (*i.e.*, squares), negative variances are theoretically not expected. However, whenever negative estimates of variance components are obtained, it is better to regard them as not existing. In the present parental population, only additive genetic variance appears to be responsible for inheritance of grain yield. This variation can be exploited through conventional breeding procedures, such as pedigree method, to realise substantial genetic grain.

There is no evidence of dominance variance in the population. However, only for the sake of illustration, average degree of dominance will be calculated. Thus $\bar{a}$

$$\sqrt{\frac{2[M_{12}(1+f)-M_{11}-fM_{13}]}{M_{11}-M_{12}}}$$

$$= \sqrt{\frac{2[588.6185(1+3)-2181.5231-3(80.2497)]}{2181.5231-588.6185}}$$

$$= \sqrt{\frac{-135.5964}{1592.9078}}$$

$$= \sqrt{-0.085}$$

$$= -0.2917$$

The value of $\bar{a}$ is negative and very low. Hence there is no indication of dominance variance for the expression of the character being investigated. It does not mean that there is no dominance at any of the loci which govern the inheritance of this character. Balancing of dominance effects may also give such results.

5.3 North Carolina Design II

Base population for developing the experimental material of this design is F_2 generation (resulting from hybridisation of two true breeding lines). North Carolina design II is a modification of design I, which can be suitably employed for the estimation of average degree of dominance of multiflowered crop species, like cotton, safflower, niger, tobacco, linseed, etc.

Experimental material is produced by mating randomly chosen *sm* plants used as pollen parents with randomly selected *f* plants employed as seed parents. All the *sm* pollen parents are mated to all the *f* seed parents, resulting in *smf* progeny families. For example, if 16 plants are chosen as males and mated to 16 plants selected as females, there will be 256 biparental progeny families.

Field arrangement is similar to that for North Carolina Design I. Four male groups, for example, might form one set. Each set comprises of *mf* progeny families, which is the experimental material for distinct unit of experiment and is planted in a randomised block design with *r* replications. If *k* plants of each progeny family are raised in each of the *r* "plots" and observations are recorded on plant basis, the structure of analysis of variance would be as shown in Table 5.5 (Comstock and Robinson, 1948). However, when observations are recorded on plot basis a different format for analysis of variance is available (Table 5.6).

TABLE 5.5 : Format for ANOVA for NC II (plants basis)

Source	*df*	Expectation *MS**
Sets	(s – 1)	
Replications in sets	$s\,(r-1)$	
Males in sets	$s\,(m-1)$	$\sigma_e^2 + k\sigma_p^2 + rk\sigma_{mf}^2 + rkf\sigma_m^2$
Females in sets	$s\,(f-1)$	$\sigma_e^2 + k\sigma_p^2 + rk\sigma_{mf}^2 + rkm\sigma_f^2$
Males × females in sets	$s\,(m-1)\,(f-1)$	$\sigma_e^2 + k\sigma_p^2 + rk\sigma_{mf}^2$
Plots in progenies	$smf\,(r-1)$	$\sigma_e^2 + k\sigma_p^2$
Within plots	$smfr\,(k-1)$	σ_e^2

* σ_{mf}^2 is progeny variance arising from interaction of male and female parents.

TABLE 5.6 : Analysis of variance for North Carolina Design II (plot basis)

Source	*df*	MS	Expectation M.S.
Sets	$(s-1)$		
Rplications in sets	$s\,(r-1)$		
Males in sets	$s\,(m-1)$	M_{21}	$\sigma_e^2 + r\sigma_{mf}^2 + rf\sigma_m^2$
Females in sets	$s\,(f-1)$	M_{22}	$\sigma_e^2 + r\sigma_{mf}^2 + rm\sigma_f^2$
Males × females in sets	$s\,(m-1)\,(f-1)$	M_{23}	$\sigma_e^2 + r\sigma_{mf}^2$
Remainder	$s\,(mf-1)\,(r-1)$	M_{24}	σ_e^2

This experimental design is factorial type with respect to the male and female effects. However, in part, the classification is also hierarchical.

5.3.1. *Estimation of Components of Variance*

After setting up an analysis of variance table, *F* test is applied to various mean squares. First of all significance of mean square for males × females in sets is tested. Appropriate denominator for this F test is obviously remainder mean square. Thus,

$$F_{(m \times f)} = \frac{M_{23}}{M_{24}}$$

The null hypothesis (H_0) is that $\sigma^2_{mf} = 0$ and the alternate hypothesis (H_1) is that $\sigma^2_{mf} \neq 0$. Significance of mean square for males × females indicates that the behaviour of different males is not consistent over different females and *vice versa*. If the mean square for males × females in sets is significant, M_{23} should be chosen as a denominator for F test of males in sets and females in sets mean square. Thus, when null hypothesis (H_0) is $\sigma^2_m = 0$, F test would be:

$$F_{(\text{Males})} = \frac{M_{21}}{M_{23}}$$

The null hypothesis is accepted if the ratio is equal to unity, within the limits of sampling variation (*i.e.* value of this ratio is smaller than the F value in table). Alternate hypothesis, H_1, is accepted if the ratio is greater than unity. Significance of this mean square implies that there are differences!amoog!the half-sib progenies of males because of the significant genetic differences among the plants chosen as pollen parents. Significance of the mean square for females in sets is likewise tested. Thus,

$$F_{(\text{Females})} = \frac{M_{22}}{M_{23}}$$

If the ratio is significant at $s\,(f-1)$ and $s\,(m-1)\,(f-1)$ degrees of freedom, alternate hypothesis (H_1) is accepted that $\sigma^2_f \neq 0$. Significance of females mean square is an indication of significant genetic differences among the plants employed as seed parents.

In case the mean square for males × females is non-significant, sum of squares for males × females is pooled with sum of squares for remainder, accompanied with similar pooling of their degrees of freedom. Mean square obtained in this way is the new remainder mean square. It is used as denominator for the F test of males and females mean square.

Since each male plant is crossed to f female plants, the progenies belonging to each male are half-sibs. By similar analogy, progenies of each of the female are also half-sibs. The variance of half-sibs is also the covariance of half-sibs, which was shown to be $\frac{1}{4}\sigma^2_A$ (section 4.6). Hence, the significance of mean squares of males as well as females provides a direct test of significance of additive genetic variance. Since the genetic expectation for heritable variation of biparental (S_3) progenies is $\frac{1}{2}\sigma_A^2 + \frac{1}{4}\sigma_D^2$, in the absence of non-allelic interaction and linkage, expectation of heritable variance of males × females interaction will be:

$$\frac{1}{2}\sigma_A^2 + \frac{1}{4}\sigma_D^2 - \frac{1}{4}\sigma_A^2 - \frac{1}{4}\sigma^2$$

$$= \frac{1}{4}\sigma_D^2$$

Thus σ_{mf}^2 is a measure of $\frac{1}{4}\sigma_D^2$. Significance of mean square for males × females, therefore, provides a direct test of significance of dominance variance.

The genetic expectation of variations of males and females are theoretically identical (*i.e.* $\frac{1}{4}\sigma_A^2$). When both the mean squares are significant, it is desirable to obtain an average estimate of $\frac{1}{4}\sigma_A^2$ over males and females. When the numbers of males and females are same, *i.e.* $m = f$, mean squares for both may be added together and averaged without weight to get M_{20} (the average mean square). Thus M_{20} is calculated as:

$$\frac{M_{21} + M_{22}}{2}$$

However, when $m \neq f$, a weighted estimate of M_{20} is desired. It is calculated as:

$$M_{20\,(\text{weighted})} = \frac{(m-1)\,M_{21} + (f-1)\,M_{22}}{(m+f)-2}$$

Estimate of $\sigma_f^2 = \sigma_m^2 = \frac{1}{4}\sigma_A^2$ is then calculated as :

$$\frac{M_{20} - M_{23}}{rn}$$

where n is number of males (= number of females).

Following the notations suggested by Comstock and Robinson (1948), $\frac{1}{4}\sigma_A^2 = \frac{1}{8}\Sigma\mu_i^2$ and $\frac{1}{4}\sigma_D^2 = \frac{1}{16}\Sigma a_i^2\mu_i^2$. Hence the weighted estimate of average degree of dominance for this experimental design is got as:

$$\sqrt{\frac{2n[M_{23} - M_{24}]}{M_{20} - M_{23}}}$$

5.4 Line × Tester Mating Design

Experimental progeny families for the North Carolina design II are derived from a base population which is an F_2 generation resulting from a cross between two inbreds. Kempthorne (1957) proposed a mating design analogous to North Carolina mating design II, which could be employed equally efficiently to self-pollinated and cross-pollinated crop species. In plants, it is possible by selfing the individuals (or sib-mating) to produce inbreds. In this mating design randomly chosen *m* inbreds (used as males and called as lines) are mated to each of the randomly selected *f* inbreds, used as females (designated as testers). Since the base population is inbreds for this mating design, it is possible to mate all the *m* inbred lines to all the *f* testers. Hence this mating design is not restricted, like the North Carolina design II, to the multiflowered crop species. This mating design is popularly known in India as line × tester. Line × tester is useful in deciding the relative ability of number of female and male inbreds to produce desirable hybrid combinations. This mating design can also provide information regarding the usefulness of male and female inbreds as parents for hybridisation to generate segregating population which is expected give superior segregates.

Whereas for the North Carolina design II, Comstock and Robinson (1952) adopted a random effects model, the line × tester design used in India assumes a fixed effects model. However, mating design initially proposed by Kempthorne (1957) is based on random effects model. Observation recorded on $i \times j$th cross grown in kth replication can be linearly expressed as shown below for this design (Arunachalam, 1974):

$$Y_{ijk} = \mu + g_i + g_j + s_{ij} + r_k + e_{ijk},$$

where Y_{ijk} is mean value of a character measured on cross $i \times j$ in kth replication: g_i = *g.c.a.* effect of ith parent, g_j = *g.c.a.* effect of the parent j, s_{ij} = *s.c.a.* effect of cross $i \times j$, r_k = replication effect, e_{ijk} environmental effect peculiar to (ijk)th individual, and μ = population mean effect.

Structure for the analysis of variance and expectation of mean sum of squares for line × tester design is presented in Table 5.7.

The field arrangement of experimental material, comprising of *mf* progeny families, is not similar to that described for North Carolina designs. The experimental material is not divided into sets. Usually the *mf* progeny families are grown in a randomised block design with *r* replications. Various sum of squares are calculated as:

Replication sum of squares:

$$\frac{\Sigma Y^2{}_{..k}}{mf} - \frac{Y^2{}_{...}}{rmf}$$

TABLE 5.7 : ANOVA for line × tester mating design

Source	df	M.S.	Expectation mean square: Random model	Expectation mean square: Fixed model
Replications	$(r-1)$			
Lines	$(m-1)$	M_1	$\sigma_e^2 + rV_{sca} + rfV_{gca(m)}$	$\sigma_e^2 + rf\frac{1}{m-1}\sum_i g_i^2$
Testers	$(f-1)$	M_2	$\sigma_e^2 + rV_{sca} + rmV_{gca(f)}$	$\sigma_e^2 + rm\frac{1}{f-1}\sum_j g_j^2$
Lines × testers	$(m-1)(f-1)$	M_3	$\sigma_e^2 + rV_{sca}$	$\sigma_e^2 + r\frac{1}{(m-1)(f-1)}\sum_i \sum_j s_{ij}^2$
Residual error	$(r-1)(mf-1)$	M_4	σ_e^2	σ_e^2

where r = number of replications
m = number of male parents (lines)
f = number of females (testers)
$Vgca$ = Covariance half-sibs
$Vsca$ = [Cov. Full sibs- 2Cov. Half-sibs].

for $(r-1)$ degrees of freedom, where $\Sigma Y_{..k}$ is sum of all the genotypes (*mf* genotypes) over all the replications. $Y_{...}$ is grand total of the character observed over all genotypes and replications.

Lines *s.s.*

$$\frac{\Sigma Y_i^2{}_{..}}{rf} - \frac{Y^2{}_{...}}{rmf}$$

for $(m-1)$ degrees of freedom. $\Sigma Y^2{}_{i..}$ is sum of squares of all the crosses involving *i*th line as one parent over all the testers and replications. This sum of square is obtained easily from two-way table.

Tester sum of squares:

$$\frac{\Sigma Y_{.j.}^2}{rm} - \frac{Y^2...}{rmf}$$

for $(f-1)$ degrees of freedom. $\Sigma Y_{.j.}^2$ is sum of squares of crosses involving *j*th tester as one parent over all lines and all replications. This sum of square is also calculated from two-way table.

Lines × testers S.S.

$$\frac{\Sigma Y_{ij.}^2}{r} - \frac{\Sigma Y_i^2..}{rf} - \frac{\Sigma Y_{.j.}^2}{rm} + \frac{Y^2...}{rmf}$$

for $(m-1)(f-1)$ degrees of freedom. $\Sigma Y_{ij.}^2$ is sum of squares of all crosses over all replications, $\frac{\Sigma Y_{i..}^2}{rf}$ and $\frac{\Sigma Y_{.j}^2}{rm}$ are crude sum of squares for lines and testers, respectively.

This is usually computed as a difference. Thus $L \times T$ sum of squares:

Treatment *s.s.* – Lines *s.s.* – Tester *s.s.*

Error sum of squares is obtained in usual way, *i.e.* by subtracting replication, lines, testers and lines × testers sums of squares from total sums of squares.

Individuals within each of the *mf* progeny families are full-sibs. Heritable variation of the *mf* progeny families is, therefore, covariance of full-sibs. *i.e.* $\frac{1}{2}\sigma_A^2 + \frac{1}{4}\sigma_D^2$, if non-allelic interaction is assumed to be absent. Since each line is crossed to all the testers, progeny families belonging to each line are half-sibs. Variation of lines is, therefore, covariance of half-sibs, *i.e.* $\frac{1}{4}\sigma_A^2$. Likewise, variation of progeny families of different testers is covariance of half-sibs, *i.e.* $\frac{1}{4}\sigma_A^2$. Therefore, variation attributable to lines × testers is got as a difference. Thus,

$$\frac{1}{2}\sigma_A^2 + \frac{1}{4}\sigma_D^2 - \frac{1}{4}\sigma_A^2 - \frac{1}{4}\sigma_A^2$$

$$= \frac{1}{4}\sigma_D^2.$$

Significance of mean square for lines × testers provides a direct test of significance of dominance variance. Significance of σ_A^2 is provided by significance of lines and testers mean squares.

F tests are applied to the various mean squares as already described for North Carolina design II.

In the earlier days, breeders used to select parents for hybridisation either on the basis of their *per se* performance or sometimes arbitrarily. Consequently, some crosses appeared to 'nick' well and others did not. Ability of a genotype to transmit desirable performance to its progeny was not given due importance till 1942. Sprague and Tatum (1942) introduced the concept of general and specific combining ability. Combining ability is the relative ability of a biotype to transmit desirable performance to its crosses. According to them general combinng ability is the average performance of a strain in a series of crosses. The term "specific combining ability is used to designate those cases in which certain combinations do relatively better or worse than would be expected on the basis of average performance of the lines involved". This aspect will be discussed at length while dealing with the diallel mating designs.

Diallel mating design, to be described in chapter 7, also facilitates identification of superior combiners and specific cross combinations. If n inbred lines are involved, at least $\frac{n(n-1)}{2}$ crosses have to be effected in diallel analysis. With large number of genotypes, therefore, number of crosses to be effected increases correspondingly. However, information is available only for n parents and $\frac{n(n-1)}{2}$ F_1 crosses. On the other hand, if m genotypes, used as lines, are crossed to f genotypes employed as testers, mf hybrids are produced which provide information about the *g.c.a.* effects of $m + f$ genotypes and *s.c.a.* effects of mf crosses. This is an advantage of line × tester mating design. In crops, such as sorghum and pearl millet, where male-sterile lines are available, $L \times T$ mating design permits testing of a large number of genotypes.

Likewise in crops such as wheat, maize and cotton, where emasculation and pollination is not difficult, line × tester design could be employed to screen a large number of genotypes for their combining ability.

The concept of general and specific combining ability is of practical importance to the breeders. It is, therefore, in the interest of breeders to know how the two combining abilities are related to various components of heritable variations. General combining ability is the average performance of progeny of a genotype which it is mated randomly to a number of genotypes. The progeny so produced is half-sib progeny. The variation of half-sib progeny is measured in terms of covariance of half-sibs, which was shown in section 4.6.1. to be equal to $\frac{1}{4}\sigma^2_A$. What we call as general combining ability, animal geneticists call as breeding value. Kempthorne (1957) has shown that variances of general and specific combining ability effects are related to components of heritable variance as:

$$\sigma^2_{gca} = Cov(H.S)$$

and since Cov (*H.S.*) is equal to $\left(\frac{1+F}{4}\right)^i \sigma^2_A, \sigma^2_{gca}$ can be expressed as

$$\frac{1}{4}\sigma^2_A + \frac{1}{16}\sigma^2_{AA} + \frac{1}{64}\sigma^2_{AAA} \;.......$$

if $F = 0$, and for a random mating population as :

$$\frac{1}{2}\sigma^2_A + \frac{1}{4}\sigma^2_{AA} + \frac{1}{8}\sigma^2_{AAA} \quad ....$$

F is the coefficient of inbreeding. Coefficient of inbreeding is the probability that two genes at any locus in an individual are identical by descent.

Likewise σ^2_{sca} = (Cov *FS* – 2Cov *HS*).

Because Cov (*FS*) = $\left(\frac{1+F}{2}\right)^{i+2j} \sigma^2_A + \sigma^2_D$, it is equal to

$$\frac{1}{2}\sigma^2_A + \frac{1}{4}\sigma^2_D + \frac{1}{4}\sigma^2_{AA} + \frac{1}{8}\sigma^2_{AD} + \frac{1}{16}\sigma^2_{DD} \;........$$

if $F = 0$, and equal to

$$\sigma^2_A + \sigma^2_D + \sigma^2_{AA} + \sigma^2_{AD} + \sigma^2_{DD} \;........$$

if $F = 1$.

Hence, σ^2_{sca}, when $F = 0$ is

$$\frac{1}{4}\sigma_D^2 + \frac{1}{8}\sigma_{AA}^2 + \frac{1}{8}\sigma_{AD}^2 + \frac{1}{16}\sigma_{DD}^2 \ldots\ldots$$

and equal to

$$\sigma_D^2 + \frac{1}{2}\sigma_{AA}^2 + \sigma_{AD}^2 + \sigma_{DD}^2 \ldots\ldots$$

provided $F = 1$.

The covariance of half-sibs for males as well as females is equal to $\frac{1}{4}\sigma_A^2$. When mean squares for males, females and males × females are significant, covariance of half-sibs for males and females is calculated as:

$$\text{Cov }(H.S.)\text{ males} = \frac{M_1 - M_3}{rf} = \frac{1}{4}\sigma_A^2 = \sigma_{gca}^2$$

$$\text{Cov }(H.S.)\text{ females} = \frac{M_2 - M_3}{rm} = \frac{1}{4}\sigma_A^2 = \sigma_{gca}^2.$$

And σ_{mf}^2 is obtained as:

$$[\text{Cov }(F.S.) - 2\text{ Cov }(H.S.)] = \sigma_{sca}^2.$$

However, when both the males and females mean squares are significant, an average estimate of Cov ($H.S.$) is desirable which is calculated as (Kempthrone, 1957 p. 470):

$$\frac{1}{r[2mf - m - f]}\left[\frac{(m-1)M_1 + (f-1)M_2}{m + f - 2} - M_3\right]$$

However, some researchers follow King *et al.*, (1961). According to King *et al.*, (1961), average Cov ($H.S.$) over males and females may be computed as:

$$\frac{M_1 + M_2 - 2M_3}{r(m + f)}$$

It should be pointed out that two estimates of average *Cov*($H.S.$) so obtained do not tally.

According to King *et al.*, (1961), *Cov*($F.S.$) may be got as:

$$\frac{1}{3r}[M_1 + M_2 + M_3 - 3M_4 + ry(6 - m - f)]$$

where y is the average estimate of Cov ($H.S.$).

Estimates of general combining ability effects of testers and lines are calculated from the two way table, as:

$$\hat{g}_{j(tester)} = \frac{Y_{.j.}}{rm} - \frac{Y_{...}}{rmf}$$

and

$$\hat{g}_{(\text{lines})} = \frac{Y_{i..}}{rf} - \frac{Y_{...}}{rmf}$$

where $\hat{g}_i$ and $\hat{g}_j$ represent the estimates of *g.c.a.* (general combining ability) effects of *i*th line and *j*th tester, respectively.

Estimate of specific combining ability (*s.c.a.*) effect ($\hat{S}_{ij}$) of $i \times j$th cross is obtained as:

$$\hat{S}_{ij} = \frac{Y_{ij.}}{r} - \frac{Y_{i..}}{rf} - \frac{Y_{.j.}}{rm} + \frac{Y_{...}}{rmf}.$$

Since the g_is and g_js are calculated as deviations from the population mean, sum of g_is and also sum of g_js are equal to zero. The g_is are obtained from the marginal totals of the lines. The precision of each g_i, therefore, depends upon the number of testers included in the study. Larger the number of testers, the more precise will be the estimate of *g.c.a.* effect of *i*th line. Similarly the precision of g_j, the *g.c.a.* effect of *j*th tester, is a function of the number of lines involved in the mating programme. For example, if number of testers is four and lines are fifteen, g_js will be measured relatively more precisely than the g_is.

The estimates of g_i s and g_j s are tested for their significance. The null hypothesis (H_0) being that $\hat{g}_i$ or $\hat{g}_j = 0$ (as case may be). The standard errors for $\hat{g}_i$s and $\hat{g}_j$s are computed as:

$$S.E._{\hat{g}i} = \left(\frac{M_4}{rf}\right)^{\frac{1}{2}}, i = 1, .., .., .., .., m$$

$$S.E._{\hat{g}j} = \left(\frac{M_4}{rm}\right)^{\frac{1}{2}}, j = 1, .., .., .., .., f$$

Significance of g is tested by means of a '*t*' test. Thus,

$$t_g = \frac{g - 0}{S.E._g}$$

The value of the ratio so obtained is referred to the '*t*' table for error degrees of freedom. For testing g_j, $S.E._{gj}$ is employed whereas for testing g_i, $S.E._{gi}$ is used.

After finding out which *g.c.a* effects deviate significantly from zero, we test the significance of difference between *g.c.a.* effects of two lines (or testers). The idea is to identify significantly superior line (or tester). Standard error for difference is calculated for lines and testers as

$$S.E.\ (\hat{g}_i - \hat{g}_j)\ \text{lines} = \left(\frac{2M_4}{rf}\right)^{\frac{1}{2}}$$

$$S.E.\ (\hat{g}_i - \hat{g}_j)\ \text{testers} = \left(\frac{2M_4}{rm}\right)^{\frac{1}{2}}$$

Standard error for the estimate of *s.c.a.* effects is calculated as:

$$S.E.\hat{s}_{ij} = \left(\frac{M_4}{r}\right)^{\frac{1}{2}}$$

and the significance of S_{ij} may be tested by an appropriate *t* test.

Significance of *s.c.a.* effect suggests that *s.c.a.* effect of the cross under consideration deviates significantly from zero. The next step is to find out which is a significantly superior cross combination, among those crosses which registered significant *s.c.a.* effects. Standard error for difference of *s.c.a.* effects of two crosses is calculated as:

$$S.E._{(\hat{s}_{ij} - \hat{s}_{kl})} = \left(\frac{2M_4}{r}\right)^{\frac{1}{2}}$$

The experimental material for the mating design proposed by Kempthorne (1957) comprises of the *mf* progeny families only. However, many research workers are tempted to raise parental lines along with *mf* progeny families in a bid to get a single degree of freedom for the contrast "parents *vs.* hybrids" (Table 5.8). Significance of mean square for parents *vs.* hybrids is taken to indicate presence of heterosis. Although, this method is statistically valid, conclusion regarding heterosis may not be reliable and useful. It is a comparison of mean of the parents as a group with the mean of hybrids as a group. Significance could result even when mean of hybrids as a group is smaller than mean of parental lines as a group. Moreover, when there is significance, it is quite likely that many hybrids do not show heterosis but significance is caused by only a few highly heterotic hybrids. Further, the tests using *F*-ratio with one degree of freedom are known to be less efficient than those with large degrees of freedom.

Arunachalam (1974) calls the mating design in which parents ($m + f$) are raised along with hybrids (mf) as a modified line × tester (MLT). In his opinion, the way MLT is used and analysed is erroneous. Linear mathematical model for the line × tester design given earlier is:

$$Y_{ijk} = \mu + g_i + g_j + s_{ij} + r_k + e_{ijk}.$$

However, when data based on mf entries are analysed from an experiment in which ($m + f + mf$) genotypes are raised in r replications, different model is required. According to Arunachalam (1974) a linear mathematical model for MLT is:

$$Y_{ijk} = \mu + \alpha m_i + \beta f_j + \gamma (g_i + g_j + S_{ij}) + r_k + e_{ijk}$$

where f_j and m_i are the effects of jth tester and ith line respectively, $\alpha = 1$, $\beta = 0$ and $\gamma = 0$ for combinations (ii_k); $\alpha = 0$, $\beta = 1$ and $\gamma = 0$ for combinations (jjk) and $\alpha = 0$, $\beta = 0$ and $\gamma = 1$ for combinations (ijk), $i \neq j$. While model for LT is simple, MLT has accommodated two parameters for each parent, *e.g.* f_j and g_j for the females, m_i and g_i for the males. Arunachalam (1974) is of the opinion that using the data of hybrids alone for LT analysis when the experimental material has been actually planted as per MLT is erroneous because it is equivalent to a field design with gaps corresponding to the parental lines in each replication. This does not conform to the basic requirements of a layout of a design. Moreover, in MLT the error mean square is based on relatively larger degrees of freedom than for LT. This will result in a biased conclusion.

TABLE 5.8 : ANOVA for modified line × tester.

Sl. No.	Source			*df*
1.	Replications			$(r-1)$
2.	Genotypes			$(g-1)$
	(a)	Parents		$(p-1)$
		(i)	Males	$(m-1)$
		(ii)	Females	$(f-1)$
		(iii)	Males *vs.* females	1
	(b)	Hybrids		$(h-1)$
		(i)	Lines	$(l-1)$
		(ii)	Testers	$(t-1)$
		(iii)	Lines × testers	$(l-1)(t-1)$
	(c)	Parents *vs.* hybrids		1
3.	Error			$(r-1)(g-1)$

where $g = (m + f + mf)$, $p = (m + f)$, $h = mf$ (or lt).

5.4.1 *Worked Example*

Three true breeding strains of cotton, *viz.* MS Khandwa 2, BN and GS 23, were crossed as testers with 13 true breeding strains as lines. The 38 hybrid combinations so produced were planted in a randomised block design with four replications. Number of nodes/plant were recorded on each cross combination per replication (Table 5.9).

TABLE 5.9: Node number per plant* in cotton

S.N.	Hybrids			Replications				Total
				1	2	3	4	
1.	Khandwa 2	×	Acala	4.8	6.0	4.8	5.0	20.6
2.	BN	×	Acala	6.0	5.8	5.8	5.4	23.0
3.	GS23	×	Acala	5.8	6.3	5.8	4.8	22.7
4.	Khandwa 2	×	9030	4.8	5.2	6.0	5.6	21.6
5.	BN	×	9030	5.2	6.5	5.8	6.0	23.5
6.	GS23	×	9030	6.0	6.0	5.6	7.5	25.1
7.	Khandwa 2	×	TM1	5.8	6.0	5.0	5.8	22.6
8.	BN	×	TM1	5.2	5.6	5.4	6.0	22.2
9.	GS23	×	TM1	5.0	6.0	4.8	5.6	21.4
10.	Khandwa 2	×	Reba B50	5.4	5.0	5.0	5.4	20.8
11.	BN	×	Reba B50	5.0	5.3	5.8	5.0	21.1
12.	Khandwa 2	×	KH33/1146	5.4	5.4	6.0	5.4	22.2
13.	BN	×	KH33/1146	6.6	6.0	5.6	5.8	24.0
14.	GS23	×	KH33/1146	5.4	6.4	6.0	5.4	23.2
15.	Khandwa 2	×	BS117	5.4	5.4	5.8	6.0	22.6
16.	BN	×	BS117	7.2	6.8	6.2	5.8	26.0
17.	GS23	×	BS117	6.0	5.6	5.8	6.3	23.7
18.	Khandwa 2	×	IST-11	5.8	5.3	5.4	4.8	21.3
19.	BN	×	IST-11	5.3	6.5	5.8	6.4	24.0
20.	GS23	×	IST-11	5.8	5.3	5.6	6.2	22.9
21.	Khandwa 2	×	J34	5.8	5.6	5.4	5.0	21.8
22.	BN	×	J34	6.7	6.2	6.2	6.2	25.3
23.	GS23	×	J34	7.2	5.8	7.0	6.0	26.0
24.	Khandwa 2	×	IC 1036	5.2	5.0	5.0	5.2	20.4
25.	BN	×	IC 1036	5.8	6.0	5.4	6.8	24.0
26.	GS23	×	IC 1036	6.8	6.6	6.8	6.6	26.8
27.	Khandwa 2	×	No 442	5.8	4.8	5.0	4.6	20.2
28.	BN	×	No 442	5.0	5.6	4.8	5.3	20.7
29.	GS23	×	No 442	4.8	4.6	5.0	5.2	19.6
30.	Khandwa 2	×	K2MB	5.0	5.3	4.8	5.5	20.6
31.	BN	×	K2MB	6.0	5.8	5.4	5.3	22.5
32.	GS23	×	K2MB	5.8	5.3	6.0	6.0	23.1
33.	Khandwa 2	×	Okra 97	6.0	5.5	4.8	5.6	21.9
34.	BN	×	Okra 97	5.4	6.0	5.4	5.8	22.6
35.	GS23	×	Okra 97	5.8	5.6	5.4	5.4	22.2
36.	Khandwa 2	×	72IH	5.2	4.8	4.4	4.8	19.2
37.	BN	×	72IH	5.3	5.4	4.4	5.3	20.4
38.	GS23	×	72IH	5.4	6.0	5.0	4.8	21.2
	Total			221.2	221.7	213.8	219.2	875.9

* Data kindly provided by Mr. K.S. Panwar.

The correction factor is calculated as:

$$\frac{(875.9)^2}{39 \times 4 = 156} = 4917.9539$$

Total *s.s.* $= (4.8^2+6.0^2+5.8^2+4.8^2+.......+5.3^2+4.8^2) - CF$
$= 4971.35 - 4917.9539$
$= 53.3961$

Hybrids *s.s.* $= \frac{1}{4}(20.6^2 + 23.0^2 + ...+20.4^2+21.2^2) - CF$
$= 30.9860$

Replication *s.s.* $= \frac{1}{39}(221.2^2+221.7^2+213.8^2+219.2^2) - CF$
$= 1.0053$

Error *s.s* $= 53.3961 - 30.986 - 1.0053$
$= 21.4048$

An analysis of variance table is now set up as shown in Table 5.10. *F* tests are then applied to various mean squares.

TABLE 5.10: Analysis of variance for node number in cotton (LT)

Source	*df*	*S.S.*	MS	*F*
Replications	3	1.0053	0.3351	1.78
Hybrids	38	30.9860	0.8154**	4.34
Error	114	21.4048	0.1877	

The *F* test for hybrids is:

$$F = \frac{0.8154}{0.1877} = 4.34.$$

Since the value of this ratio is larger than the table value of *F* for 38 and 114 degrees of freedom, it is safe to conclude that there are significant differences among 39 hybrids for node number/plant. If and only if the hybrid mean square is significant, one should proceed for line × tester analysis. From the hybrid totals of Table 5.9, set up a two-way table (Table 5.11).

The tester *s.s* is obtained from marginal totals of Table 5.11. Thus tester *s.s.* is:

TABLE 5.11: Two-way table for node number per plant (totals over 4 replications)

Testers	Lines													$Y_{.j.}$
	Acala	9030	TM1	Reba B50	KII33 /1146	BS 117	IST11	J34	IC 1036	No. 442	*K2MB*	Okra 97	72III	
Khandwa 2	20.6	21.6	22.6	20.8	22.2	22.6	21.3	21.8	20.4	20.2	20.6	21.9	19.2	275.8
BN	23.0	23.5	22.2	22.9	24.0	26.0	24.0	25.3	24.0	20.7	22.5	22.6	20.4	301.1
GS23	22.7	25.1	21.4	21.1	23.2	23.7	22.9	26.0	26.8	19.6	23.1	22.2	21.2	299.0
$Y_{i..}$	66.3	70.2	66.2	64.8	69.4	72.3	68.2	73.1	71.2	60.5	66.2	66.7	60.8	875.9

$$\frac{1}{13\times4}(275.8^2+301.1^2+299.0^2)-CF$$
$$=\frac{1}{52}(256127.85)-4917.9539$$
$$=7.5816.$$

Sum of squares for lines is got as :

$$\frac{1}{3\times4}(66.3^2+70.2^2+...+60.8^2)-CF$$
$$=\frac{1}{12}(59201.37)-4917.9539$$
$$=15.4936.$$

The sum of squares for lines × testers are found as a difference between hybrid sum of squares on one hand and sum of testers *s.s.* and lines *s.s.* on the other. Thus lines × tester *s.s.*

$$30.9860-(7.5816+15.4936)=7.9108.$$

Analysis of variance for line × tester is now set up as in Table 5.12.

TABLE 5.12: Analysis of variance for node number in cotton

Source	*df*	*SS*	MS	*F*
Replications	3	1.0053	0.3351	1.78
Hybrids	38	30.9860	0.8154**	4.34
Lines	12	15.4936	1.2911**	3.91
Testers	2	7.5816	3.7908**	11.50
Lines × testers	24	7.9108	0.3296*	1.75
Error	114	21.4048	0.1877	

The *F* test for lines × testers mean square is applied as:

$$F=\frac{0.3296}{0.1877}=1.75$$

When this value is referred to the *F* table, significance is indicated. Thus the lines do not appear to behave consistently over different testers and *vice versa.*

Mean square for lines × testers is now used as a denominator for *F* tests of testers and lines. Thus,

$$F_{\text{lines}}=\frac{1.2911}{0.3296}=3.91$$

and

$$F_{\text{testers}} = \frac{3.7908}{0.3296} = 11.50$$

Both the mean squares are found to be significant suggesting genetic differences among testers as well as lines for number of nodes/ plant.

Since the mean squares for testers as well as lines are significant, we would like to estimate the magnitude of σ^2_A responsible for the node number. As a first step, we calculate an estimate of Cov (*H.S.*). Thus,

$$\text{Cov}(H.S.)_{\text{testers}} = \frac{3.7908 - 0.3296}{4 \times 13}$$

$$= 0.0665$$

and

$$\text{Cov}(H.S.)_{\text{lines}} = \frac{1.2911 - 0.3296}{4 \times 3}$$

$$= 0.0801.$$

Since Cov (*H.S.*) accounts for one-fourth of an additive genetic variance, in the absence of non-allelic interaction, estimates, of σ^2_A are:

$$\sigma^2_{A\,(\text{testers})} = 0.0665 \times 4$$

$$= 0.266$$

and

$$\sigma^2_{A\,(\text{lines})} = 0.0801 \times 4$$

$$= 0.3204$$

As pointed out earlier, it is desirable to have an average estimate of Cov (*H.S.*) when mean squares both for testers and lines are significant.

Thus,

$$\text{Cov}(H.S.)_{\text{pooled}} = \frac{1}{r(2mf - m - f)}\left[\frac{(m-1)\,M_1 + (f-1)\,M_2}{(m+f)-2} - M_3\right]$$

$$= \frac{1}{4(2 \times 13 \times 3 - 13 - 3)}\left[\frac{12 \times 1.2911 + 2 \times 3.7908}{14} - 0.3296\right]$$

$$= \frac{1}{248}\,(1.6482 - 0.3296)$$

$$= 0.0053$$

Estimate of average σ^2_A is, therefore, 0.0212.

Average estimate of Cov (*H.S.*) following King *et al.* (1961) is computed as:

$$\frac{M_1 + M_2 - 2M_3}{r(m+f)}$$

$$= \frac{1.2911 + 3.7908 - 2(0.3296)}{4(16)}$$

$$= 0.0691.$$

Average estimate of additive genetic variance is, therefore, $0.0691 \times 4 = 0.2764$. Method of King *et al.* (1961) appears to give average estimate closer to individual estimates of Cov (*H.S.*).

Estimate of covariance of full-sibs is calculated as:

$$\frac{1}{3r}\ [M_1 + M_2 + M_3 - 3M_4 + ry\,(6-m-f)]$$

$$= \frac{1}{3 \times 4}\ [1.2911 + 3.7908 + 0.3296 - 3(0.1877) + 4(0.0691)\,(6-13-3)]$$

$$= 0.1737$$

Hence the estimate of σ^2_s could be got as:

$$[\text{Cov}\ (F.S) - 2Cov\ (H.S)]$$

$$= [0.1737 - 2(0.0691)]$$

$$= 0.0355.$$

Estimate of dominance variance (σ^2_D) would, therefore, be:

$$4 \times 0.0355$$

$$= 0.142.$$

In section 4.6.1., it was mentioned that the coefficient of inbreeding also influences the components of heritable variance. Thus, covariance of half-sibs, if $F = 1$, in the absence of non-allelic interaction would be:

$$\text{Cov}\ (H.S.) = \left(\frac{1+1}{4}\right)^i \sigma^2_A$$

$$= \frac{1}{2}\sigma^2_A$$

Estimate of additive variance for node number/plant assuming $F = 1$, is:

$$2 \times \text{Cov}\ (H.S.)$$

$$= 2 \times 0.0691$$

$$= 0.1382.$$

On the other hand, if the coefficient of inbreeding is zero (population is random mating), then covariance of half sibs is:

$$\text{Cov}(H.S.) = \left(\frac{1+0}{4}\right)^i \sigma_A^2$$

$$\frac{1}{4}\sigma_A^2$$

Hence estimate of σ_A^2 is:

$$4 \times \text{Cov}(H.S.)$$
$$= 4 \times 0.0691$$
$$0.2764.$$

The magnitudes of genetic components of variance depend upon the extent of inbreeding, because the frequencies of genotypes are influenced by the extent of inbreeding.

The ratio σ_g^2 to σ_s^2 provides information regarding the relative importance of additive genetic variance in the expression of character. In the present case the ratio is:

$$\frac{\sigma_g^2}{\sigma_s^2} = \frac{0.0691}{0.0355} = 1.946$$

The value of this ratio is greater than unity, which suggests the importance of additive genetic variance. This is a fixable component. Therefore, selection is expected to results in substantial improvement of this character.

Now, the general combining ability effects of the testers and lines have to be calculated to identify desirable combiners. Estimate of *g.c.a.* effect of *j*th tester is calculated as:

$$\hat{g}_j = \frac{Y_{.j.}}{rm} - \frac{Y_{...}}{rmf}, j = 1, 2, 3$$

Hence, $\hat{g}_1$ the estimate of *g.c.a.* effect of first tester, *i.e.* Khandwa 2, will be:

$$\frac{275.8}{52} - \frac{875.9}{156}$$
$$= -0.3108.$$

General combining ability effects of BN and GS 23 are also calculated from the marginal totals of Table 5.13 in a similar fashion.

Estimate of general combining ability effect of the *i*th line is got as:

$$\hat{g}_i = \frac{Y_i..}{rf} - \frac{Y...}{rmf}, \quad i = 1, 2, ..., 13$$

Therefore, estimate of *g.c.a.* effect of line 1 (Acala) is:

$$\hat{g}_i = \frac{66.3}{12} - \frac{875.}{156}$$
$$= -0.0897.$$

General combining ability effects of other lines are also found likewise. Estimates of *g.c.a.* effects of testers and lines employed in the present example are presented in Table 5.13.

Standard errors for testers and lines are got as:

$$S.E._{gj} = \left(\frac{0.1877}{4 \times 13}\right)^{\frac{1}{2}} = 0.06$$

and

$$S.E._{gi} = \left(\frac{0.1877}{4 \times 3}\right)^{\frac{1}{2}} = 0.125$$

Significance of *g.c.a.* effects of testers is tested as:

$$t = \frac{g_j - 0}{S.E._{gj}}$$

Therefore, the test of significance for *g.c.a.* effect of Khandwa 2 is:

$$\frac{0.3108 - 0}{0.06} = 5.18$$

When this value is referred to the '*t*' table it is found to be significant which implies departure of the *g.c.a.* effect from zero. Each *g.c.a.* effect is tested in this way. However, with increase in number of testers, this procedure will have to be repeated a number of times. An easy alternative is available. Since the error degrees of freedom are usually greater than 30, the value of calculated '*t*' is regarded as significant if it exceeds 1.96. Hence, all the *g.c.a.* effects are significant at 5 per cent level, if they are larger than the value ($S.E._{gi} \times 1.96$). By similar analogy, any *g.c.a.* effect greater than $S.E._{gi}$ (or g_j) × 2.576 is regarded as significant at 1 per cent level. Thus *g.c.a.* effects of those testers which exceed 0.06 × 1.96 = 0.1176, are significant at 5 per cent level, and those greater than 0.06 × 2.576 = 0.1545, significant at 1 per cent level. Put one asterisk for signifi-

cance at 5 per cent and two asterisks for significance at 1 per cent level on the *g.c.a.* effects. In this example, *g.c.a.* effects of all the testers are found to be significant.

TABLE 5.13: Showing *g.c.a.* effects of testers and lines for node number

Testers	*g.c.a.*	Lines	*g.c.a.*
Khandwa 2	–0.3108**	Acala	–0.0897
BN	0.1756**	9030	0.2353
GS 23	0.1353**	TM 1	– 0.0980
$S.E._{gi}$ ±	0.06	Reba B50	–0.2147
		KH33/1146	0.1686
		BS 117	0.4103**
		IST11	0.0686
		J34	0.4769**
		IC 1036	0.3186*
		No. 442	–0.5730**
		K2MB	–0.0980
		Okra 97	–0.0563
		72IH	–0.5480**
		$S.E._{gi}$ ±	0.1250

*,** Significant at 5 and 1 per cent levels, respectively.

The *g.c.a.* effects of those males which exceed 0.245 and 0.322 are regarded as significant at 5 and 1 per cent level, respectively.

In cotton, number of nodes per plant is a measure of earliness. Less number of nodes is desirable. A parent which transmits genes for lesser number of nodes to its progeny is regarded as a desirable combiner. Thus, parental strains with significant and negative *g.c.a.* effects are desirable combiners. Present analysis revealed that among the testers BN and GS23 and among the lines J34, BS 117 and IC 1036 are undesirable combiners for this attribute. On the other hand, Khandwa 2, No. 442, and 72IH with significant and negative *g.c.a.* effects are desirable combiners.

When *g.c.a.* effects of two or more testers are in desirable direction and significant it is useful to identify best combiners in the lot. Standard error of differences of *g.c.a.* effects, *viz.* $S.E._{(gi - gj)}$, where g_i is the estimate of *g.c.a.* effect of one genotype and g_j that of another, is helpful in this screening process. Thus a '*t*' test

$$\frac{g_i - g_j}{S.E._{(g_i - g_j)}}$$

will indicate the most desirable combiner. $S.E._{(gi-gj)}$, for testers is got as:

$$\left(\frac{2\text{ Error mean square}}{rm}\right)^{\frac{1}{2}}$$

Thus $S.E._{(g_i-g_j)}$, for testers in the worked example is

$$\left(\frac{2\times 0.1877}{4\times 13}\right)^{\frac{1}{2}}$$

$$= 0.0849.$$

Likewise, standard error of difference of *g.c.a.* effects for lines is calculated as:

$$\left(\frac{2\text{ Error mean square}}{rf}\right)^{\frac{1}{2}}$$

which for the present example is:

$$\left(\frac{2\times 0.1877}{4\times 3}\right)^{\frac{1}{2}}$$

$$= 0.1768.$$

If the difference between *g.c.a* effects of two testers is more than $0.0849 \times 1.96 = 0.1664$, tester with large *g.c.a* effect could be regarded as significantly superior than the other. Likewise, if the difference between *g.c.a.* effects of two lines exceeds $(0.1768 \times 1.96) = 0.3465$, the line with larger *g.c.a.* effects is regarded as superior combiner than the other. In the present example, testers BN and GS 23 are equally undersirable because difference between their *g.c.a* effects is non-significant. Among the lines, *g.c.a* effect of J34 is significant and positive, however, it is statistically *at par* with BS117 and IC1036. Lines No.442 and 72IH are equally desirable.

One thing needs to be mentioned regarding general combining ability effects. Breeders usually attempt to identify superior varieties for most of the characters of economic interest. For example, a variety might be high yielding in a geographic region for which the breeder is evolving varieties. When employed as a parent in crosses, this variety may emerge as a poor combiner. In other words, this line does not appear to transmit desirable genes for better performance to its progeny. Such a behaviour could result from intra- and/or inter-allelic interaction of genes concerned with the character. Thus superior performance of a variety is not always reflected in its combining ability. In general, there is a close agreement between the *per se* performance and the *g.c.a* effect of a given genotype.

Superiority of cross combinations could be inferred from their specific combining ability effects. *s.c.a* effects are computed as:

$$s_{ij} = \frac{Y_{ij\cdot}}{r} - \frac{Y_{i\cdot\cdot}}{rf} - \frac{Y_{\cdot j\cdot}}{rm} + \frac{Y_{\cdots}}{rmf}$$

s.c.a effect of cross Khandwa 2 × Acala is, therefore, got as:

$$\frac{20.6}{4} - \frac{66.3}{12} - \frac{275.8}{52} + \frac{875.9}{156} = -0.0641.$$

Specific combining effects of rest of the crosses are presented in Table 5.14.

TABLE : 5.14 : Showing *s.c.a.* effects of cross combinations for node number

	Testers		
Lines	Khandwa 2	BN	GS23
Acala	–0.0641	0.1494	0.0147
9030	–0.1372	–0.1506	0.2897
TM 1	0.4468*	–0.1416	–0.3013
Reba B 50	0.1128	0.1494	–0.2603
KH33/1146	0.0798	0.0414	–0.1183
BS 117	–0.0622	0.2994	–0.2353
IST 11	–0.0452	0.1414	–0.0933
J 34	–0.3288	0.0578	0.2731
IC 1036	–0.5202*	–0.1086	0.6317**
No. 442	0.3218	–0.0416	–0.2763
K2MB	–0.0532	–0.0666	0.1237
Okara 97	0.2298	–0.0836	–0.1433
72 IH	0.098	–0.1423	0.0442

$S.E._{sij}$ ± 0.2166.

*, ** Significant at 5 and 1 per cent levels, respectively.

For testing the significance of *s.c.a* effects we need standard error for *s.c.a.* effects. Thus,

$$S.E._{s_{ij}} = \left(\frac{\text{Error mean square}}{r}\right)^{\frac{1}{2}}$$

$$= (0.1877/4)^{1/2}$$

$$= 0.2166$$

Significance of *s.c.a.* effects is tested by a '*t*' test. Thus 't' test for *s.c.a.* effect of Khandwa 2 × Acala would be:

$$t = \frac{-0.0641}{0.2166} = 0.295$$

This value is found to be non-significant and hence it is safe to conclude that the estimate of *s.c.a.* effect of this cross equals zero, within the limits of sampling variation. Significance may alternatively be tested as described for *g.c.a.* effects. Thus *s.c.a.* effect of any cross which exceeds 0.2166 × 1.96 = 0.4245 and 0.2166 × 2.576 = 0.5579 could be regarded as significant at 5 and 1 per cent levels, respectively. In the present example *s.c.a.* effects of GS23 × IC 1030, Khandwa 2 × IC 1036 and Khandwa 2 × TM 1 have been found to be significant. However, among these crosses only one *viz.*, Khandwa 2 × IC 1036 has *s.c.a* effect in desirable direction. This cross is, therefore, desirable cross combination from the point of view of node number per plant.

At times geneticists encounter an interesting situation. Crosses selected on the basis of their *s.c.a.* effects do not appear to be in agreement with superior crosses selected on the basis of their *per se* performance.

5.5 North Carolina Design III

Like the North Carolina designs I and II, base population for this design is F_2 generation resulting from hybridisation of two inbreds. Unlike the two earlier designs, however, experimental material for this design is produced by mating randomly selected *sm* plants from F_2 (employed as pollen parents) to both the inbreds from which F_2 was generated. This results in 2 *sm* matings.

The 2 *sm* progeny families are divided into *s* sets for field planning. Each set comprises of *m* pairs of progeny families. Members of each pair have one parent (male parent) in common but the female parents are different *i.e.* two inbreds. Field arrangement is similar to North Carolina designs I and II, where set is the unit of experiment. The 2*m* progeny families, belonging to a given set, are planted in a randomised block design with *r* replications. Although the male parents for this design are randomly chosen from F_2, the female parents are fixed. Hence the effects for inbreds are regarded as fixed effects.

TABLE 5.15 : Analysis of variance for NC III

Source	*df*	MS	Expectation M.S.
Sets	$(s-1)$		
Replications in sets	$s(r-1)$		
Inbreds in sets	s^*		
F_2 parents in sets	$s(m-1)$	M_{31}	$\sigma_e^2 + 2r\sigma_m^2$\$
F_2 parents × inbreds in sets	$s(m-1)$	M_{32}	$\sigma_e^2 + r\sigma_{ml}^2$
Remainder	$s(2m-1)(r-1)$	M_{33}	σ_e^2

σ_{ml}^2 is variation of progeny families due to interaction of genotypes of F_2 parents and inbreds

* The degree of freedom is s because, $s(l-1) = s(2-1) = s$

\$$2r\sigma_m^2$ because $r.l\,\sigma_m^2 = r.2.\,\sigma_m^2$, since inbreds are 2.

The structure for analysis of variance for this design is presented in Table 5.15. Significance of various mean squares is tested by means of *F* test. Remainder mean square is employed to test the significance of F_2 parents × inbreds mean square. Thus,

$$F = \frac{M_{32}}{M_{33}},$$

where the null hypothesis (H_0) is $\sigma_{ml}^2 = 0$

Appropriate denominator for *F* test of F_2 parents is M_{33}. Thus *F* test for F_2 parents is:

$$F = \frac{M_{31}}{M_{33}},$$

where null hypothesis (H_0) is that $\sigma_m^2 = 0$. Significance of this mean square implies genetic differences among the F_2 parents.

5.5.1. *Estimation of Variance Components and Average Degree of Dominance*

Since the plants chosen as male parents are mated to both the inbreds, experimental progenies are not biparental progenies like the NC I and II. Hence genetic expectation of total variation of the progenies is different from the earlier two designs. Individuals from two progeny families of each male parent are half-sibs, because each male is mated to two inbreds. Therefore, variation of progenies of males is equal to the covariance of half-sibs. Thus variance of males is equal to $\frac{1}{4}\sigma_A^2$. Significance of F_2 parents, therefore, provides a direct test of significance of additive genetic variance.

In this mating design, seed parents are the two parental inbred lines. Thus the form of analysis of this experiment is of 2 × *s* kind. Interaction variance of F_2 pollen parents with inbreds can, therefore, be obtained as variance of one-half the difference of progenies over 2 inbreds. Derivation of the genetic expectation for σ_{ml}^2 has been given by Comstock and Robinson (1952 pp. 506 and 507), which is $pq\ \Sigma a_i^2 \mu_i^2$. If $p = q = \frac{1}{2}$, as is assumed in these designs, σ_{ml}^2 reduces to $\frac{1}{4}\Sigma a_i^2 \mu_i^2$. According to Comstock and Robinson (1948), $\frac{1}{4}\Sigma a_i^2 \mu_i^2$ is equal to σ_D^2 and therefore, $\sigma_{ml}^2 = \sigma_D^2$. Significance of mean square for F_2 parents × inbreds thus provides a direct test of significance of dominance variance.

If the mean sum of squares for F_2 parents is found to be significant, estimate of σ_m^2 is calculated as:

$$\sigma_m^2 = \frac{M_{31} - M_{33}}{2r}$$

Estimate of additive variance is, therefore, got as $4\,\sigma_m^2$.

If the mean square for F_2 parents × inbreds is significant, σ_{ml}^2 is calculated as:

$$\frac{M_{32} - M_{33}}{r}$$

Average degree of dominance involved in the action of genes may be calculated for this experiment as:

$$\bar{a} = \sqrt{\frac{M_{32} - M_{33}}{M_{31} - M_{33}}}$$

5.5.2 *Worked Example*

Sixteen plants of wheat were tagged in F_2 generation and employed as pollen parents. Each pollen parent was crossed to the 2 inbreds which produced the F_2 generation. Resulting 32 progenies were divided into 4 sets. Each set comprised of 4 male groups having 8 progeny families. The experimental material of each set was planted in a randomised block design with 2 replications. Observations were recorded on grain yield/ plot (Table 5.16).

TABLE 5.16 : Kernel yield/plant (g) in wheat

Sets	Males	Rep.I		Rep.II		Inbreds		Total
		P_1	P_2	P_1	P_2	P_1	P_2	
		$\bar{L}_{1i}$	$\bar{L}_{2i}$	$\bar{L}_{1i}$	$\bar{L}_{2i}$			
I	1	9.2	9.2	7.2	10.6	16.4	19.8	36.2
	2	12.8	14.6	8.0	12.4	20.8	27.0	47.8
	3	9.0	15.2	5.4	10.4	14.4	25.6	40.0
	4	13.8	14.0	8.0	8.8	21.8	22.8	44.6
	Male total	44.8	53.0	28.6	42.2	73.4	95.2	-
	Rep. total	–	97.8	–	70.8	–	–	168.6
II	1	7.2	11.2	6.4	9.0	13.6	20.2	33.8
	2	6.4	12.0	10.2	14.8	16.6	26.8	43.4
	3	8.2	11.0	9.4	13.0	17.6	24.0	41.6
	4	7.6	8.8	8.2	11.8	15.8	20.6	36.4
	Male total	29.4	43.0	34.2	48.6	63.6	91.6	-
	Rep. total	–	72.4	–	82.8	–	–	155.2
III	1	10.6	18.2	10.8	11.2	21.4	29.4	50.8
	2	7.6	10.5	6.0	9.2	13.6	19.7	33.3
	3	7.4	9.2	8.0	10.0	15.4	19.2	34.6
	4	10.2	16.2	12.6	13.2	22.8	29.4	52.2
	Male total	35.8	54.1	37.4	43.6	73.2	97.7	–
	Rep. total	–	89.9	–	81.0	–	–	170.9
IV	1	10.2	16.0	11.6	13.0	21.8	29.0	50.8
	2	11.2	14.4	10.0	13.2	21.2	27.6	48.8
	3	13.0	15.2	14.2	14.6	27.2	29.8	57.0
	4	11.0	11.8	8.4	9.4	19.4	21.2	40.6
	Male total	45.4	57.4	44.2	50.2	89.6	107.6	-
	Rep. total	–	102.8	–	94.4	–	–	197.2
	Grand total							691.9

As a first step for analysis calculate the correction factor as:

$$\frac{(GT)^2}{s \times r \times m \times f} = \frac{(691.9)^2}{4 \times 2 \times 4 \times 2}$$

$$= 7480.0877$$

Total sum of squares is got as :

$$(9.2^2 + 12.8^2 + 9.0^2 + \ldots + 14.6^2 + 9.4^2) - CF$$

$$= 7981.89 - CF$$
$$= 501.8023$$

Sum of squares for sets

$$= \frac{(168.6^2 + 155.2^2 + 170.9^2 + 197.2^2)}{r \times m \times f = 2 \times 4 \times 2 = 16} - CF$$

$$= 7537.9781 - 7480.0877$$
$$= 57.8904$$

Sum of squares for replications in sets

$$= \frac{(97.8^2 + 72.4^2 + \ldots\ldots + \ldots\ldots + 94.4^2)}{m \times f = 4 \times 2 = 8} - \text{Crude } S.S. \text{ for sets}$$

$$= 7599.6613 - 7537.9781$$
$$= 61.6831$$

Since within each set there are two replications (*i.e.* hierarchical classification) correction factor for replication sum of squares is crude sum of squares for sets. Likewise crude S.S. for sets is used as a correction factor for sum of squares for inbred lines and F_2 parents in sets. Sum of squares for inbreds in sets

$$= \frac{(73.4^2 + 63.6^2 + 73.2^2 + \ldots + 97.7^2 + 107.6^2)}{r \times m = 2 \times 4 = 8} - \text{Crude } S.S. \text{ sets}$$

$$= 7674.4463 - 7537.9781$$
$$= 136.4681$$

Sum of squares for F_2 parents in sets

$$= \frac{(36.2^2 + 47.8^2 + 40.0^2 + \ldots + 57.0^2 + 40.6^2)}{r \times f = 2 \times 2 = 4} - \text{Crude S.S. sets}$$

$$= 7684.2325 - 7537.9781$$
$$= 146.2544$$

Sum of squares for $F_2 \times$ inbreds interaction is got as :

$$\frac{(16.4^2 + 20.8^2 + 14.4^2 + \ldots + 29.8^2 + 21.2^2)}{r = 2} -$$

crude SS F_2 parents – crude SS inbreds + crude SS for sets

$$= 7846.745 - 7684.2325 - 7674.4463 + 7537.9781$$
$$= 26.0443$$

Sum of squares for error =

Total $S.S.$ – ($S.S.$ sets + $S.S.$ replications + $S.S.$ inbreds + $S.S.F._2$ parents + $S.S.F._2$ × inbreds)

$= 501.8023 - (57.8904 + 61.6831 + 136.4681 + 146.2544 + 26.0443)$

$= 73.462$

Now the analysis of variance table is set up as shown in table 5.17.

TABLE 5.17 : ANOVA for Kernel yield/plant (g) of wheat (North Carolina design III)

Source	*df*	S. S.	*M.S.*	*F*
Sets	3	57.8904	19.2968**	
Replications in sets	4	61.6831	15.4208**	
Inbreds in sets	4	136.4681	34.1170**	
F_2 parents in sets	12	146.2544	12.1879**	4.64
F_2 parents × inbreds in sets	12	26.0443	2.1704	0.82
Error	28	73.4620	2.6236	

** Significant at 1 percent level

F tests for various mean squares are carried out as described in section 5.5 Thus F test for F_2 parents × inbreds in sets would be:

$$\frac{2.1704}{2.6236} = 0.82$$

When the value of this ratio is referred to F table for 12 and 28 degrees of freedom, it is found to be non-significant. This suggests that the F_2 parents do not express differential behaviour. In other words, dominance variance is not involved in the inheritance of this character. However, mean square for F_2 parents in sets is highly significant. There are significant genetic differences among the 16 plants randomly selected from F_2 generation as pollen parents. This also suggests that additive genetic variance is the only component of genotypic variance which is responsible for inheritance of this trait. Magnitude of σ^2_A is then obtained as $4\,\sigma^2_m$, and σ^2_m is got as:

$$\frac{12.1879 - 2.6236}{2r = 2 \times 2 = 4}$$

$$= 2.3910$$

$$\therefore \sigma^2_A = 2.3910 \times 4$$

$$= 9.564$$

5.6 Triple Test-Cross

Although the North Carolina mating design III is recognised as most efficient among the three designs (Mather and Jinks, 1982) the estimates of dominance variance obtained are less precise. In mating designs it is assumed that infinitely large number of families of infinitely large size would be produced as experimental material. However, it is seldom practiced and consequently sampling variance influences the reliability of estimates computed. Kearsey and Jinks (1968) pointed out three difficulties encountered while attempting to estimate additive, dominance and environmental components of variance of a quantitative character based on the second degree statistics. These are:

(i) Non-allelic interaction is assumed to be absent, although valid test to show its absence is seldom provided by many of the mating designs. Two tests have, however, been proposed by Hayman (1954) in diallel analysis to detect non-allelic interaction.

(ii) The estimates of dominance variance are usually associated with larger standard errors as compared with corresponding values for additive genetic variance, and lastly

(iii) Estimates of additive genetic variance and dominance variance are differentially influenced by the distribution of genes with increasing and decreasing effects on the quantitative traits.

An extension of North Carolina mating design III was proposed by Kearsey and Jinks (1968) which is popularly known as "Triple Test-Cross". It provides an unambiguous test for detection of non-allelic interaction and in addition permits testing the significance and estimation of additive genetic and dominance variance. This mating design combines the scaling test approach of Mather (1949) to detect non-allelic interaction, with the mating design approach of Comstock and Robinson (1952).

The experimental material for the triple test-cross, as the name implies, is produced by randomly selecting n plants from F_2 generation (like Comstock and Robinson's 1952 mating designs) and each is crossed to the three testers, *viz*., the two inbred parents (P_1 and P_2) and the F_1 produced by crossing P_1 and P_2. In this way $3n$ progeny families are produced as experimental material. The $3n$ progeny families are planted in randomized block design with r replications. Within each replication each of the progeny family of each set will have k plants on which observations will be recorded. The 3 progeny families are denoted by L_{1i}, L_{2i} and L_{3i}, suggesting that these are the families produced by crossing *i*th F_2 plant to P_1, P_2 and F_1, respectively. The k plants of each of the progeny family could be completely randomized within a replicate which provides an estimate of within family error mean square for k-1 degrees of freedom. And because there will be $3n$ progeny families per replicate, mean within family error mean square can be computed for $3nr$ (k–1) degrees of freedom (over replications).

The analysis can be divided into two parts for convenience, *viz*., first concerned with the detection of non-allelic interaction and second with testing the significance of additive genetic and dominance variance and computing their estimates. Several modifications were subsequently proposed in this triple test-cross approach (Perkins and Jinks 1970; Jinks and Perkins, 1970; Jinks and Virk, 1977; Chahal and Jinks, 1978 and others). However, in the present text we shall confine to the modification proposed by Jinks and Perkins (1970), and Perkins and Jinks (1970).

5.6.1 *Detection of non-allelic interaction*

The kinds of gametes produced by F_1 represent a mixture of equal parts of the gametes produced by the two inbred parents, so long as genes are independent in transmission. Hence Kearsey and Jinks (1968) proposed a scaling test $\bar{L}_{1i} + \bar{L}_{2i} - 2\bar{L}_{3i} = 0$. This relationship would be equal to zero within the limits of sampling variation. $\bar{L}_{1i}$, $\bar{L}_{2i}$ and $\bar{L}_{3i}$ refer to mean measurements of progeny families produced by crossing *i*th randomly selected plant from F_2 generation to P_1, P_2 and F_1, respectively. This is demonstrated for parents differing at two loci each with two alleles in table 5.18. The nine genotypes from F_2 generation when crossed to AABB (P_1), aabb (P_2) and AaBb (F_1), produce progeny families with

TABLE 5.18 : $\bar{L}_{1i}$, $\bar{L}_{2i}$, $\bar{L}_{3i}$ and $\bar{L}_{1i} + \bar{L}_{2i} - 2\bar{L}_{3i}$ for arbitrary case of F_2

Genotypes of F_2 plants	$\bar{L}_{1i}$ AABB(P_1)	$\bar{L}_{2i}$ aabb(P_2)	$\bar{L}_{3i}$ AaBb(F_1)	$\bar{L}_{1i} + \bar{L}_{2i} - 2\bar{L}_{3i}$
AABB	da + db	ha + hb	½(da + db + ha + hb)	da + db + ha + hb– da –db –ha–hb = 0
AABb	½(da + db + da + hb)	½(ha + hb + ha –db)	½(da +ha + hb)	da + ha + hb–da– ha–hb = 0
AAbb	da + hb	ha –db	½(da – db + ha + hb)	da – db +ha + hb – da +db–ha –hb = 0
AaBB	½(da + db + ha + db)	½(ha + hb –da + hb)	½(da + ha + hb)	db + ha + hb –db –ha –hb = 0
AaBb	½(da + db + ha + hb)	–½da –½db +½ha + ½hb	½ha +½hb	ha+hb– ha–hb=0
Aabb	½da + ½ha + hb	–½da – db + ½ha	–½db + ½ha + ½hb	–db + ha + hb + db –ha –hb = 0
aaBB	ha + db	–da + hb	–½da +½db + ½ha + ½hb	–da + db + ha + hb + da –db –ha –hb = 0
aaBb	½db + ha + ½hb	–da–½db+ ½hb	–½da + ½ha + ½hb	–da + ha + hb + da –ha –hb = 0
aabb	ha + hb	–da–db	–½da –½db + ½ha + ½hb	–da –db + ha + hb + da + db–ha –hb = 0

means as shown in this table. The scaling tests $\bar{L}_{1i} + \bar{L}_{2i} - 2\bar{L}_{3i}$ are zero in all the cases.

Bias due to correlated gene distribution has been described by Kearsey and Jinks (1968).

The test for non-allelic interaction proposed by Kearsey and Jinks (1968) could be carried out for individual F_2 plants or alternatively a combined analysis of variance could be carried out for n such comparisons together. This test is equally applicable when the genes are associated in the parents or dispersed between them. However, it would be desirable to choose homozygous parents which differ at maximum number of loci governing the inheritance of a quantitative trait being investigated.

A modification in the triple test cross was proposed by Perkins and Jinks (1970). A statistic $\dfrac{\sum_{i=1}^{n}(\bar{L}_{1i} + \bar{L}_{2i} - 2\bar{L}_{3i})^2}{6nr}$ is computed for n

degrees for freedom and tested for its significance against its own replicate error mean square. The statistic mentioned above is the mean squared deviation from zero. In other words, it is the sum of $(\overline{L}_{1i} + \overline{L}_{2i} - \overline{L}_{3i})^2$ for all n such comparisons (over replications). The squared sum is then divided by $6nr$ where n is number of F_2 plants used to produce experimental progeny families and r is number of replications. According to Perkins and Jinks (1970) variation due to this contrast measures $\frac{1}{32}J + \frac{1}{64}L + \frac{1}{16}[i]^2$ for the F_2 sample when non-allelic interaction is present. Where $J = \Sigma j^2$, $L = \Sigma l^2$

From the total of $(\overline{L}_{1i} + \overline{L}_{2i} - 2\overline{L}_{3i})$ over n such values, another statistic could be computed (*i.e.* squared mean deviation)

$$\frac{\left[\sum_{i=1}^{n}(\overline{L}_{1i} + \overline{L}_{2i} - 2\overline{L}_{3i})\right]^2}{6nr}$$

The divisor is 6 because for any sum of squares the divisor is sum of the squares of the coefficients. The coefficients associated with the contrast $(\overline{L}_{1i} + \overline{L}_{2i} - 2\overline{L}_{3i})$ are, 1, 1 and 2, respectively and consequently the divisor for this contrast would be $1^2 + 1^2 + 2^2 = 6$.

In simple words $\left[\sum_{i=1}^{n}(\overline{L}_{1i} + \overline{L}_{2i} - 2\overline{L}_{3i})\right]^2$ is square of grand total of $\overline{L}_{1i} + \overline{L}_{2i} - 2\overline{L}_{3i}$ values over the n F_2 plants and over replications. This statistic, when non-allelic interaction is present, is a measure of i type digenic non-allelic interaction. It is associated with one degree of freedom, which is also nonsignificant when tested against its own replicate error mean square in the absence of non-allelic interaction. But its significance suggests the presence of $\frac{1}{16}[i]^2$ in F_2 sample. Estimate of $\frac{1}{32}J + \frac{1}{64}L$ could be then obtained by subtraction. Thus:

$$\frac{\sum_{i=1}^{n}(\overline{L}_{1i} + \overline{L}_{2i} - 2\overline{L}_{3i})^2}{6nr} - \frac{\left[\sum_{i=1}^{n}(\overline{L}_{1i} + \overline{L}_{2i} - 2\overline{L}_{3i})\right]^2}{6nr}$$

The estimate of $J+L$ is associated with $(n-1)$ degrees of freedom. Hence the non-allelic component of variation for the F_2 sample could be partitioned into that due to i type interaction and that due to $j + l$ type non-allelic interactions. This could be explained with the help of a worked example.

5.6.2 *Worked Example*

Two true breeding varieties of wheat were crossed and the F_2 generation of this cross was grown. From the F_2 generation, 16 plants were randomly chosen and crossed as pollen parents to P_1, P_2 and F_1. The 48 (=3*n*) progeny families were grown in randomized block design with two replications. Within each replication, 5 plants of each progeny family were grown on which observations were recorded on kernel yield per plant (g). The data are presented in table 5.19. Variation in kernel yield per plant around mean of each progeny family was computed for each of the 48 progeny families. Thus there were 16 values each for within family variation for VL_{1i}, VL_{2i} and VL_{3i}. These 16 values were pooled for each of these 3 kinds of progeny families. Since each within family variance was based on $k-1 = 4$ degrees of freedom, $V_{L_{1i}}$, $V_{L_{2i}}$ and $V_{L_{3i}}$ are each associated with 64 degrees of freedom. The pooled, *i.e.* $V_{L_{1i}}$, $V_{L_{2i}}$ and $V_{L_{3i}}$ values are:

$$V_{L_{1i}} = 0.886$$

$$V_{L_{2i}} = 1.275$$

$$V_{L_{3i}} = 1.960$$

Since the analysis of variance is based on mean values of 5 plants/plot, the estimates of these variances are also averaged over 5 plants. Thus

$$\frac{0.886 + 1.275 + 1.960}{5 \times 3} = 0.2747$$

TABLE 5.19 : Values of the contrast $\overline{L}_{1i} + \overline{L}_{2i} - 2\,\overline{L}_{3i}$ for 16 F_2 plants (kernel yield/plant, *g*)

SNo.	Replication 1			Replication 2			$\overline{L}_{1i} + \overline{L}_{2i} - 2\overline{L}_{3i}$		
	$\overline{L}_{1i}$	$\overline{L}_{2i}$	$\overline{L}_{3i}$	$\overline{L}_{1i}$	$\overline{L}_{2i}$	$\overline{L}_{3i}$	Rep. 1	Rep. 2	Total
1	9.2	9.2	10.1	7.2	10.6	11.5	−1.8	−5.2	−7.0
2	12.8	14.6	15.7	8.0	12.4	12.0	−4.0	−3.6	−7.6
3	9.0	15.2	13.2	5.4	10.4	12.6	−2.2	−9.4	−11.6
4	13.8	14.0	13.2	8.0	8.8	8.4	1.4	0.0	1.4
5	11.2	14.4	12.1	10.0	13.2	11.7	1.4	−0.2	1.2
6	10.2	16.0	13.5	11.6	13.0	11.9	−0.8	0.8	0.0
7	13.0	15.2	13.2	14.2	14.6	13.9	1.8	1.0	2.8
8	11.0	11.8	10.4	8.4	9.4	8.7	2.0	0.4	2.4
9	10.2	16.2	12.5	12.6	13.2	12.7	1.4	0.4	1.8
10	7.4	9.2	8.6	8.0	10.0	9.8	−0.6	−1.6	−2.2
11	7.6	10.5	9.7	6.0	9.2	9.0	−1.3	−2.8	−4.1
12	7.2	11.2	10.9	6.4	9.0	9.1	−3.4	−2.8	−6.2
13	6.4	12.0	11.1	10.2	14.8	13.5	−3.8	−2.0	−5.8
14	8.2	11.0	9.7	9.4	13.0	11.4	−0.2	−0.4	−0.6
15	7.6	8.8	7.9	8.2	11.8	9.9	0.6	0.2	0.8
16	10.6	18.2	13.9	10.8	11.2	10.7	1.0	0.6	1.6
						Total	−8.5	−24.6	−33.1

The grand total of this table is really speaking $\left[\sum_{i=1}^{n}(\overline{L}_{1i} + \overline{L}_{2i} - 2\overline{L}_{3i})\right]$, and the correction factor for this analysis (or the contrast) is got as:

$$\frac{\left[\sum_{i=1}^{n}(\overline{L}_{1i} + \overline{L}_{2i} - 2\overline{L}_{3i})\right]^2}{6nr}$$

$$= \frac{(-33.1)^2}{6 \times 16 \times 2} = 5.706$$

And this squared mean deviation is as we know a measure of *i* type non-allelic interaction for 1 degree of freedom. The total sum of squares are computed as:

$$\frac{(-1.8)^2 + (-4.0)^2 + (-2.2)^2 + \ldots (0.2)^2 + (0.6)^2}{6} - CF$$

$$= \frac{220.45}{6} - CF$$

$$= 36.741 - 5.706 = 31.035$$

The sum of squares for epistasis (non-allelic interaction in broadest sense) is got as:

$$\frac{\sum_{i=1}^{n} (\bar{L}_{1i} + \bar{L}_{2i} - 2\bar{L}_{3i})^2}{6nr}.$$

In other words, this is the mean of squared deviations from zero. Thus s.s. epistasis :

$$\frac{(-7.0)^2 + (-7.6)^2 + (-11.6)^2 + \ldots + (0.8)^2 + (1.6)^2}{6 \times 2}$$

$$= \frac{358.85}{12} = 29.904$$

This measures $J + L + [i]^2$ in the presence of non-allelic interaction. The sum of squares attributable to $J + L$ is then calculated as:

$$29.904 - 5.706$$
$$= 24.198$$

The analysis of variance can now be set up as in table 5.20.

TABLE 5.20 : ANOVA for triple test-cross (Kernel yield/plant)

Source	*df*	*S.S.*	*M.S.*	*F*
Non-allelic interaction	16 (n)	29.904	1.869**	6.82
Overall $[i]^2$	1	5.706	5.706**	20.8
$J + L$	15 ($n - 1$)	24.198	1.613**	5.87
Within progeny families	192	–	0.274	

** Significant at 1 per cent level.

From this analysis of variance table it is clear that non-allelic interaction has significant role in the variation observed for kernel yield/plant. The additive × additive type of non-allelic interaction as well as the combine $J + L$ (*i.e.* additive × dominance and dominance × dominance kinds of non-allelic interaction) also govern the variability of kernel yield in the material being investigated.

5.6.3. *Testing significance of additive genet:c and dominance variance and estimation of D and H components*

If the triple test-cross indicates absence of non-allelic interaction, significance of additive genetic variance (D) and dominance variance (H) can be tested as is done in the standard North Carolina mating design III. Like the non-allelic interaction the estimates of D and H will refer to those loci at which the testers (*i.e.* parental lines) differ.

The format for analysis of variance, based on the mean measurements of L_{1i} and $L2i$ as suggested by Kearsey and Jinks (1968) is presented in Table 5.21. This was modified by Jinks and Perkins (1970) who suggested inclusion of data recorded on L_{3i} generation also for computation of D (Table 5.22).

TABLE 5.21 : Format for ANOVA suggested by Kearsey and Jinks (1968)

Source of variation	*df*	Expectation Mean squares	
Sums ($\bar{L}_{1i} + \bar{L}_{2i}$)	$(n-1)$	$\sigma^2 + 2r\sigma^2_m$	Ms
Differences ($\bar{L}_{1i} - \bar{L}_{2i}$)	$(n-1)$	$\sigma^2 + 2r\sigma^2_{ml}$	Md
Within crosses	$n(r-1)$	σ^2	Me

TABLE 5.22 : Format for ANOVA suggested by Jinks and Perkins (1970)

Source of variation	*df*	Expectation Mean squares	
Sums ($\bar{L}_{1i} + \bar{L}_{2i} + \bar{L}_{3i}$)	$(n-1)$	$\sigma^2 + 3r\sigma^2_m$	Ms
Differences ($\bar{L}_{1i} - \bar{L}_{2i}$)	$(n-1)$	$\sigma^2 + 2r\sigma^2_{ml}$	Md
Error	$n(r-1)$	σ^2	Me

According to Kearsey and Jinks (1968) as well as Jinks and Perkins (1970) expectations of σ^2_m and σ^2_{ml} are $\frac{1}{8}D$ and $\frac{1}{8}H$, respectively. However, according to Falconer (1960) covariance of half-sibs equals $\frac{1}{4}V_A$. Similarly σ^2_{ml} according to Comstock and Robinson (1952) equals dominance variance (V_D). Before we deal with the approach of Kearsey and Jinks (1968) and also Jinks and Perkins (1970) it would be in the interest of reader to show how $\sigma^2_m = \frac{1}{8}D$ and $\sigma^2_{ml} = \frac{1}{8}H$

Following the terminology of Mather and Jinks (1982) the mean measurements of progeny produced by random mating of plants from F_2 generation to the 3 testers, *viz.*, P_1, P_2 and F_1, would be as shown in Table 5.23, assuming single locus with 2 alleles (A, a). Variance of half the sums, *i.e.* ½ ($\bar{L}_{1i}$ + $\bar{L}_{2i}$), represents variance of half sib progeny families obtained by crossing randomly selected plants from F_2 to the two testers P_1 and P_2.

TABLE 5.23: Mean measurements of progeny families produced by crossing of F_2 plants to P_1. P_2 and F_1.

Genotypes of testers		Genotypes of F_2 plants			Array Mean
		AA ¼	*Aa* ½	*aa* ¼	
AA		*AA*	½*AA* + ½ *Aa*	*Aa*	
	$\bar{L}_{1i}$	*d*	½*d* + ½*h*	*h*	½*d* + ½*h*
aa		*Aa*	½*Aa* + ½*aa*	*aa*	
	$\bar{L}_{2i}$	*h*	½*h* – ½*d*	–*d*	½*h* – ½*d*
Aa		½*AA* + ½*Aa*	¼*AA* + ½*Aa* + ¼*aa*	½*Aa* + ½*aa*	
	$\bar{L}_{3i}$	½ (*d* + *h*)	(½*h*)	(½*h* – ½*d*)	½*h*

From the table 5.23 the total (and also the mean) of entire progeny generated by crossing plants from F_2, *viz.*, *AA*, *Aa* and *aa*, to both the parents *AA* and *aa*, is got as:

Half the sums $\left(\frac{\bar{L}_{1i} + \bar{L}_{2i}}{2}\right)$ for each of the family are,

$\frac{1}{2}(d+h), \frac{1}{2}h, \frac{1}{2}(h-d)$, respectively.

Total of these, taking into consideration the proportions in which the families appear, would be :

$$\tfrac{1}{4}(\tfrac{1}{2}d + \tfrac{1}{2}h) + \tfrac{1}{2}(\tfrac{1}{2}h) + \tfrac{1}{4}(\tfrac{1}{2}h - \tfrac{1}{2}d)$$
$$= \tfrac{1}{2}h$$

Contribution of this locus to the variance of half the sums is, therefore, obtained as:

$$\frac{1}{4}\left(\frac{1}{2}d+\frac{1}{2}h\right)^2+\frac{1}{2}\left(\frac{1}{2}h\right)^2+\frac{1}{4}\left(\frac{1}{2}h-\frac{1}{2}d\right)^2-\left(\frac{1}{2}h\right)^2$$

$$=\frac{1}{8}d^2$$

When several loci are considered, then this would be $\frac{1}{8}\Sigma d^2$ in the absence of non-allelic interaction. This could be written as $\frac{1}{8}D$, following Mather and Jinks (1982).

Variance of half the difference represents interaction of F_2 plants with two testers, *viz.*, P_1 and P_2. It is computed as shown below:

Half the difference of three progeny families from table 5.23 is :

$$\left(\frac{1}{2}d-\frac{1}{2}h\right), \frac{1}{2}d, \left(\frac{1}{2}h+\frac{1}{2}d\right)$$

The total (and equally the mean) would be :

$$\frac{1}{4}\left(\frac{1}{2}d-\frac{1}{2}h\right)+\frac{1}{2}\left(\frac{1}{2}d\right)+\frac{1}{4}\left(\frac{1}{2}h+\frac{1}{2}d\right)$$

$$=\frac{1}{2}d$$

Contribution of this locus to variance of half the difference could be obtained as:

$$\frac{1}{4}\left(\frac{1}{2}d-\frac{1}{2}h\right)^2+\frac{1}{2}\left(\frac{1}{2}d\right)^2+\frac{1}{4}\left(\frac{1}{2}h+\frac{1}{2}d\right)^2-\left(\frac{1}{2}d\right)^2$$

$$=\frac{1}{8}h^2$$

Considering several loci, it would be $\frac{1}{8}\Sigma h^2$ or $\frac{1}{8}H$, in the absence of non-allelic interaction.

Hence, after entering the values of sum of squares in the table of ANOVA, significance of mean squares for sums (either $\overline{L}_{1i}+\overline{L}_{2i}$ or $\overline{L}_{1i}+\overline{L}_{2i}+\overline{L}_{3i}$) is tested against error. The value of this ratio is then referred to the F table for corresponding degrees of freedom. Significance of this mean square suggests significant differences among n plants selected randomly from F_2 generation and crossed to the two/three testers. Alternatively this provides a direct test of significance for additive genetic variance. Its significance is an indication that additive genetic variance is an important cause of variation observed for the character being investigated. Estimate of σ^2_A is computed as:

$$8\sigma^2_m=8\left[\frac{Ms-Me}{3r/2r}\right].$$

Significance of mean square for difference points to the differential behaviour of n F_2 plants, relative to each other, over the testers. This also suggests significant role of dominance variance in the inheritance of character being studied. Estimate of dominance variance (σ^2_D or H) is obtained as:

$$8\sigma^2_{ml}=8\left[\frac{Md-Me}{2r}\right]$$

The average degree of dominance is then computed as:

$$\sqrt{\frac{D}{H}}$$

Whereas in the analysis of variance approach suggested by Kearsey and Jinks (1968) additive variance is based only on L_{1i} and L_{2i}, in the modified procedure suggested by Jinks and Perkins (1970) all the items in following comparisons are orthogonal and provide estimates of additive and dominance variance:

Comparisons	$\bar{L}_{1i}$	$\bar{L}_{2i}$	$\bar{L}_{3i}$	Testing for
1	1	1	1	Additive variance
2	1	–1	–	Dominance variance
3	1	1	–2	Non-allelic interaction

Variance of comparison 2 over all *n* sets of progeny families ($i=1$ to n) can be used to detect and estimate dominance variance (Comstock and Robinson, 1952 and Kearsey and Jinks, 1968). Squared deviations of comparison 3 added over all the *n* sets may be employed to detect and estimate non-allelic interaction component of heritable variation (Kearsey and Jinks, 1968). Variance of comparison 1 over *n* sets may be used to detect and to estimate the additive component of genotypic variation.

6

THE DIALLEL MATING DESIGN (Graphical and Numerical Approach)

6.1 Diallel Mating

Breeders cross two or more varieties or inbred lines in order to create variability for a character which they wish to improve. In this process they have to take decisions regarding the choice of parents to be employed for hybridisation and the choice of cross (crosses) to be advanced from among the several crosses effected by them. For simply inherited characters the choice of parents for hybridisation may not pose a serious problem. However, the task becomes difficult when the principal character is one such as grain yield. It was recognised by the earlier breeders that for quantitative characters parents cannot be selected with confidence on the basis of their own performance. In several cases it is observed that certain parents "nick" well when crossed and produce a large number of superior segregates. On the other hand, certain crosses between equally desirable parents produce an array of disappointing progeny. Hence breeders used to handle several segregating populations simultaneously. It was possible to identify a superior cross only when several generations were raised and much time, efforts and money wasted. There was an urgent need, therefore, to develop a technique which could permit identification of superior varieties to be used as parents for hybridisation and also pin-point cross-combinations likely to yield desirable segregates so that crosses having low probability of producing high performance segregates could be discarded.

The object of hybridisation in several crops, such as maize, sorghum, cotton *etc.* is also to exploit hybrid vigour. On the other hand, breeders of many self-pollinated crops are not primarily interested in hybrid performance. Their object of hybridisation is to combine in a single genotype the desirable genes that are found in two or more genotypes.

The *per se* performance of neither the parents nor the hybrids is likely to provide reliable indication regarding the possibility of isolating superior segregates from hybrid swarm. The cross combinations which appear promising in F_1 need not necessarily give large proportion of high manifestation selections in later inbred generations. The F_1s may exhibit superior performance due to dominance and/or non-allelic interactions. As the generations are advanced linkages break and new combinations are formed. This leads to dissipation of the superiority because the degree of dominance observed in F_1 declines and combinations which bestowed superiority due to non-allelic interaction do not exists as such. However, if information could be obtained about the genetic systems governing the inheritance of attributes to be improved it should be possible to assess the potential of different crosses in F_1 and F_2 generations and predict their performance in subsequent generations. One of the techniques which is widely used for this purpose is the diallel analysis.

The term 'diallel' was introduced by Schmidt (1919) which is a Greek word and implies all possible crosses among a collection of male and female animals. Hayman (1954) defined "diallel cross" as the set of all possible matings between several genotypes. The genotypes may be individuals, clones, homozygous lines *etc.* and if there are n of them, there are n^2 mating combinations, counting reciprocals separately. Like the other mating designs considered in chapter 5, diallel mating design also permits estimation of the magnitude of additive and non-additive components of heritable variance. Some other genetic properties of parental lines can also be studied from this design.

Hinklemann (1977) classified the diallel mating systems into various types as:

(i) *Diallel Mating Type I*

This is also referred to as a 'factorial' mating design. North Carolina II is an example of this type. In this mating design m plants are mated to randomly chosen f plants.

(ii) *Diallel Mating Type II*

It involves mating of monoecious individuals or inbred lines. If n individuals are chosen there will be n^2 matings.

There are four sub-types of this mating design depending upon which progeny families constitute the experimental material. These are:

(a) All n^2 combinations

(b) $\frac{n(n-1)}{2}$ F_1s and n parental lines

(c) $\frac{n(n-1)}{2}$ F_1s and $\frac{n(n-1)}{2}$ reciprocal F_1s, and

(d) Only $\frac{n(n-1)}{2}$ F_1s.

These sub-types refer to Griffing's (1956) methods 1, 2, 3 and 4, respectively.

(iii) *Partial Diallel Crosses*

This design was proposed by Kempthorne and Curnow (1961). When n becomes large, experimental material becomes unmanageable. On the other hand, if n is reduced sampling error becomes larger. In order to overcome this difficulty it was necessary to develop a design based on a sample of crosses from matings of a large number of inbred lines. According to Kempthorne and Curnow (1961) it is possible to draw valid inferences from 's' crosses, sampled from crosses where n lines are involved in a diallel mating. In diallel mating any given line is involved in $(n - 1)$ matings. The value of s is so chosen that it is less than $(n - 1)$. Thus, from the total crosses only $\frac{ns}{2}$ crosses are selected for analysis.

(iv) Two levels diallel crosses (Hinklemann, 1974), and

(v) Various combinations of pure forms given above.

The concept of Diallel Mating design II has been extended further to:

(i) Three-way design or the triallel mating design (Rawlings and Cockerham, 1962a). With n inbred lines there will be $\frac{n(n-1)(n-2)}{6}$ different three-way matings.

(ii) Four-way mating design or quadriallel was also proposed by Rawlings and Cockerham (1962b). There will be $\frac{n(n-1)(n-2)(n-3)}{12}$ four-way matings if n parents are used.

(iii) Partial triallel and partial four-way crosses (Hinklemann, 1965, 1968).

The data recorded on progeny families can be analysed in various ways. However, in this chapter we wii· consider the analysis proposed by Hayman (1954a). When n inbred lines are crossed in diallel fashion n^2 progeny families are produced. We can adopt the graphical and/or numerical approach proposed by Hayman (1954a) to analyse and interpret the results. Several assumptions are involved in this approach in order to simplify the genetic situation. These assumptions are:

(i) Diploid segregation,
(ii) No difference between reciprocal crosses,
(iii) Independent action of non-allelic genes, and in the diallel cross,
(iv) No multiple allelism,
(v) Homozygous parents, and
(vi) Genes independently distributed between the parents.

6.2 Graphical Analysis

Let us begin with a simple situation of a single locus with two alleles, *viz.* A and a to understand the basic principles underlying Hayman's (1954a) diallel analysis. With respect to this locus there will be two inbred lines in the population. If we also assume that frequencies of these genotypes are equal in the population *i.e.*, $\frac{1}{2}$, diallel mating will produce progeny families as shown in Table 6.1. There are two arrays corresponding to each common parent. An array is one parent and all the crosses involving it. Two kinds of progeny families comprise the AA array. The frequency of AA progeny in the array involving AA as common parent is ½. Likewise the frequency of Aa progeny family is ½. Values associated with genotypes AA and Aa are d and h, respectively, expressed as deviation from mid-point. Therefore, the mean of AA array is ½ $(d + h)$. By same analogy mean of array aa is ½ $(h - d)$.

TABLE 6.1: Diallel mating of two inbred lines, means, variances (V_r) and covariances (W_r) of arrays

		Female inbred line				
		AA	aa		V_r	W_r
	Value	d	$-d$	Mean of		
	Frequency	½	½	array		
	AA	AA	Aa			
Male	d	d	h	$\frac{1}{2}(d+h)$	$\frac{1}{4}(d-h)^2$	$\frac{1}{2}d(d-h)$
inbred	$\frac{1}{2}$					
line	aa	Aa	aa			
	$-d$					
	$\frac{1}{2}$	h	$-d$	$\frac{1}{2}(h-d)$	$\frac{1}{4}(d+h)^2$	$\frac{1}{2}d(d+h)$

Now let us derive the overall mean of progeny families produced by diallel mating of two inbred lines. The frequency of each progeny family in the entire population is product of frequencies of inbred lines, *i.e.*, $\frac{1}{4}$. Hence the overall mean is:

$$\frac{1}{4}(d)+\frac{1}{4}(h)+\frac{1}{4}(h)+\frac{1}{4}(-d)$$

$$=\frac{1}{2}(h)$$

Variance of progeny family means within an array around the array mean (V_r) is also shown in Table 6.1. For array AA, it is obtained as:

$$V_{r_A}=\frac{1}{2}(d)^2+\frac{1}{2}(h)^2-\left(\frac{1}{2}d+\frac{1}{2}h\right)^2$$

$$=\frac{1}{4}d^2-\frac{1}{2}dh+\frac{1}{4}h^2$$

$$=\frac{1}{4}(d-h)^2$$

Variance of progeny family means for aa array derived in similar fashion is $\frac{1}{4}$ $(d + h)^2$. In the absence of dominance, *i.e.*, $h = 0$, V_{rA} and V_{ra} are identical, *i.e.*, $\frac{1}{4}d^2$.

We can also derive covariance of progeny family means within an array with means of non-common parents of that array (Wr). The covariance for *AA* array can be derived as:

$$W_{r_A} = \left[\frac{1}{2}(d \times d) + \frac{1}{2}(-d \times h)\right]$$

$$= \frac{1}{2}d^2 - \frac{1}{2}dh$$

$$= \frac{1}{2}d\,(d - h).$$

Since the sum of means of two inbred lines is zero, correction factor to be deducted from sum of cross products is also zero. Hence sum of cross products over two progenies yields covariance. Covariance of progeny family means within *aa* array with means of corresponding non-recurrent parents is $\frac{1}{2}d\,(d + h)$. Like the V_rs, W_{rA} and W_{ra} are identical in the absence of dominance. Thus $W_{rA} = W_{ra} = \frac{1}{2}d^2$ when $h = 0$.

Values of V_{rA} and V_{ra} can be used to derive mean variance over arrays, *i.e.*, $\overline{V}_r$.

$$\frac{1}{2}\left[\frac{1}{4}(d-h)^2 + \frac{1}{4}(d+h)^2\right]$$

$$= \frac{1}{4}(d^2 + h^2)$$

Mean covariance ($\overline{W}_r$) is derived as shown below:

$$\frac{1}{2}\left[\frac{1}{2}d^2 - \frac{1}{2}dh + \frac{1}{2}d^2 + \frac{1}{2}dh\right]$$

$$= \frac{1}{2}d^2$$

We can also derive from this table variance of array means around overall mean ($V_{\bar{r}}$) as:

$$V_{\bar{r}} = \frac{1}{2}\left(\frac{1}{2}d + \frac{1}{2}h\right)^2 + \frac{1}{2}\left(\frac{1}{2}h - \frac{1}{2}d\right)^2 - \left(\frac{1}{2}h\right)^2$$

$$= \frac{1}{2}\left(\frac{1}{4}d^2 + \frac{1}{2}dh + \frac{1}{4}h^2\right) + \frac{1}{2}\left(\frac{1}{4}h^2 - \frac{1}{2}dh + \frac{1}{4}d^2\right) - \frac{1}{4}h^2$$

$$= \frac{1}{4}d^2 .$$

There is a definite relationship between V_{rA} and V_{ra} and W_{rA} and W_{ra}.

Thus,

$$W_{ra} - W_{rA} = V_{ra} - V_{rA} .$$

How? Let us see. Substitute the values derived for covariances and variances in expression given above. Thus,

$$\frac{1}{2}d^2 + \frac{1}{2}dh - \frac{1}{2}d^2 + \frac{1}{2}dh = \frac{1}{4}d^2 + \frac{1}{2}dh + \frac{1}{4}h^2 - \frac{1}{4}d^2 + \frac{1}{2}dh - \frac{1}{4}h^2$$

$$= dh.$$

Another relationship is

$W_{rA} - V_{rA} = W_{ra} - V_{ra}$.

Substituting the values for covariances and variances we find:

$$\frac{1}{2}d^2 - \frac{1}{2}dh - \frac{1}{4}d^2 + \frac{1}{2}dh - \frac{1}{4}h^2$$

$$= \frac{1}{4}d^2 - \frac{1}{4}h^2$$

Since $W_{ra} - W_{rA} = V_{ra} - V_{rA}$, regression of W_r on V_r (b_{wr}/V_r) will be unity. Regression line of W_r on V_r will also be of unit slope because change in the value of W_r, if common parent *AA* is substituted for *aa*, is equal to change observed for V_r, *i.e.*, $\Delta W_r = \Delta V_r$. From basic statistics we know that linear regression equation is expressed as:

$$\overline{Y} = a + b\overline{X}$$

where a is the origin (or the point on Y axis where the regression line intercepts it) and b is the regression coefficient (and measures the slope of line). In the present context 'a' can be obtained by substituting $\overline{W_r}$ for $\overline{Y}$ and $\overline{V}_r$ for $\overline{X}$. Thus,

$$a = \overline{W}_r - b\overline{V}_r \text{, and since } b = 1,$$

$$\frac{1}{2}d^2 - \frac{1}{4}d^2 - \frac{1}{4}h^2$$

$$= \frac{1}{4}d^2 - \frac{1}{4}h^2 \text{ or } \frac{1}{4}(d^2 - h^2)$$

The regression line will pass through points $\overline{W}_r\left(\frac{1}{2}d^2\right), \overline{V}_r\left(\frac{1}{4}d^2 + \frac{1}{4}h^2\right)$. **We have derived expression for '*a*' – the** point of interception, which is $\frac{1}{4}(d^2 - h^2)$. The point, where line with unit slope cuts the W_r axis, provides an indication regarding the degree of dominance involved in the action of genes. Thus when d^2 is larger in magnitude than h^2, regression line cuts the W_r axis on positive side, *i.e.*, above the origin. Regression line intercepts W_r axis below the origin when $h^2 > d^2$, *i.e.*, when there is overdominance. Line will pass through the origin (*i.e.* 0) when $d^2 = h^2$. This implies complete dominance and suggests that both the additive and dominance components of heritable variance are equally responsible for the inheritance of character being studied.

Reader should note that when dominance is present the magnitude of V_{rA} is less than that of V_{ra}. Similarly W_{rA} is less than W_{ra} when $h^2 \neq 0$. Hence point for the array whose common parent bears dominant gene (with positive or negative effects) will occupy position near the origin. On the other hand, point for the array whose common parent possesses recessive gene will find its position far away from the origin on W_r, V_r graph. If dominance is absent $V_{rA} = V_{ra}$ and $W_{rA} = W_{ra}$ and the two array points coincide.

In this example we imagined a single gene difference. Hence there was no need to consider non-allelic interaction and linkage. As the next simple case let us consider a diallel cross involving four inbred lines which represent all possible combinations of two gene differences, *i.e.*, *A*, *a* and *B*, *b*. The means of arrays (four in this case, corresponding to *AABB*, *AAbb*, *aaBB* and *aabb* inbred lines), variances (V_rs) and covariances (W_rs) are presented for this diallel cross in Table 6.2.

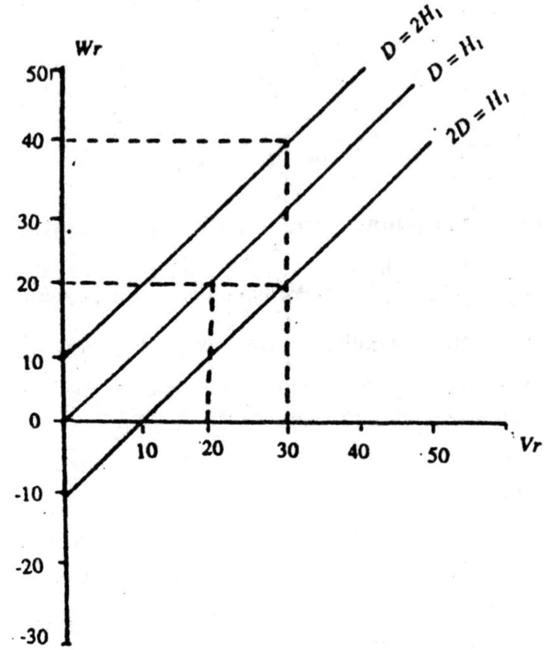

V_r, W_r Graph

FIG. 6.1: *V_r. W_r graph. Linear regression line of W_r. V_r passes through the origin when $D = H_1$ (i.e., complete dominance), above the origin when $D > H_1$ (i.e., partial dominance), and below the origin when $H_1 > D$ (i.e., overdominance). In this figure D is assumed to be equal to $2H_1$ for partial dominance and $D = ½H_1$ for overdominance.*

TABLE 6.2: **Array means, variances (*Vrs*) and covariances (*Wrs*) for diallel (Two gene difference)**

Arrays	Means	*Vrs*	*Wrs*
AABB	$\frac{1}{2}(d_a+h_a)+\frac{1}{2}(d_b+h_b)$	$\frac{1}{4}[(d_a-h_a)^2+(d_b-h_b)^2]$	$\frac{1}{2}[d_a(d_a-h_a)+d_b(d_b-h_b)]$
AAbb	$\frac{1}{2}(d_a+h_a)+\frac{1}{2}(h_b-d_b)$	$\frac{1}{4}[(d_a-h_a)^2+(d_b+h_b)^2]$	$\frac{1}{2}[d_a(d_a-h_a)+d_b(d_b+h_b)]$
aaBB	$\frac{1}{2}(h_a-d_a)+\frac{1}{2}(d_b+h_b)$	$\frac{1}{4}[(d_a+h_a)^2+(d_b-h_b)^2]$	$\frac{1}{2}[d_a(d_a+h_a)+d_b(d_b-h_b)]$
aabb	$\frac{1}{2}(h_a-d_a)+\frac{1}{2}(h_b-d_b)$	$\frac{1}{4}[(d_a+h_a)^2+(d_b+h_b)^2]$	$\frac{1}{2}[d_a(d_a+h_a)+d_b(d_b+h_b)]$

It is assumed that frequencies of all the genes are equal and that genes are independent in their action and inheritance. In this case we find that the V_r and W_r for array *aabb* are larger in magnitude than those derived for array *AABB*. Substitution of common parent *AABB* for *aabb* will change the value of V_r (ΔV_r) and W_r (ΔW_r). Thus,

$$\Delta V_r = aabb - AABB$$

$$= \frac{1}{4}d_a^2 + \frac{1}{2}d_a h_a + \frac{1}{4}h_a^2 + \frac{1}{4}d_b^2 + \frac{1}{2}d_b h_b + \frac{1}{4}h_b^2$$

$$- \frac{1}{4}d_a^2 + \frac{1}{2}d_a h_a - \frac{1}{4}h_a^2 - \frac{1}{4}d_b^2 + \frac{1}{2}d_b h_b - \frac{1}{4}h_b^2$$

$$= d_a h_a + d_b h_b.$$

Likewise ΔW_r is

$$\frac{1}{2}d_a^2 + \frac{1}{2}d_a h_a + \frac{1}{2}d_b^2 + \frac{1}{2}d_b h_b - \frac{1}{2}d_a^2 + \frac{1}{2}d_a h_a - \frac{1}{2}d_b^2 + \frac{1}{2}d_b h_b$$

$$= d_a h_a + d_b h_b.$$

Similarly moving from *AABB* to array *AAbb* gives ΔV_r and ΔW_r as shown below:

$$\Delta V_r = \frac{1}{4}d_a^2 - \frac{1}{2}d_a h_a + \frac{1}{4}h_a^2 + \frac{1}{4}d_b^2 - \frac{1}{2}d_b h_b + \frac{1}{4}d_b^2$$

$$- \frac{1}{4}d_a^2 + \frac{1}{2}d_a h_a - \frac{1}{4}h_a^2 - \frac{1}{4}d_b^2 - \frac{1}{2}d_b h_b - \frac{1}{4}d_b^2$$

$$= -d_b h_b$$

$$\Delta W_r = \frac{1}{2}d_a^2 - \frac{1}{2}d_a h_a + \frac{1}{2}d_b^2 - \frac{1}{2}d_b h_b - \frac{1}{2}d_a^2 + \frac{1}{2}d_a h_a$$

$$- \frac{1}{2}d_b^2 - \frac{1}{2}d_b h_b$$

$$= -d_b h_b$$

So if we plot the four array points on a graph, all the array points will fall on a straight line of unit slope in the absence of non–allelic interaction and linkage. Since the array *aabb* has larger values for V_r

and W_r it will occupy a position far away from the origin. On the other hand, point for array *AABB* will be nearer to the origin. Array points *AAbb* and *aaBB* will be intermediate in their position. This is as per expectation because the difference between V_rs for *aabb* and other arrays equals difference between W_rs for *aabb* array and the other arrays. For rectilinear relationship it is essential that $\Delta V_r = \Delta W_r$ for the arrays under consideration.

Here also we find that the point of origin, *i.e.*, *a* is equal to $\frac{1}{4}\left(d_a^2 - h_a^2\right) + \frac{1}{4}\left(d_b^2 - h_b^2\right)$. The regression line will pass through $\overline{W}_r\left(= \frac{1}{2}d_a^2 + \frac{1}{2}d_b^2\right)$ and $Vr\left(= \frac{1}{4}d_a^2 + \frac{1}{4}h_a^2 + \frac{1}{4}d_b^2 + \frac{1}{4}h_b^2\right)$.

In this way when two gene pairs are involved, relationship between W_r and V_r provides a test for adequacy of additive–dominance model. If non-allelic interaction is involved, as will be shown later, ΔW_r does not equal ΔV_r and the rectilinear relationship is lost. The regression of W_r on V_r will not be a straight line with unit slope. Same thing holds true for linkage (rather association and dispersion of genes among the parents).

In the two examples considered in preceding paragraphs it was assumed that genotypes of inbred lines were known and frequencies of these genotypes were equal in the population. As a matter of fact genotypes of inbred lines are not always known. This is particularly true for quantitative characters. In addition, we do know whether the two alleles (assuming that there are only two alleles at a locus) at a locus are equally common among the parents. Further, we cannot be sure that the pairs of alleles at different loci are randomly distributed relative to each other. The genes may be associated or dispersed in the inbred lines.

Let us look at the consequences of unequal gene frequencies. If we consider a single locus with two alleles, *viz.* *A* and *a*, there will be two inbred lines with respect to this locus. Let the frequencies of *AA* and *aa* be *p* and *q*, respectively. Diallel mating between these two inbred lines will result in three kinds of progeny families (Table 6.3). The *AA* array comprises of two kinds of progeny families, *viz.* *AA* and *Aa*. Frequencies of these progeny families in the overall population are p^2 and pq respectively. However, total of the frequencies of progeny families of this array is $p^2 + pq = p\,(p + q) = p$. Therefore, the proportions of progeny families *AA* and *Aa* within *AA* array are *p* and

q, respectively. Since the values of genotypes AA and Aa are d and h, respectively the mean of this array is $pd + qh$. Mean for aa array can be derived similarly.

TABLE 6.3: Diallel mating of two inbred lines with unequal gene frequencies

		Female inbred lines		Mean	V_r	W_r
	Genotype	AA	aa			
	Frequency	p	q			
	value	d	$-d$	$(pd - qd)$		
	AA	AA	Aa			
Male	p	p	q	$(pd + qh)$	$pq\,(d - h)^2$	$2pqd\,(d - h)$
inbred	d	d	h			
lines	aa	Aa	aa			
	q	p	q			
	$-d$	h	$-d$	$(ph - qd)$	$pq\,(d + h)^2$	$2pqd\,(d + h)$

Variance of the progeny family means within an AA array around array mean is derived as:

$$V_{rA} = p\,(d)^2 + q(h)^2 - [pd + qh]^2$$
$$= pd^2 + qh^2 - p^2d^2 - 2pqdh - q^2h^2$$
$$= pd^2\,(1 - p) + qh^2\,(1 - q) - 2pqdh$$

Since $1 - p = q$ and $1 - q = p$,

$$= pqd^2 + pqh^2 - 2pqdh$$
$$= pq\,(d^2 + h^2 - 2dh)$$
$$= pq(d - h)^2.$$

Variance for the aa array can be similarly obtained. Total heritable variation of the progeny families resulting from diallel mating is:

$$p^2\,(d)^2 + pq(h)^2 + pq(h)^2 + q^2\,(-d)^2 - [d\,(p - q) + 2pqh]^2$$
$$= 2pq\,[d + h\,(q - p)]^2 + 4p^2q^2h^2.$$

This is equal to $2pq\alpha^2 + 4p^2q^2d^2$, *i.e.*, $\sigma_A^2 + \sigma_D^2$ in Falconer's (1960) notations.

The covariance of progeny family means within each array with the means of their non-common parents is also shown for two arrays in Table 6.3. Let us derive W_r for aa array. Thus W_{ra} is:

$$pd\,(h) + q\,(-d)\,(-d) - [(pd - qd)\,(ph - qd)]$$
$$= pdh + qd^2 - p^2dh + pqd^2 + pqdh - q^2d^2$$
$$= pdh\,(1 - p + q) + qd^2\,(1 + p - q),$$ Since $1 - p = q$, and $1 - q, = p$,

$$= pdh\,(2q) + qd^2\,(2p)$$

$= 2pqdh + 2pqd^2$
$= 2pqd\,(d + h).$

Even when frequencies of genes A and a in the population are unequal, relationships shown earlier between W_rs and V_rs hold true. Thus,

$$W_{ra} - W_{rA} = V_{ra} - V_{rA}$$
$$= 2pqd^2 + 2pqdh - 2pqd^2 + 2pqdh$$
$$= 4pqdh.$$

Another interesting relationship is:

$$W_{ra} - V_{ra} = W_{rA} - V_{rA}$$
$$= 2pqd^2 + 2pqdh - pqd^2 - 2pqdh - pqh^2$$
$$= pqd^2 - pqh^2$$
$$= pq\,(d^2 - h^2).$$

Relationship between W_r and V_r shown in the preceding paragraphs suggests that the difference between two W_rs (ΔW_r) is equal to the difference between two V_rs (ΔV_r). Hence if we plot the array points on W_r, V_r graph and join them we get a straight line of unit slope (*i.e.*, making an angle of 45° to the base). Thus even when the frequencies of genes are unequal the relationship between W_r and V_r is similar to that described for equal gene frequencies. This line will pass through $\overline{W_r}$ and $\overline{V_r}$.

Let us now generalise the theory given above to several loci influencing a given character. We assume that how the two alleles at a locus are distributed among the parents is unknown and that non-allelic interaction is absent. The variance and covariance of array whose common parent bears most of the dominant genes will be relatively smaller in magnitude than the array whose common parent carries most of the recessive genes. Hence point for the array whose common parent bears most of the dominant genes will be located on W_r, V_r graph near the origin. On the other hand, point for the array having common parent with most of the recessive genes will find its place far away from the origin. However, the line connecting the two array points will be straight with unit slope only in the absence of non-allelic interaction and independence of genes in inheritance. If there is no dominance, all the array points will cluster at one point (within the limits of sampling variation).

Let us now revert to the case of a single locus with two alleles.

When the regression of W_r on V_r is unity, mathematical relationship between W_r and V_r can be expressed as:

$$\overline{W}_r = a + b\overline{V}_r$$

In this expression '*a*' provides information about the degree of dominance. We need genetic expectations for $\overline{W}_r$ and $\overline{V}_r$. Thus $\overline{W}_r$ is got as:

$$\begin{aligned} & p[2pqd^2 - 2pqdh] + q\,[2pqd^2 + 2pqdh] \\ &= 2p^2q^2d^2 - 2p^2qdh + 2pq^2d^2 + 2pq^2dh \\ &= 2pqd^2\,(p+q) - 2pqdh\,(p-q), \text{ and since } (p+q) = 1 \\ &= 2pqd^2 - 2pq\,(p-q)dh. \end{aligned}$$

For several loci the expression for $\overline{W}_r$ following notations of Mather and Jinks (1971) is:

$$\begin{aligned} & S2pqd^2 - S2pq(p-q)dh \\ &= \frac{1}{2}D - \frac{1}{4}F. \end{aligned}$$

The mean variance ($\overline{V}_r$) over two arrays is derived as:

$$\begin{aligned} \overline{V}_r &= p[pq(d-h)^2] + q\,[pq\,(d+h)^2] \\ &= p^2qd^2 - 2p^2qdh + p^2qh^2 + pq^2d^2 + 2pq^2dh + pq^2h^2 \\ &= pqd^2\,(p+q) + pqh^2\,(p+q) - 2pqdh\,(p-q) \\ &= pqd^2 + pqh^2 - 2pq\,(p-q)dh. \end{aligned}$$

For several loci the genetic expression for $\overline{V}_r$ could be written as:

$$Spqd^2 + Spqh^2 - S2pq\,(p-q)dh$$

or

$$\frac{1}{4}D + \frac{1}{4}H_1 - \frac{1}{4}F$$

Substituting the values obtained for $\overline{W}_r$ and $\overline{V}_r$ we get '*a*', the point where regression line cuts the W_r axis, as:

$$a = \overline{W}_r - b\overline{V}_r, \text{ and because } b = 1,$$

$$= \frac{1}{2}D - \frac{1}{4}F - \frac{1}{4}D - \frac{1}{4}H_1 + \frac{1}{4}F$$

$$= \frac{1}{4}D - \frac{1}{4}H_1 \text{ or } \frac{1}{4}(D - H_1)$$

The V_r, W_r graph, even if we imagine several loci and unequal gene frequencies, provides information on following aspects, provided assumptions listed in section 6.1 are satisfied:

1. In the absence of non-allelic interaction and random distribution of genes, regression line of W_r on V_r will be linear and of unit slope. Regression line of W_r on V_r is, therefore, used to detect the adequacy of additive-dominance model, especially when experiment is not replicated. When experiment is replicated, adequacy of additive-dominance model is tested through the analysis of $(W_r - V_r)$ values for each array.
2. Regression line will intercept W_r axis above the origin if D is larger in magnitude than H_1. This implies importance of additive genetic variance for inheritance of the character. If D is equal to H_1, regression line will pass through the origin indicating that both the components of genotypic variance are equally important for inheritance of character. When H_1 is larger in magnitude than D, regression line will intercept W_r axis below the origin. This situation is known as overdominance and suggests that dominance variance is relatively more important for the expression of character being investigated.

   Thus, the point of interception depends upon overall level of dominance. This inference is valid only if additive-dominance model is satisfactory.
3. If the common parent of an array contains most of the dominant genes (irrespective of positive or negative effect), V_r and W_r of this array will be relatively smaller in magnitude as compared with V_r and W_r for an array whose common parent bears most of the recessive genes. Hence, array point near the origin represents that array whose common parent contains most of the dominant genes. On the other hand, array point far away removed from the origin refers to the array whose common parent possesses most of the recessive genes.

   Points between these extremes represent those arrays which possess different proportions of dominant and recessive genes in that order. Thus array point closer to the point for most dominant array has relatively more dominant and less recessive genes and so on.

Hayman (1954a) suggested that the array points should fall around the regression line but not beyond the limits of parabola given by relationship :

$$W_{ri} = (V_{ri} \cdot V_p)^{1/2}$$

6.3 Numerical Analysis

In chapter 5 various mating designs were described. These designs offer a test of significance for additive and dominance components of heritable variance. It is also possible to obtain the estimates of additive and dominance components from the mean squares of these mating designs. The graphical approach to diallel analysis described in section 6.2 provides information about the adequacy of additive-dominance model, the average degree of dominance and characterises parents containing most of the dominant and recessive genes. Many useful properties of the parental lines can be learned from numerical approach to diallel analysis.

When n inbred lines are crossed in a diallel fashion, n^2 progeny families are produced.

Usually the experimental design adopted to plant the progeny families developed as a result of diallel mating is randomised blocks with r replications. The method of diallel cross analysis has been extensively used for estimation of second degree genetic parameters. There is a range of alternative methods of partitioning the total variation (Jinks and Hayman 1953; Jinks 1954; Hayman 1954; Griffing 1956) where parental lines are inbreds. Dickinson and Jinks (1956) gave method for analysis where parents are heterozygous. There are also several alternative ways of deriving variance components from the mean squares according to whether maternal or reciprocal effects are present or not (Griffing 1956; Wearden 1964) and whether the parental lines are fixed sample or a random sample of a population of inbreds (Griffing 1956; Wearden 1964).

The diallel analysis proposed by Hayman (1954) is applicable essentially to full diallel, *i.e.*, n^2 progeny families comprising of n parents, $\frac{n(n-1)}{2}$ F_1s and $\frac{n(n-1)}{2}$ reciprocal F_1s. The analysis involves averaging of the values of crosses and their reciprocals and using their averages for calculation of statistics such as variance of parents, variance of each array, and the covariance of an array with its non-recurrent parents. However, several times it is observed that only n parents and

$\frac{n(n-1)}{2}$ crosses are grown and the data used to estimate various statistics. Singh (1981) is of the opinion that this is erroneous. He calls the experimental material comprising of n parents and $\frac{n(n-1)}{2}$ F_1s as half diallel. According to Singh (1981) correct analysis of half-diallel set may be performed by substituting the value of a cross for its reciprocal to complete the two-way table and using the correct error components in the expectations of second degree statistics.

If the mean squares for genotypes are found to be significant, a diallel table is prepared separately for each replication. A diallel table is an arrangement in a square of n^2 measurements corresponding one-to-one to the mating combinations of a diallel cross, each row and column of the square corresponding to offspring with a common parental genotype (Hayman, 1954a). The off-diagonal elements comprise of average of a cross and its reciprocal. From the diallel table, variance of progeny family means within an array (V_r), covariance of progeny family means within an array on the means of non-common parents of that array (W_r), are found for each array in addition to the variance of parents (V_p), variance of array means around overall mean $(V_{\bar{r}})$, $\bar{V}_r$, $\bar{W}_r$ and $(m_{LI} - m_{L0})^2$. $(m_{LI} - m_{L0})$ represents difference between the mean of n parents (m_{L0}) and the mean of their n^2 progeny families (m_{LI}). These statistics are calculated as shown below:

V_{ri}, which is the variance of ith array, is calculated as:

$$\frac{1}{n-1}\sum_{i=1}^{n} x_i^2 - \frac{(\Sigma x_i)^2}{n}$$

Where Σx_i^2 is the sum of squared progeny family means within ith array, $(\Sigma x_i)^2$ is the square of ith array total and n is the number of parents (and also the progeny families within an array).

Covariance of progeny family means within ith array with the means of non-recurrent parents of this array (W_{ri}) is got as:

$$\frac{1}{n-1}\sum_{i=1}^{n} x_i y_i - \frac{\Sigma x_i \Sigma y_i}{n}$$

Where x_i is the mean of non-common parent of ith array and Σx_i is total of the means of parents. y_i denotes the progeny family mean of ith array and Σy_i is the total of ith array.

Mean variance ($\overline{V_r}$) is computed as:

$$\frac{\sum_{i=1}^{n} V_{ri}}{n}$$

and similarly $\overline{W_r}$ is found as:

$$\frac{\sum_{i=1}^{n} W_{ri}}{n}$$

Where ΣV_{ri} and ΣW_{ri} represent totals of V_r and W_r, respectively over arrays.

Variance of parents is calculated as variance of diagonal elements of the diallel table.

Instead of using the array means, array totals are employed to calculate the variance of array means ($V_{\bar{r}}$) as shown below:

$$\left(\frac{1}{n}\right)^2\left[\frac{1}{n-1}\left(\sum_{i=1}^{n} Y_{i\cdot}^2 - \frac{1}{n}Y_{\cdot\cdot}^2\right)\right]$$

Where $Y_{i\cdot}$ is total of ith array, $Y_{\cdot\cdot}$ is grand total. Statistic $(m_{L1} - m_{L0})^2$ is obtained as:

$$\left(\frac{1}{n}\right)^2\left[\left(\frac{1}{n}Y_{\cdot\cdot}\right) - \sum_{i=1}^{n} y_{ii}\right]^2$$

Where $\sum_{i=1}^{n} y_{ii}$, represents sum of n parental values in the diallel table.

Before we proceed to the numerical analysis, it is necessary to detect the adequacy of additive-dominance model. Mather (1949) developed simple scaling tests to detect whether non-allelic interaction plays a significant role in the determination of mean expressions of various generations. For second degree statistics such a test is provided by the relationship between the expected values of V_r and W_r of different arrays.

Let us return to the case of single locus diallel described in section 6.2. It was shown that the genetic expectations of W_{rA} and W_{ra} are

$\frac{1}{2}d(d-h)$ and $\frac{1}{2}d(d+h)$, respectively. Variances, V_{rA} and V_{ra}, were shown to be $\frac{1}{4}(d-h)^2$ and $\frac{1}{4}(d+h)^2$ respectively. It was shown earlier that $W_{rA}-V_{rA}=\frac{1}{4}d^2-\frac{1}{4}h^2$ and $W_{ra}-V_{ra}=\frac{1}{4}d^2-\frac{1}{4}h^2$.

Thus

$$W_{rA}-V_{rA}=\frac{1}{2}d^2-\frac{1}{2}dh-\frac{1}{4}d^2+\frac{1}{2}dh-\frac{1}{4}h^2$$

$$=\frac{1}{4}d^2-\frac{1}{4}h^2$$

and

$$W_{ra}-V_{ra}=\frac{1}{2}d^2+\frac{1}{2}dh-\frac{1}{4}d^2-\frac{1}{2}dh-\frac{1}{4}h^2$$

$$=\frac{1}{4}d^2-\frac{1}{4}h^2$$

For unequal frequencies of genes also this relationship is found to be true. Thus

$$W_{rA}-V_{rA}=2pqd^2-2pqdh-pqd^2+2pqdh-pqh^2$$
$$=pqd^2-pqh^2,$$

which summing over all the loci would be $Spqd^2-Spqh^2$. This can be alternatively expressed as $\frac{1}{4}(D-H_1)$. Similarly, $W_{ra}-V_{ra}$ would be ¼ $(D-H_1)$. Hence, in the absence of non-allelic interaction and independent distribution of genes among the parents W_r-V_r should be identical, within the limits of sampling variation, for all the arrays. Heterogeneity would upset this constancy. Homogeneity of W_r-V_r, provides evidence in support of adequacy of the additive-dominance model. Homogeneity of W_r-V_r over arrays, however, may several times result from balancing of these values.

Provided that the experiment is replicated, variance of (W_r-V_r) is analysed for lines and block difference (Hayman, 1954a, *pp.* 799-800). A significant lines effect suggests failure of the additive-dominance hypothesis. It should be noted that the (W_r-V_r) values of n arrays may be correlated. If the experiment is not replicated, graph of W_r, V_r provides a basis to test the validity of this assumption. In case of failure of this hypothesis, the regression line may not be linear and of a unit slope (*i.e.*, W_r-V_r is not constant over arrays).

Since the experiments are usually replicated, $W_r - V_r$ values are obtained for each of the *n* arrays in each replication. $(W_r - V_r)$ values are analysed in a customary fashion recommended for randomised block design with *r* replications (Table 6.4).

TABLE 6.4: Format for $(W_r - V_r)$ analysis of variance

Source	*df*	*MS*
Replications	$(r-1)$	
$(W_r - V_r)$	$(n-1)$	M_1
Error	$(r-1)(n-1)$	M_2

Homogeneity of $(W_r - V_r)$ over arrays is tested by *F* test as:

$$F = \frac{M_1}{M_2}$$

Significance of the *F* ratio implies heterogeneity of $(W_r - V_r)$ values over arrays. It is desirable in these circumstances to drop those arrays which exhibit non-allelic interaction. This can be accomplished by dropping one array at a time and analysing $(W_r - V_r)$ values till the mean square for lines $(W_r - V_r)$ turns out to be non-significant. Estimates of various parameters are not valid if assumptions are not satisfied.

Provided, the additive-dominance model is satisfactory, values of $Vr, \overline{W}_r, V_p, V_{\bar{r}}, (m_{L1} - m_{L0})^2$ obtained for each replication are averaged over the replications. Estimate of environmental component of variation is provided by the error mean square.

Using these statistics the estimates of components of variation are obtained as shown below (following perfect fit solutions provided by Hayman, 1954a):

$$\hat{E} = E$$

$$\hat{D} = V_p - \hat{E}$$

$$\hat{H}_1 = 4\overline{V}_r + V_p - 4\overline{W}_r - \left(\frac{3n-2}{n}\right)\hat{E}$$

$$\hat{H}_2 = 4\overline{V}_r - 4V_{\bar{r}} - 2\hat{E}$$

$$\hat{F} = 2V_p - 4\overline{W}_r - \frac{2(n-2)}{n}\hat{E}$$

and $$\hat{h}^2 = 4(m_{L1} - m_{L0})^2 - \frac{4(n-1)}{n^2}\hat{E}$$

Readers will recall that as pointed out in section 4.5, additive genetic variance of the random mating population (D_R), comprises of four components. Expansion of $D_R = S4pq[d + h(q - p)]^2$ gives following components:

$$D = S4pqd^2$$
$$H_1 = S4pqh^2$$
$$H_2 = S16p^2q^2h^2 = H_R$$
$$F = S8pq(p - q)\,dh.$$

D measures additive effects, and equals $S(d^2)$, *i.e.*, additive variance described for selfing series, if $p = q = ½$. H_1 is a measure of dominance effects like the H_2. If and only if $p = q = 0.50$, $H_1 = H_2 = S(h^2)$. F measures the average covariation of additive and dominance effects over all the arrays. If $p = q = 0.50$, $F = 0$. However, in the absence of equal gene frequencies, the sign and magnitude of F can be used to determine relative frequencies of dominant and recessive genes in the parental population. Thus, if increasing alleles are in overall excess in the parental population, *i.e.*, $p > q$, at most of the loci, and if increasing alleles are dominant, sign of F will be positive. Similarly if decreasing alleles are in overall excess, *i.e.*, $q > p$, at most of the loci and decreasing alleles are dominant to increasing alleles, sign of h will be negative and consequently sign of F will be positive. For this reason whenever dominant alleles are more frequent among the parental lines, sign of F is positive. h^2 is a measure of dominance effects. These dominance effects are available as algebraic sum over all the loci, which are in heterozygous phase in all the crosses.

Although no worthwhile estimates of the errors of these components are available, consistency of their relative magnitudes, if not their absolute magnitudes over replications is satisfactory for interpretation (Mather and Jinks, 1971, 1982). However, Hayman (1954a, *pp.* 797) described a basis for estimation of standard errors of these parameters. When the experiment is not replicated, estimate of mean square (S^2) may be obtained as:

$$\frac{1}{2} V_{ar}(W_r - V_r)$$

and the diagonal elements of a covariance matrix given by Hayman (1954a) may be used to estimate standard errors of these components

(Askel and Johnson, 1963). Diagonal elements, which are the multipliers for estimation of variances of components, are:

$$D = \frac{n^5 + n^4}{n^5}$$

$$H_1 = \frac{n^5 + 41n^4 - 12n^3 + 4n^2}{n^5}$$

$$H_2 = \frac{36n^4}{n^5}$$

$$F = \frac{4n^5 + 20n^4 - 16n^3 + 16n^2}{n^5}$$

$$h^2 = \frac{16n^4 + 16n^2 - 32n + 16}{n^5}$$

$$E = \frac{n^4}{n^5}$$

On the other hand, when the experiment is replicated, sum of squares of deviations observed from expected values of V_r, W_r, V_p, $V_{\bar{r}}$, $(m_{L1} - m_{L0})^2$ are used to calculate S^2. Expected values of W_r and V_r are obtained as (Hayman, 1954a, *p*. 799):

$$\hat{W}_{ri} = \frac{1}{2}(\overline{W}_r - \overline{V}_r + W_{ri} + V_{ri})$$

and $$V_{ri} = \frac{1}{2}(-\overline{W}_r + \overline{V}_r + W_{ri} + V_{ri})$$

where $\hat{W}_{ri}$ and $\hat{V}_{ri}$ are the expected values of covariance and variance, respectively, of *i*th array. Expected values of $V_{\bar{r}}$, V_p and $(m_{L1} - m_{L0})^2$ are obtained as means of their values over *r* replications. Sum of squares of deviations for V_p, $V_{\bar{r}}$, W_r, V_r and $(m_{L1} - m_{L0})^2$ are calculated for each replication separately and then added. Since information from *r* replications is used to calculate total sum of squares, latter is divided by the number of replications. From the data in each replication we calculate values of *n* W_rs, *n* V_rs and one each of $V_{\bar{r}}$, V_p and $(m_{L1} - m_{L0})^2$. In other words, *r* (2*n* + 3) statistics are obtained from *r* replications. However, we estimate *D*, H_1, H_2, h^2, *E* and *n* F_rs (Mean of

$n\ F_r s$ gives F. Actually we calculate F and not the $F_r s$), hence the degrees of freedom equals number of constants minus number of statistics, *i.e.*, $r\,(2n + 3) - (5 + n)$. Division of sum of squares by the degrees of freedom provides S^2. Standard errors for D, H_1, H_2, F, E and h^2 are then obtained as:

$$S.E._D = \left(\frac{n^5 + n^4}{n^5} S^2\right)^{\frac{1}{2}}$$

$$S.E._{H_1} = \left(\frac{n^5 + 41n^4 - 12n^3 + 4n^2}{n^5} S^2\right)^{\frac{1}{2}}$$

$$S.E._{H_2} = \left(\frac{36n^4}{n^5} S^2\right)^{\frac{1}{2}}$$

$$S.E._{h^2} = \left(\frac{16n^4 + 16n^2 - 32n + 16}{n^5} S^2\right)^{\frac{1}{2}}$$

$$S.\ E._F = \left(\frac{4n^5 + 20n^4 - 16n^3 + 16n^2}{n^5} S^2\right)^{\frac{1}{2}}$$

and $$S.E._E = \left(\frac{n^4}{n^5} S^2\right)^{\frac{1}{2}}$$

where n is the number of inbred lines.

Significance of the components of variation is tested by means of 't' test. For example 't' test for $\hat{D}$ would be:

$$t_{\hat{D}} = \frac{\hat{D} - 0}{S.E._{\hat{D}}}$$

If the estimates of D, H_1, H_2, F, h^2 and E are significant, following ratios may be obtained, which furnish information on various aspects of inheritance pattern of the metric character being investigated:

1. Since the coefficients of D and H_1 are equal, the ratio

$$\sqrt{\frac{H_1}{D}}$$

provides information regarding average degree of dominance involved in the action of genes. If the ratio equals unity, complete dominance is indicated. On the other hand, values of ratio > 1 and < 1 suggest overdominance and partial dominance, respectively.

2. Since the genetic expectation of H_1 is $S4pqh^2$ and that of H_2 is $S16p^2q^2h^2$, following ratio is employed to determine the relative distribution of increasing (positive) and decreasing (negative) genes among the common parents of arrays (irrespective of whether they are dominant or recessive).

$$\frac{H_2}{4H_1},$$

This ratio will attain a maximum value of 0.25 if the increasing and decreasing genes are symmetrically distributed, on an average, among the inbred lines. Deviation of the value from 0.25 implies asymmetrical distribution of genes with positive and negative effects among the parents.

3. Relative distribution of dominant and recessive genes among the parental strains (Hayman, 1954, p. 795) can be inferred from ratio:

$$\frac{\sqrt{4(DH_1)}+F}{\sqrt{4(DH_1)}-F}$$

If the dominant and recessive genes are symmetrically distributed among the parental lines, this ratio equals unity, within the limits of sampling variance.

4. $$\frac{\left(\frac{1}{2}F\right)^2}{D(H_1-H_2)}=1=\frac{16p^2q^2(p-q)^2d^2h^2}{16p^2q^2(p-q)^2d^2h^2}$$

If the ratio of h to d is constant over all the loci, this expectation will hold good for any number of genes. However, if values of d and h (taking signs into account) vary independently over loci, this ratio will have a value of zero. Hence, irrespective of dominance level this ratio can be used to measure the extent to which dominance level varies from one locus to another.

5. Following Mather and Jinks (1971) narrow sense heritability is obtained as:

$$\frac{\frac{1}{2}D_R}{\frac{1}{2}D_R+\frac{1}{4}H_R+E}\times 100$$

which is really a measure of

$$\frac{\frac{1}{2}D+\frac{1}{2}H_1-\frac{1}{2}H_2-\frac{1}{2}F}{\frac{1}{2}D+\frac{1}{2}H_1-\frac{1}{4}H_2-\frac{1}{2}F+E}\times 100$$

On the other hand, broad sense heritability may be found as:

$$\frac{\frac{1}{2}D_R+\frac{1}{4}H_R}{\frac{1}{2}D_R+\frac{1}{4}H_R+E}\times 100$$

6. Dominance and recessive nature of genes with increasing and decreasing effects can be inferred from the sign of coefficient of correlation between $(W_r + V_r)$, known as the parental order of dominance for each array, and $\overline{Y}_r$, mean of common parent of the array. Negative correlation coefficient suggests that increasing genes contained in the parental strains are dominant. Why? We know that for the array whose common parent contains most of the dominant genes, W_r and V_r values are lowest as compared to the array whose common parent possesses most of the recessive genes. By similar reasoning we infer that the increasing genes are recessive if the correlation coefficient is positive. If the correlation coefficient is non-significant, we conclude that dominant genes contained in the parental strains are equally positive and negative.

Provided that the correlation coefficient between $(W_r + V_r)$ and $\overline{Y}_r$ is significant, a graph can be plotted from the standardized values of $\overline{Y}_r$ and $(W_r + V_r)$. We use average values of parental means and $(W_r + V_r)$ for each array over replications. The standardised values (z_i) for n parental means is calculated, following Johnson and Askel (1959), as:

$$z_i = \frac{x_i - \overline{x}}{s}$$

where s is the standard deviation of n parental means, $\overline{x}$ is the average of n parental means and x_i is the mean value of ith parent over replications. z values for all the n parents are calculated in this fashion.

Standardised values of $W_r + V_r$ are also obtained similarly for n arrays.

Standardised values of $W_r + V_r$ are plotted against corresponding standardised values of $\overline{Y}_r$. Values of $\overline{Y}_r$ take position on the x axis and $W_r + V_r$ on the y axis. Since quadrants 1 and 2 have positive values of $W_r + V_r$, points of arrays falling in these quadrants will indicate presence of recessive genes in the common parent of array (Fig. 6.2).

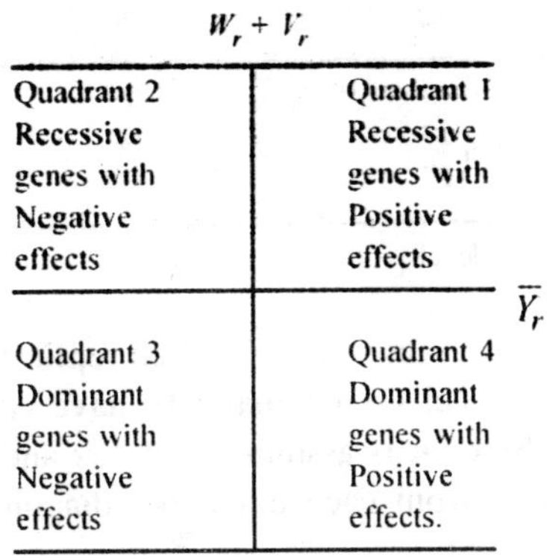

FIG. 6.2: *Standardised deviation graph*

By same analogy array points occupying positions in 3rd and 4th quadrants, refer to those arrays whose common parents possess most of the dominant genes. Mean performance of the common parents of arrays falling in quadrants 1 and 4 will be superior to those in quadrants 2 and 3. Hence, array points falling in quadrants 1 and 4 indicate that common parents of these arrays have most of the increasing (positive) genes, contrary to those falling in quadrants 2 and 3, which possess most of the decreasing (negative) genes. Thus, an array whose common parent bears predominantly dominant genes with increasing effects will find its place in the fourth quadrant. On the other hand, if common parent of an array carries dominant genes having negative effects, it will fall in the third quadrant.

6.4 Worked Example

Seven true breeding genotypes of sorghum were crossed in a diallel fashion, excluding reciprocals. The 21 F_1s and 7 parental lines were planted in a randomised block design with two replications. Observations were recorded on 1000-grain weight in grammes.

Data was subjected to analysis of variance procedure recommended for randomised block design. Analysis revealed significant differences among 28 sorghum genotypes for 1000-grain weight (Table 6.5).

TABLE 6.5: ANOVA for 1000-grain weight (7 × 7 diallel)

Source	*df*	*SS*	Mean square
Replications	1	0.3536	0.3536
Genotypes	27	578.8924	21.4405**
Error	27	73.9452	2.7387

** Significant at 1 per cent level.

Prepare two diallel tables, one for each replication (Table 6.6 and 6.7). Each table has 49 cells. Diagonal cells have values of 1000-grain weight for parents. Since it is assumed that F_1s and reciprocal F_1s do not differ significantly from each other, off–diagonal cells are mirror images.

From each diallel table calculate variances of progeny family means within an array around the array mean (V_r) for each array. For example V_{r1}, the variance for 1st array in replication 1 is calculated as:

$$\frac{1}{6}\ [(18.44^2 + 22.13^2 + 27.91^2 + 25.29^2 + 28.95^2$$

$$+ 27.85^2 + 29.41^2) - \frac{(179.98)^2}{7}\ ]$$

$$= \frac{1}{6}\ (99.452886)$$

$$= 16.7555.$$

Calculate in similar fashion V_{r2}, V_{r3}, V_{r4}, V_{r5}, V_{r6} and V_{r7}. Also compute seven V_rs for seven arrays of replication two (Table 6.8).

From the seven values of the V_rs of replication 1, calculate mean variance, $\overline{V}_r$ as shown below:

$$\frac{1}{7}\ (16.5755 + 15.8645 + 9.6783 + 11.4156 + 4.2030$$

$$+ 1.4703 + 5.9067)$$

$$= 9.3019.$$

TABLE 6.6: 1000-grain weight of sorghum (Rep.1)

	1	2	3	4	5	6	7
1.	18.44	22.13	27.91	25.29	28.95	27.85	29.41
2.	22.13	17.14	23.00	22.11	25.64	25.90	29.87
3.	27.91	23.00	22.56	19.78	24.29	27.78	27.24
4.	25.29	22.11	19.78	16.13	24.99	24.41	24.17
5.	28.95	25.64	24.29	24.99	22.56	26.47	23.96
6.	27.85	25.90	27.78	24.41	26.47	25.79	26.89
7.	29.41	29.87	27.24	24.17	23.96	26.89	26.28
Total	179.98	165.79	172.56	156.88	176.86	185.09	187.82

Perental total 148.90, Grand total 1224.98

TABLE 6.7: 1000-grain weight of sorghum (Rep.2)

	1	2	3	4	5	6	7
1.	22.51	23.07	23.74	23.07	26.27	29.70	29.77
2.	23.07	18.53	20.77	25.59	26.47	27.67	29.88
3.	23.74	20.77	20.93	25.17	25.30	26.82	26.96
4.	23.07	25.59	25.17	16.39	20.39	20.91	24.18
5.	26.27	26.47	25.30	20.39	22.73	26.24	25.87
6.	29.70	27.67	26.82	20.91	26.24	27.20	28.21
7.	29.77	29.88	26.96	24.18	25.87	28.21	27.05
Total	178.13	171.98	169.69	155.70	173.27	186.75	191.92

Parental total 155.34, Grand total 1227.44

Value of the $\overline{V}_r$ for replication 2 is obtained likewise. It is 8.6353.

Covariance of progeny family means within an array with means of their non-common parents (W_r) is calculated for each of the seven arrays in both the replications. Thus W_{r1}, the covariance for array 1 in replication 1 is found as:

$$\frac{1}{6}[(18.44^2 + 22.13 \times 17.14 + 27.91 \times 22.56 + 25.29 \times 16.13 + 28.95 \times 22.56 + 27.85 \times 25.79 + 29.41 \times 26.28) - \frac{(179.98 \times 148.90)}{7}]$$

$$= \frac{1}{6}(3901.1774 - 3828.4317) = 12.1242.$$

Note that means of non-recurrent parents of array 1 for replication 1 are 18.44, 17.14, 22.56, 16.13, 22.56, 25.79 and 26.28. Calculate the covariances for other arrays of replication 1 in similar fashion (Table 6.8). Seven W_rs are also obtained for replication 2 in a like manner.

From seven values of W_r in replication 1, calculate mean covariance ($\overline{W_r}$). Thus values of $\overline{W_r}$ for replication 1 and 2 are found to be 5.4203 and 6.4875, respectively.

TABLE 6.8: Showing V_r and W_r values for seven arrays

	V_r		W_r	
Arrays	Replication 1	Replication 2	Replication 1	Replication 2
1.	16.5755	10.0489	12.1242	11.0765
2.	15.8645	15.9380	13.6940	10.4770
3.	9.6783	6.5483	7.7639	6.3390
4.	11.4156	10.6123	7.1934	3.6068
5.	4.2030	5.3559	−2.7337	5.1006
6.	1.4703	7.7030	1.6263	6.7393
7.	5.9067	4.2411	−1.7254	2.0738

Another statistic that is obtained from diallel table is the variance of array means around overall mean ($V_{\bar{r}}$). For each replication $V_{\bar{r}}$ is calculated. For example, $V_{\bar{r}}$ for replication 1 is calculated as:

$$\left(\frac{1}{n}\right)^2\left[\frac{1}{n-1}\left(\Sigma \text{ array total}^2 - \frac{1}{n}\text{Grand total}^2\right)\right]$$

$$= \frac{1}{49}\Big[\frac{1}{6}(179.98^2 + 165.79^2 + 172.56^2 + 156.88^2 + 176.86^2 + 185.09^2 + 187.82^2) - \frac{1}{7}(1224.98)^2\Big]$$

$$= \frac{1}{49}\left[\frac{1}{6}(215081.51 - 214368.00)\right]$$

$$= \frac{1}{49}\left[\frac{1}{6}(713.51)\right]$$

$$= 2.4269.$$

$V_{\bar{r}}$ for replication 2 calculated in similar fashion is 2.8778.

Estimate of $(m_{L1} - m_{L0})^2$ is got from the grand total and the parental total in each replication. Thus $(m_{L1} - m_{L0})^2$ for replication 1 is calculated as:

$$\left(\frac{1}{n}\right)^2\left[\left(\frac{1}{n}\text{Grand total}\right) - \text{Parental total}\right]^2$$

$$= \frac{1}{49}\left[\left(\frac{1}{7} \times 1224.98\right) - 148.90\right]^2$$

$$= \frac{1}{49}\ (174.9971 - 148.90)^2$$

$= 13.8991.$

Value of $(m_{L1} - m_{L0})^2$ for replication 2 is 8.1702.

In the diallel table, diagonal elements represent parental entries. Variance of parents (V_P) is, therefore, found from the diagonal entries of each diallel table. For example, V_P for replication 1 is got as:

$$\frac{1}{6}\ [(18.44^2 + 17.14^2 + 22.56^2 + 16.13^2 + 22.56^2$$

$$+25.79^2 + 26.28)^2 - \frac{(148.90)^2}{7}]$$

$$= \frac{1}{6}(3267.6598 - 3167.3157)$$

$= 16.7240.$

Variance of parents in replication 2 is found to be 16.2895.

Before we proceed ahead with the numerical analysis, validity of the assumption regarding adequacy of additive-dominance model should be tested. As mentioned previously, two tests are available to verify this assumption. Firstly, we will describe $(W_r - V_r)$ analysis. Joint regression of W_r on V_r will be explained while dealing with graphical analysis. From Table 6.8, $(W_r - V_r)$ values are obtained for each array in each of the two replications (Table 6.9). Analysis of $(W_r - V_r)$ values proceeds along the conventional lines recommended for randomised block design.

TABLE 6.9: ($W_r - V_r$) values for 2 replications

Array	Replication 1	Replication 2	Total
1	-4.4513	1.0276	-3.4237
2	-2.1705	-5.4610	-7.6315
3	-1.9144	-0.2093	-2.1237
4	-4.2222	-7.0055	-11.2277
5	-6.9367	-0.2553	-7.1920
6	0.1560	-0.9637	-0.8077
7	-7.6321	-2.1673	-9.7994
Total	-27.1712	-15.0345	-42.2057

Correction Factor $= 127.23722$

Total S.S. $= [(-4.4513)^2 + (-2.1705)^2 \ldots + (-2.1673)^2] - CF$

$= 238.0985 - 127.23722$

$= 110.86128$

Treatment *S.S.* $$= \left[\frac{(-3.4237)^2 + (-7.6315)^2 + \ldots + (-9.7994)^2}{2}\right] - CF$$

$$= \frac{348.93832}{2} - 127.23722$$

$= 47.23194$

Replication S.S. $$= \frac{(-27.1712)^2 + (-15.0345)^2}{7} - CF$$

$= 10.52139$

Error *S.S.* $= 110.86128 - (47.23194 + 10.52139)$

$= 53.10795.$

From these sums of squares, set up an analysis of variance table (Table 6.10).

TABLE 6.10: ANOVA for ($W_r - V_r$)

Source	*df*	*SS*	*MS*	*F*
Replications	1	10.52139	10.52139	1.18
($W_r - V_r$)	6	47.23194	7.87199	0.88
Error	6	53.10795	8.85132	

$W_r - V_r$ mean square is found to be non-significant when tested against error mean square. Hence, values of $W_r - V_r$ could be regarded as consistent over arrays, which implies that additive-dominance model is satisfactory. Now we proceed to the numerical and then graphical analysis.

Arrange the values of $V_r, \overline{W}_r, V_p, V_{\bar{r}}$ and $(m_{L1} - m_{L0})^2$ for each replication in a tabular form (Table 6.11).

TABLE 6.11: Values of statistics for 1000-grain weight in sorghum

Statistics	Replication		Mean
	1	2	
V_p	16.7240	16.2895	16.5067
$\overline{V}_r$	9.3019	8.6353	8.9686
$\overline{W}_r$	5.4203	6.4875	5.9539
$V_{\bar{r}}$	2.4269	2.8778	2.6523
$(m_{L1} - m_{L0})^2$	13.8991	8.1702	11.0346

It was pointed out earlier that error mean square itself is an estimate of error variance in the grouped randomisation. Thus $\hat{E} = 2.7387$.

Components of variance are now got from the mean values of six statistics by means of a perfect fit solution. Thus,

$$\hat{D} = V_p - \hat{E}$$
$$= 16.5067 - 2.7387$$
$$= 13.7680$$

$$\hat{H}_1 = V_p + 4\overline{V}_r - 4\overline{W}_r - \frac{(3n-2)}{n}\hat{E}$$
$$= 16.5067 + 4\,(8.9686) - 4\,(5.9539) - \frac{19}{7}\,2.7387$$
$$= 16.5067 + 35.8744 - 23.8156 - 7.4336$$
$$= 21.1319$$

$$\hat{H}_2 = 4\overline{V}_r - 4V_{\bar{r}} - 2\hat{E}$$
$$= 4(8.9686) - 4(2.6523) - 2(2.7387)$$
$$= 35.8744 - 10.6092 - 5.4774$$
$$= 19.7878$$

$$\hat{F} = 2V_p - 4\overline{W}_r - \frac{2(n-2)}{n}\hat{E}$$
$$= 2(16.5067) - 4(5.9539) - \frac{2(5)}{7}\,2.7387$$

$$= 33.0134 - 23.8156 - 3.9124$$
$$= 5.2854$$
$$\hat{h}^2 = 4\,(m_{L1} - m_{L0})^2 - \frac{4(n-1)}{n^2}\,\hat{E}$$
$$= 4(11.0346) - \frac{24}{49}\; 2.7387$$
$$= 44.1384 - 1.3414$$
$$= 42.797.$$

In order to find the accuracy of these components of variation we need standard errors. When experimental material is replicated, standard errors are based on mean square calculated from expected and observed values of W_r, V_r, $V_{\bar{r}}$, V_P and $(m_{L1} - m_{L0})^2$ over replications.

Expected value of V_r for *i*th array in each replication is found as:

$$\hat{V}_{ri} = \frac{1}{2}(-\overline{W}_r + \overline{V}_r + W_{ri} + V_{ri}),$$

where W_{ri} and V_{ri} are the observed values of W_r and V_r respectively for *i*th array. $\overline{W}_r$ and $\overline{V}_r$ are average values of W_r and V_r respectively.

Expected value of W_r for *i*th array in each replication is calculated as:

$$\hat{W}_{ri} = \frac{1}{2}(\overline{W}_r - \overline{V}_r + W_{ri} + V_{ri}).$$

Thus expected W_r for array 1 in replication 1 is obtained as:

$$W_{r1} = \frac{1}{2}\;(5.4203 - 9.3019 + 12.1242 + 16.5755)$$
$$= 12.4090.$$

In a similar manner, expected values of rest of the W_rs are calculated for replications 1 and 2.

Expected V_r for array 1 in replication 1 is got as:

$$V_{r1} = \frac{1}{2}(-5.4203 + 9.3019 + 12.1242 + 16.5755)$$
$$= 16.2906$$

Now find the deviations of V_r, W_r, $V_{\bar{r}}$, V_P and $(m_{L1} - m_{L0})^2$ as (observed value – expected value) for each array in each replication. Summation of the deviation squared, *viz.* (observed – expected)^2, for each statistic in each replication gives sum of squares (Table 6.12).

Since this sum of squares is a total over two replications, sum of squares averaged over replications will be 70.0610/2 = 35.03.

Data were recorded on 28 progeny families grown in two replications. Following statistics were calculated from this data:

V_rs	14	(7 for each replication)
W_rs	14	(7 for each replication)
V_ps	2	(one for each replication)
$V_{\bar{r}}$	2	(one for each replication)
$(m_{l1} - m_{l0})^2$	2	(one for each replication)
Total	34	

TABLE 6.12: Calculation of sum of squares

S.S. due to	Replication 1	Replication 2	Total
W_r	11.7351	16.5826	28.3177
V_r'	11.7353	13.3498	25.0851
$V_{\bar{r}}$	0.0508	0.0508	0.1016
V_p	0.0730	0.0730	0.1460
$(m_{L1} - m_{L0})^2$	8.2053	8.2053	16.4106
Total			70.0610

Out of thirtyfour degrees of freedom twelve have been utilised to calculate estimates of 12 constants, *viz.* D, H_1, H_2, h^2, E and 7 F_rs we are, therefore, left with 22 degrees of freedom. Hence the mean deviation squared (S^2) is got as:

$$\frac{35.03}{22} = 1.5922$$

This mean square is employed to find the standard errors of estimates of components of variance. For example, $S.E._D$ is found as:

$$\left(\frac{n^5 + n^4}{n^5} S^2\right)^{\frac{1}{2}}$$

$$= \left(\frac{19208}{16807} 1.5922\right)^{\frac{1}{2}}$$

$$= (1.1428 \times 1.5922)^{1/2}$$

$$= 1.3488.$$

Estimates of the components of variance, along with their standard errors, are shown below:

Components	Estimates	Standard errors
$\hat{D}$	13.7680**	1.3488
$\hat{H}_1$	21.1319**	3.2474
$\hat{H}_2$	19.7878**	2.8614
$\hat{F}$	5.2854	3.2359
$\hat{h}^2$	42.7970**	1.8828
$\hat{E}$	2.7387**	0.4768

From the estimates of components it is apparent that the variation observed for 1000-grain weight is determined by additive and dominance components of genotypic variance. Although the sign of F is positive, which suggests that the dominant genes are preponderant, the estimate is non-significant. Hence conclusion drawn from this component regarding dominance properties of genes is not valid.

These components can be used for calculation of various ratios (described in section 6.3) as shown below:

1. $$\sqrt{\frac{H_1}{D}}$$

$$= \sqrt{\frac{21.1319}{13.768}}$$

$$= 1.238$$

Average degree of dominance involved in the action of genes is in overdominance range . The ratio suggests that although both additive and dominance components of genotypic variance govern the expression of this character, dominance component is relatively more important. This is a fixed effects model and hence conclusions refer to the parental lines used for diallel mating. When overdominance is involved, gene action can be best exploited by production of hybrids for commercial planting. Alternatively, either biparental mating or recurrent selection in segregating material followed by conventional selection scheme is likely to lead to substantial improvement in the character.

2. $$\frac{H_2}{4H_1}$$

$$= \frac{19.7878}{4 \times 21.1319}$$

$$= 0.23.$$

Since the value of this ratio is close to 0.25, it seems that the genes with increasing and decreasing effects are symmetrically distributed among the parental lines.

3. $$\frac{\sqrt{4DH_1} + F}{\sqrt{4DH_1} - F}$$

$$= \frac{\sqrt{(4 \times 13.768 \times 21.1319)} + 5.2854}{\sqrt{(4 \times 13.768 \times 21.1319)} - 5.2854}$$

$$= \frac{34.1141 + 5.2854}{34.1141 - 5.2854}$$

$$= 1.3666.$$

Provided that the dominant and recessive genes are symmetrically distributed among the parental genotypes, this ratio equals unity. Ratio calculated above leads to the conclusion that dominant and recessive genes are asymmetrically distributed among the parental strains. Dominant genes are probably more preponderant (because the sign of F is positive).

4. $$\frac{\frac{1}{2}D + \frac{1}{2}H_1 - \frac{1}{2}H_2 - \frac{1}{2}F}{\frac{1}{2}D + \frac{1}{2}H_1 - \frac{1}{4}H_2 - \frac{1}{2}F + E} \times 100$$

$$= \frac{\frac{1}{2}(13.768) + \frac{1}{2}(21.1319) - \frac{1}{2}(19.7878) - \frac{1}{2}(5.2854)}{\frac{1}{2}(13.768) + \frac{1}{2}(21.1319) - \frac{1}{4}(19.7878) - \frac{1}{2}(5.2854) + 2.7387} \times 100$$

$$= \frac{4.9133}{12.5990} \times 100$$

$$= 38.99\%.$$

This ratio indicates that large part of the variability observed for this character is non-additive in nature. Only 39% variation is heritable in nature and is governed by additive genetic variation.

5. Information provided in Table 6.13 is used to compute the coefficient of correlation between the parental means ($\overline{Y}_r$) and the parental order of dominance ($W_r + V_r$).

TABLE 6.13: Showing $\overline{Y}_r$ and ($W_r + V_r$) values for 7 arrays averaged over 2 replications

Array	Parental mean ($\overline{Y}_r$)	($W_r + V_r$)
1	20.475	24.9125
2	17.835	27.9867
3	21.745	15.1647
4	16.260	16.414
5	22.645	5.9628
6	26.495	8.7694
7	26.665	5.2481
Total	152.120	104.4582

$$r_{\overline{Y}_r (W_r + v_r)} = \frac{Cov_{\overline{Y}_r (W_r + V_r)}}{\sigma_{\overline{Y}_r} . \sigma_{W_r + V_r}}$$

$$Cov_{\overline{Y}_r (W_r + V_r)} = \frac{1}{6} \Big[(20.475 \times 24.9125) + (17.835 \times 27.9867) + (21.745 \times 15.1647) + (16.260 \times 16.414) + (26.665 \times 5.9628) + (26.495 \times 8.7694) + (26.665 \times 5.2481) - \frac{(152.120 \times 104.4582)}{7} \Big]$$

$$= \frac{1}{6} (2113.1875 - 2270.0258)$$

$$= - 26.1397.$$

Variance of the parental means is found to be 15.7606, therefore, the standard deviation would be 3.9699. Similarly standard deviation for ($W_r + V_r$) is found to be 8.9859. Thus, coefficient of correlation is:

$$\frac{-26.1397}{3.9699 \times 8.9859} = -0.7327.$$

Significance of correlation coefficient is tested as:

$$t = \frac{r}{\sqrt{1 - r^2}} \sqrt{n - 2}$$

$$= \frac{-0.7327}{\sqrt{1 - (-0.7327)^2}} \sqrt{5}$$

$$= \frac{-0.7327 \times 2.236}{0.6805}$$

$$= 2.4075.$$

This value is found to be non-significant for (7 – 2) = 5 degrees of freedom. Hence, we infer that dominant genes contained among the parental lines are equally increasing and decreasing in their effect.

Now let us turn to the graphical analysis. It was mentioned in the earlier section that joint regression of W_r on V_r provides a test to detect validity of hypothesis that additive-dominance model is satisfactory. From the average values of V_r and W_r over two replications, regression of W_r on V_r is calculated (Table 6.14).

TABLE 6.14: Vr and W_r values for seven arrays (mean over 2 replications), and $\bar{Y}_r$ for later use

Array	W_r	V_r	$\bar{Y}_r$
1	11.6003	13.3122	20.475
2	12.0855	15.9012	17.835
3	7.0514	8.1133	21.745
4	5.4001	11.0139	16.260
5	1.1834	4.7794	22.645
6	4.1828	4.5866	26.495
7	0.1742	5.0739	26.665
Total	41.6777	62.7805	152.120
$\bar{x}$	5.9539	8.9686	21.7314
σ^2	21.7148	20.6270	15.7606
σ	–	–	3.9699

We need covariance of W_r with V_r, ($Cov_{W_r V_r}$) to find the regression of W_r on V_r, ($b_{W_r V_r}$). Covariance is obtained as:

$$\frac{1}{6}\Big[\ (11.6003 \times 13.3122 + 12.0855 \times 15.9012$$
$$+ 7.0514 \times 8.1133 + 5.4001 \times 11.0139$$
$$+ 1.1834 \times 4.7794 + 4.1828 \times 4.5866$$
$$+ 0.1742 \times 5.0739 - \frac{(41.6777 \times 62.7805)}{7}\Big]$$
$$= \frac{1}{6}\ [489.01038 - 373.7924]$$
$$= 19.2029.$$

Variance of V_r is obtained in usual manner. It is presented in Table 6.14. Thus regression of W_r on V_r is:

$$\frac{19.2029}{20.627} = 0.9309.$$

In order to test the significance of regression coefficient 't' test is applied as:

$$t_b = \frac{b-0}{S.E._b}.$$

If this ratio is found to be significant at (n –2) degrees of freedom, we conclude that the calculated regression value is significantly different from zero. This is followed by another 't' test, *viz.*

$$t_b = \frac{1-b}{S.E._b}$$

The value of calculated t so obtained is referred to the 't' table for $n-2$ degrees of freedom. Non-significance of this ratio implies that the calculated value of b equals unity. We, therefore, need an estimate of standard error of b, which is calculated as:

$$S.E._b = \left[\frac{\Sigma(y-\bar{y})^2 - b\Sigma(y-\bar{y})(x-\bar{x})}{(n-2)\Sigma(x-\bar{x})^2}\right]^{\frac{1}{2}}$$

Where $\Sigma(y-\bar{y})^2$ is sum of square of W_r values. $\Sigma(x-\bar{x})^2$ is

S.S. of V_r values. $\Sigma(y-\bar{y})(x-\bar{x})$ is sum of cross products of W_r, V_r values. Thus,

$$S.E._{b} = \left(\frac{130.2889 - 0.9309(115.2179)}{5(123.7625)}\right)^{\frac{1}{2}}$$

$$= \left(\frac{23.03256}{618.8125}\right)^{\frac{1}{2}}$$

$$= 0.1929.$$

Significance of '*b*' is found as:

$$t = \frac{0.9309 - 0}{0.1929}$$

$$= 4.82.$$

This value is found to be highly significant which implies that calculated value of *b* is significantly different from zero. Hence, second *t* test is applied to detect whether *b* deviates from unity or not. Thus,

$$t = \frac{1 - 0.9309}{0.1929}$$

$$= 0.3582.$$

Calculated value of '*t*' is non-significant for 5 degrees of freedom. Hence, we conclude that the calculated value of regression coefficient does not deviate significantly from unity. Thus, our assumption regarding the adequacy of additive-dominance model is satisfied.

On the basis of ($W_r - V_r$) analysis as well as the results of joint regression analysis, inference can be drawn that non-allelic interaction is absent. Whatever non-additive variance is observed, it is entirely attributable to dominance variance.

Next step is to calculate the value of '*a*', which gives point of interception of the W_r axis by the regression line. Thus,

$$a = \overline{W_r} - b\overline{V_r}$$

$$= 5.9539 - 0.9309(8.9686)$$

$$= -2.3949.$$

In order to plot the linear regression line of unit slope (making an angle of 45° to the V_r axis) we have to find expected values of W_r for each of the seven arrays. Thus,

$$\hat{W}_{ri} = a + bV_{ri}$$

where $\hat{W}_{ri}$ is the expected value of W_r for *i*th array and V_{ri} is the observed value of V_r for *i*th array. For example, W_{r1}, the expected W_r for array 1 is found as:

$$- 2.3949 + 0.9309\ (13.3122)$$
$$= 9.9974.$$

Expected values of covariances for remaining arrays are obtained likewise (Table 6.15).

The array points are expected to remain within the limits of parabola. We, therefore, need expected values of W_r to plot points for parabola. Expected value of W_r is then obtained as:

$$W_{ri} = \sqrt{(V_p \times V_{ri})}$$

where V_p is the variance of parents (averaged over replications). Thus W_{r1}, the expected value of W_{r1} for parabola is got as:

$$W_{r1} = \sqrt{(16.5067 \times 13.3122)}$$
$$= 14.8236.$$

Remaining expected values of W_r are obtained similarly (Table 6.15).

TABLE 6.15: Observed values of V_r, W_r and expected values of W_r for seven arrays

Array	V_r	W_r		
	Observed	Observed	For regression	For parabola
1	13.3122	11.6003	9.9974	14.8236
2	15.9012	12.0855	12.4075	16.2011
3	8.1133	7.0514	5.1582	11.5725
4	11.0139	5.4001	7.8579	13.4834
5	4.7794	1.1834	2.0542	8.8821
6	4.5866	4.1828	1.8747	8.7011
7	5.0739	0.1742	2.3283	9.1517

Plotting the Graph

Following steps are involved in plotting the graph of W_r, V_r.

(i) V_r values take the position on X axis or the base. Choose an appropriate interval between observed V_r values and mark the base accordingly.

(ii) Likewise mark the Y axis with values of W_r spread at appropriate intervals.

(iii) Against the observed values of V_r plot corresponding expected values of W_r (for regression). Join the points which will give a linear regression line passing through $\overline{W}_r$ and $\overline{V}_r$.

(iv) Plot the expected values of W_r (parabola) against the observed values of V_r and join the points by a free-hand drawing. This will give a parabola.

(v) Lastly observed values of W_r are plotted against the corresponding observed values of V_r. There will be seven array points.

Such a graph has been plotted for you (Fig. 6.3).

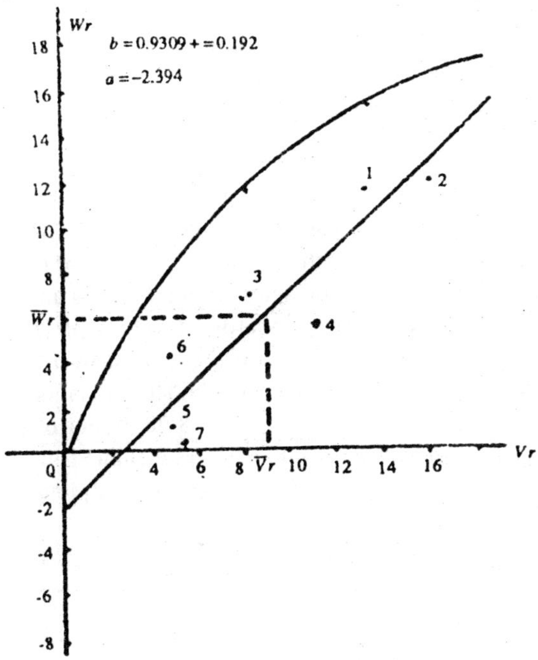

FIG. 6.3 : V_r, W_r Graph for 1000-grain weight of sorghum

From this W_r, V_r graph we can draw three valid conclusions, *viz.*

(i) Since the regression of W_r on V_r is unity, additive-dominance model is satisfactory. There is no evidence of non-allelic interaction.

(ii) Linear regression line of unit slope intercepts W_r axis below the origin. Hence, overdominance is involved in the action of genes governing inheritance of 1000-grain weight.

(iii) Array points 7 and 5 are nearer to the origin. Parental lines 7 and 5, therefore, appear to possess most of the dominant genes for this attribute. On the other hand, point for array 2 is far away from the origin (it could be verified on the basis of V_r and W_r values also given in Table 6.15). Hence parental line 2 possesses most of the recessive genes. The array points are then arranged in the decreasing order of dominance of genes contained in them. The order is 7, 5, 6, 3, 4, 1, 2.

Standardised Deviations Graph

This graph is plotted from the standardised values of parental means and $(W_r + V_r)$ values for seven arrays.

Standardised value of $\overline{Y}_r$ for the parent 1 is obtained as:

$$z_1 = \frac{20.475 - 21.731}{3.9699} = -0.3164,$$

where 20.475 is the mean of parent 1 (Table 6.14), 21.7314 is the mean of seven parents and 3.9699 is the standard deviation of means of seven parents. Standardised values for other parental means are calculated in similar fashion (Table 6.16). Standardised values of $(W_r + V_r)$ are calculated from seven $(W_r + V_r)$ values averaged over 2 replications, overall average of $(W_r + V_r)$ value and standard deviation of $(W_r + V_r)$ values. Standard deviation of $W_r + V_r$ is 8.9859 and overall mean is 14.923. Standardised values of $(W_r + V_r)$ calculated in this way, are presented in Table 6.15. Standardised graph is then plotted using these values (Fig. 6.4).

TABLE 6.16 : Standardised values of $\overline{Y}_r$ and $Wr + Vr$

Array	$\overline{Y}_r$	$(W_r + V_r)$
1	−0.3164	1.1116
2	−0.9813	1.4537
3	0.0034	0.0268
4	−1.3782	0.1659
5	0.2301	−0.9971
6	1.1999	−0.6848
7	1.2427	−1.0766

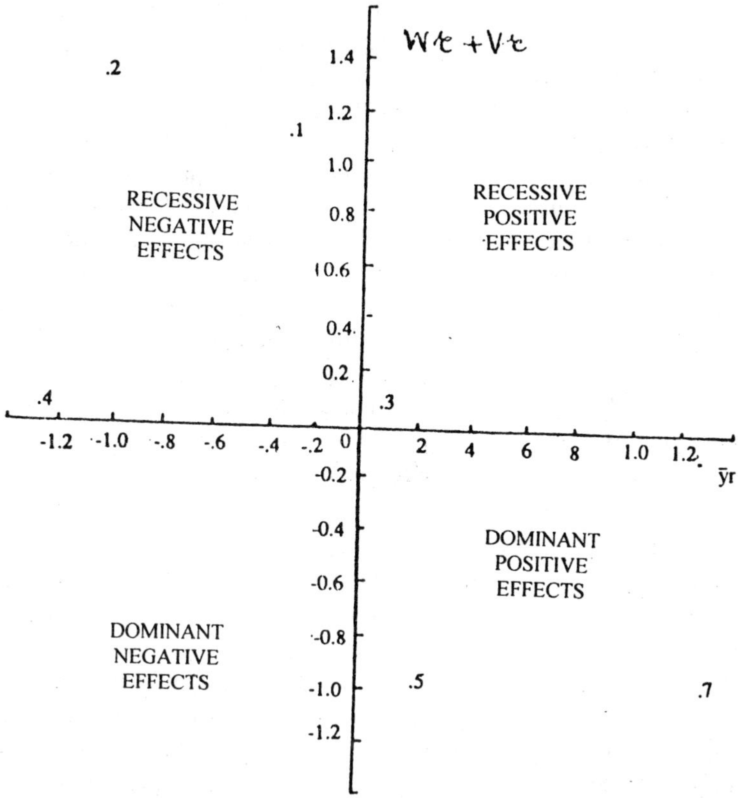

FIG. 6.4: *Standardised Deviations Graph*

The graph reveals that the parental lines 5, 6 and 7 possess most of the dominant genes with positive effects for 1000-grain weight. These lines may, therefore, be employed for hybridisation, whenever bolder seed is desired. On the other hand, parents 1, 2 and 4 possess most of the recessive genes with negative influence on the character. Parental strain 3 is a border line case. It seems that genes with positive influence possessed by this strain are dominant as well as recessive in nature.

6.5 Reference Population

Reader is aware of the fact that the gene effects are defined in context of a well specified population, which we may call as "reference population". Hence the issue concerns whether the parents of diallel should be regarded as a population about which inferences are to be made (a fixed effects model) or as a random sample from some larger population of parents (a random effects model). Some clarification regarding the latter kind of reference population is desirable. In this model, the experimental progenies developed by diallel mating are assumed to be a random sample from random mating population. This implies that the inbred lines employed for diallel mating are a random sample from a parental population of inbreds, which in turn were derived from a parent population by means of inbreeding system, free from forces which tend to change gene frequencies. Griffing (1956b) has shown that selfing the individuals from a random mating population, which is in Hardy-Weinberg equilibrium, leads to homozygous lines, however, it is possible to obtain gene frequencies in the original population by crossing these inbred lines in a diallel fashion.

The diallel analysis proposed by Hayman (1954a) is based on a fixed effects model. On the other hand, analyses proposed by Griffing (1956a), to be described in chapter 7, take care of both the fixed effects as well as the random effects situations. In the fixed effects model, interest is primarily in comparison of the combining ability effects of parents actually employed for diallel mating and also the identification of superior cross combinations. On the other hand, inferences are to be drawn about the base population from which inbred lines have been sampled when random effects model is chosen. These inferences are drawn from the estimates of components of variance. Although the procedures described for analysis of variance are similar for both fixed effects and random effects models, the parameters tested in two models are very different.

According to Hinklemann (1975) one should define whether he is dealing with exploratory diallel experiments or comparative diallel experiments in order to discuss the type of inference that can be made. The objective of exploratory diallel experiments could be to collect wider genetic information regarding various types of gene action. On the other hand, comparative experiments are aimed at comparing the lines in an experiment, such as comparing the average performance of lines in crosses or comparison among the crosses themselves. While discussing the usefulness of diallel mating designs, Hayward (1979) expressed the view that in case of cross-pollinated crops, these experimental designs are useful in the initial strategic survey stages of breeding programmes which provide information about the heritability and the genetic architecture. The strategic survey stage of breeding is followed by a second phase where elite individuals among a set of selected genotypes are identified, which may form the basic plants of synthetic variety or parents of an F_1 hybrid. Thus we are dealing with fixed effects model because the idea is to assess the specific set of individuals in relation to each other with no extrapolation to any base population. The exploratory diallel method of Hinklemann (1975) and the initial strategic survey stages of breeding programme advocated by Hayward (1979) imply the random effects model. Validity of the random effects model has been questioned while dealing with selected materials. Most of the plant material of interest to the breeder is selected for traits of economic importance (Sokol and Baker, 1977). Eberhart the Gardner (1966) expressed the view that plant breeders and geneticists are usually interested in genetic information about the parents and should ,therefore, be using a fixed effects model in most of the cases. They are of the opinion that diallel parents selected from material of interest to the breeder cannot be regarded as a random sample. Estimation of genetic variance components in self-pollinated crops, therefore, does not provide any useful information in their opinion.

6.6 Assumptions involved in the Diallel Analysis

Assumptions involved in the diallel analysis were listed in section 6.1. Valid inferences can be drawn from the diallel analysis only when these assumptions are satisfied. Bias caused by the failure of assumptions is presented in this section for appreciation of readers.

6.6.1 *Diploid Segregation*

Assumption of diploid segregation is usually made because most of our knowledge concerning gene action pertains to diploid species (Cockerham, 1963). However, certain polyploids behave as diploids during meiosis and hence they fulfil the requirement. Diallel analysis of polyploid species should, therefore, be avoided.

6.6.2 *Reciprocal Differences*

When reciprocal differences are found, two values of each statistic, such as V_r, W_r, $\overline{W}_r$, $\overline{V}_r$, $V_{\bar{r}}$, *etc.* are obtained from the table, one by using columns and the other by using rows as arrays. This ambiguity could be removed by replacing all entries in the diallel table by their mean reciprocal. If the differences are independent of genotype then the estimates of the genetical components are correct as long as E contains variation between reciprocals. If the differences depend on genotype then the genetical components are only averages in some way over maternal effects.

6.6.3 *Residual Heterozygosity in Parents*

It may not be difficult to fulfil the assumption regarding homozygous parents in case of self-pollinated crops. Even in the case of cross-pollinated crops, such as maize, adequate sib-mating is likely to yield homozygous inbred lines. Only when the genotypes employed as parents for diallel mating are drawn from early generation segregating material this assumption may not be satisfied. Dickinson and Jinks (1956) have developed a procedure for diallel analysis when the parents are heterozygous. However, the consequences of using heterozygous parents on the results of diallel analysis have been described by Hayman (1954).

Provided that all the assumptions, upon which Hayman's (1954) analysis operates, are satisfied the regression line of W_r on V_r will be a straight line of unit slope. However, if the parents are not homozygous, W_r, V_r graph is a scatter about the regression line of unit slope. Points above the line refer to heterozygous parents and those below the line to homozygous parents. In other words, the points will be distributed in a triangular fashion with homozygous parents occupying same relative positions on this line of unit slope as expected for diallel with homozygous parents. However the array points whose common parents are heterozygous fall at the apex of triangle (Hayward, 1979). As the ratio of variation between parental groups to within parental groups becomes narrower, the graph of W_r, V_r becomes less informative (Allard, 1955).

Several analyses have been proposed for various situations, *e.g.* diallel analyses of Jinks and Hayman (1953) for fully homozygous parents, method of Oake's (1967) for partially heterozygous parents and Dickinson and Jink's (1965) procedure for fully heterozygous parents.

When residual heterozygosity exists among the parents, perfect fit solutions employed to compute various components of variance will be biased and hence the average degree of dominance estimated as $\sqrt{H_1 / D}$ will be underestimated (Hayman, 1954a). Likewise the ratio $H_2/4H_1$ will provide an underestimate of average gene frequency in the parental population.

6.6.4 *Correlated Gene Distribution*

In diallel analysis it is assumed that genes are independently distributed among the parents. This implies that the presence or absence of an allele at a particular locus is statistically independent of the presence or absence of the alleles at the other loci. Failure of this assumption may result either due to linkage of genes in the population from which parents were selected, or due to the effect of sample size while choosing the parents (Baker, 1978). However, linkage as such has no effect on the results of diallel set of crosses. According to Feyt (1976), the genes at n loci cannot be independent unless a minimum of 2^n parents are used in diallel cross. Unless genes are independently distributed among the parents, valid inference cannot be drawn from diallel analysis (Kempthorne, 1956; Sokol and Baker, 1977).

Estimate of D will be zero when the genes are equally dispersed among the parental lines. On the other hand, estimate of D will be greater than Σd^2 if the genes are associated. Thus the measure of average degree of dominance, $\sqrt{H_1 / D}$, may be either inflated or reduced by the combined effects of correlation of genes on estimates of H_1 and D. For example, a particular combination of dispersion and unidirectional dominance of genes may convert partial dominance into overdominance.

The W_r, V_r graph is also disturbed due to non-independent distribution of genes (Coughtrey and Mather, 1970). Influence of correlated genes on the W_r, V_r graph may be described by considering a simple case, where the inheritance of an attribute is governed by two loci each having two alleles, *viz.* *A, a* and *B, b*. Let us also assume that genes *A* and *B* increase the expression of a character and genes *a* and *b* tend to decrease it. With respect to these loci, there will be four inbred lines *AABB*, *AAbb*, *aaBB* and *aabb* in the population. If the genes are independently distributed and frequencies of genes A, a and B, b are equal, proportions of these genotypes will be $\frac{1}{4}$ each in the population. Let us introduce a parameter c to measure the distribution of genes among the parents. It takes a value of + 1 when genes with reinforcing effects (effects in same direction) are associated in one parent. On the other hand, $c = -1$ when the genes are equally dispersed among the parents. When gene pairs are distributed among the parents independently of each other $c = 0$, and hence the frequencies of parental types will be $\frac{1}{4}$ each. When the degree of association and dispersion is taken into consideration, frequencies of the four genotypes may be expressed as shown in Table 6.16. When genes are associated completely $c = 1$. Hence the frequencies of genotypes $AABB$ and $aabb$ will be $\frac{1}{2}$ each. On the other hand, frequencies of $AAbb$ and $aaBB$ will be zero. When $c = -1$, frequencies of genotypes $AAbb$ and $aaBB$ will be $\frac{1}{2}$ each. Let us simplify the situation by assuming that $d_a = d_b = h_a = h_b = d$ and that digenic non-allelic interaction is absent, *i.e.*, $i_{ab} = j_{ab} = j_{ba} = l_{ab} = 0$. Therefore, mean expression of $AABB$ is $d_a + d_b = 2d$ expressed as deviation from mid-point. Variances and covariances are also presented in this table along with the array means. Since the means of progeny families within the $AABB$ array are identical, V_r for this array is zero. Similarly W_r for this array is zero. Let us derive V_r for $AAbb$ array. Thus V_{rAAbb} is:

$$\left(\frac{1}{4}(1+c)(2d)^2 + \frac{1}{4}(1-c)(2d)^2\right) - (d)^2$$

$$= d^2 + d^2c + d^2 - d^2c - d^2$$

$$= d^2.$$

W_r for this array is:

$$W_{rAAbb} = \left[\frac{1}{4}(1+c)(2d.2d)\right]$$

$$= \left(\frac{1}{4} + \frac{1}{4}c\right)(4d^2)$$

TABLE 6.17: Diallel mating when genes are correlated

		Male parents				Mean	V_r	W_r	$W_r - V_r$
	Genotype Frequency Mean	*AABB* ¼(1 + *c*) 2*d*	*AAbb* ¼(1 − *c*) 0	*aaBB* ¼ (1 − *c*) 0	*aabb* ¼ (1 + *c*) −2*d*	 1 0			
Genotype Frequency Mean	*AABB* ¼ (1 + *c*) 2*d*	*AABB* 2*d*	*AABb* 2*d*	*AaBb* 2*d*	*AaBb* 2*d*	2*d*	0	0	0
	AAbb ¼(1 − *c*) 0	*AABb* 2*d*	*AAbb* 0	*AaBb* 2*d*	*Aabb* 0	*d*	d^2	$d^2\ (1 + c)$	d^2c
Female Parents	*aaBB* ¼(1 − *c*) 0	*AaBB* 2*d*	*AaBb* 2*d*	*aaBB* 0	*aaBb* 0	*d*	d^2	$d^2(1 + c)$	d^2c
	aabb ¼(1 + *c*) −2*d*	*AaBb* 2*d*	*Aabb* 0	*aaBb* 0	*aabb* −2*d*	0	$2d^2(1 + c)$	$2d^2\ (1 + c)$	0

$$= d^2 + d^2c$$
$$= d^2 (1 + c).$$

Since values of V_r and W_r for *AABB* array are zero, point for this array on W_r, V_r graph will fall on origin .The values of V_r and W_r for *aabb* array are larger in magnitude than for AABB array but identical. $\Delta W_r = \Delta V_r$ for these two arrays. Hence when the two array points are joined, a linear regression line of unit slope is obtained. We get a straight line of unit slope when one unit increase on X axis is accompanied with an increase of one unit on Y axis. Change in V_r due to the substitution of *aabb* as a common parent in *AABB* array can be measured as ΔV_r. It is found to be equal to ΔW_r, which is $2d^2 (1 + c)$.

The change in V_r for *AAbb* array measured from *AABB* is d^2, which is not equal to ΔW_r. In other words, for this array ΔV_r is not equal to ΔW_r. If c is positive, *i.e* , genes are associated, magnitude of ΔW_r will be larger than ΔV_r for this array. The point for this array will, therefore, move to the left of regression line. When the three array points are joined, regression line is obtained which is concave downwards. Reader should note that ΔV_r and ΔW_r for the arrays *AAbb* and *aaBB* are identical and, therefore, give one point on W_r, V_r graph.

If the genes are dispersed, that is c is negative (but only if it is less than $-$ 1) points for *AAbb* and *aaBB* arrays will lie to the right of regression line because ΔV_r will be larger than ΔW_r. This will give a regression line which is concave upwards.

6.6.5 *Non-allelic Interaction*

It is unrealistic to assume that there is no non-allelic interaction. Gilbert (1958) and Cockerham (1959) are of the opinion that until experimentally proven otherwise absence of non-allelic interaction cannot be assumed, while dealing with quantitative characters.

Hayman (1954a) provided tests to detect presence of non-allelic interaction. However, theoretical considerations of Coughtrey and Mather (1970), and the computer simulation studies of Feyt (1976) show that Hayman's test for non-allelic interaction is reliable, only if the genes are distributed independently among the parents. Purturbations of W_r, V_r graphs may be caused by non-allelic interaction and/or correlation between genes.

TABLE 6.18: Showing effect of digenic non-allelic interaction on V_r, W_r and $W_r - V_r$ of four arrays

		Male parents				Mean	Vr	Wr	$(Wr-Vr)$
	Genotype Frequency Mean	$AABB$ ¼ $d(2+\theta)$	$AAbb$ ¼ $-d\theta$	$aaBB$ ¼ $-d\theta$	$aabb$ ¼ $d(-2+\theta)$				
Mean Frequency	$AABB$ $d(2+\theta)$ ¼	$AABB$ $d(2+\theta)$ ¼	$AABb$ $d(2+\theta)$ ¼	$AaBB$ $d(2+\theta)$ ¼	$AaBb$ $d(2+\theta)$ ¼	$d(2+\theta)$	0	0	0
Female	$AAbb$ $-d\theta$ ¼	$AABb$ $d(2+\theta)$ ¼	$AAbb$ $-d\theta$ ¼	$AaBb$ $d(2+\theta)$ ¼	$Aabb$ $-d\theta$ ¼	d	$d^2(1+\theta)^2$	$d^2(1+\theta)$	$-d^2\theta(1+\theta)$
Parents	$aaBB$ $-d\theta$ ¼	$AaBB$ $d(2+\theta)$ ¼	$AaBb$ $d(2+\theta)$ ¼	$aaBB$ $-d\theta$ ¼	$aaBb$ $-d\theta$ ¼	d	$d^2(1+\theta)^2$	$d^2(1+\theta)$	$-d^2\theta(1+\theta)$
	$aabb$ $d(-2+\theta)$ ¼	$AaBb$ $d(2+\theta)$ ¼	$Aabb$ $-d\theta$ ¼	$aaBb$ $-d\theta$ ¼	$aabb$ $d(-2+\theta)$ ¼	0	$d^2(2+\theta^2)$	$d^2(2+\theta^2)$	0

Estimates of variance components are subject to large sampling errors (Baker, 1978). Hayman (1963) concluded that estimates of variance components could not be significant estimates of population parameters, unless the number of parents exceeds 10. With fewer than 10 parents, a fixed model is recommended.

The effect of non-allelic interaction on the W_r, V_r graph has been described by Mather and Jinks (1971). They have shown that if the complementary kind of non-allelic interaction is present, the regression line is concave upward. On the other hand, with duplicate type of non-allelic interaction, the regression line is concave downwards. How? Let us see. If we assume that an attribute is determined by two gene pairs each having two alleles, *viz*. *A*, *a*, *B*, *b*, there will be four kinds of inbred lines in the population, *viz*. *AABB*, *AAbb*, *aaBB* and *aabb*. If the frequency of each of these genes is ½, proportions of four parental lines in the population will be ¼ each. Further, let us assume that $d_a = d_b = h_a = h_b = d$ and $i_{ab} = j_{ab} = j_{ba} = l_{ab} = \theta d$, where θ measures the strength of non-allelic interaction (Mather, 1967). Variances (V_r) and covariances (W_r) of the four arrays will be as shown in Table 6.17. Frequencies of genotypes and means are similar among the male and female parents.

Since V_r for the *AABB* array is identical with W_r for this array, *i.e.*, zero, the array point falls on origin of W_r, V_r graph. The change in V_r, if *aabb* is substituted as common parents in *AABB* array, is $d^2(2 + \theta^2)$. The covariance of *aabb* array deviates from the W_r of *AABB* array by an amount equal to $d^2(2 + \theta^2)$. Since $\Delta V_r = \Delta W_r$ for these two arrays, the points for the *AABB* and *aabb* arrays will give a straight line of unit slope when the points are joined. Taking *AABB* as the base, we find that ΔV_r for *AAbb* array is not equal to ΔW_r. The V_r and W_r for *AAbb* and *aaBB* arrays are, however, identical and the two array points coincide. Hence, there will be only three array points on W_r, V_r graph. According to Mather (1967), θ takes a value of + 1 when non-allelic interaction is of complementary type. Theta (θ) takes value of − 1 when the non-allelic interaction is of duplicate type, and θ = 0 when non-allelic interaction is absent. Readers can verify that when θ =1, magnitude of V_r for *AAbb* array (and also the *aaBB*) will be larger than its W_r. Hence, the array point will fall to the right of regresson line. Thus the regression line will be concave upwards when the three array points are joined. When duplicate type of non-allelic interaction is involved (provided $\theta < -1$), the regression line will be concave downwards. The reason being that the magnitude of ΔW_r will be larger than ΔV_r for *AAbb* array, when θ is < -1.

Hayman (1954a) pointed out that in the presence of complementary kind of non-allelic interaction, estimate of average degree of dominance calculated as $\sqrt{H_1 / D}$ is inflated but it has little effect on the estimators of the gene frequency. Duplicate type of non-allelic interaction, on the other hand, leaves $\sqrt{H_1 / D}$ and $H_2/4H_1$ unaltered.

7

DIALLEL MATING DESIGN (Combining Ability Analysis)

7.1 Griffing's (1956) Diallel Analysis

Hayman's (1954) graphical and numerical approach to diallel analysis provides information on several valuable aspects of the genetic make up of a quantitative character, such as the adequacy of additive-dominance model, average degree of dominance involved in the action of genes, preponderance of dominant and recessive genes among the parental lines, symmetrical or asymmetrical distribution of genes with positive and negative effects on the attribute, *etc.* It was pointed out in section 6.1 that this approach to diallel analysis operates on several assumptions. Now it will be apparent that conformity with these unrealistic restrictions will hardly be realised in practice in respect of quantitative characters. In effect, the model reduces to that of a single diallelic gene with diallel mating between the two homozygotes, say, *AA* and *aa* (where *A, a* are the alleles at a locus), mating between heterozygotes not being considered (Arunachalam, 1976). The analysis has been subsequently extended to many genes under almost impossible restrictions. It is pertinent to note that there are no built-in parameters in the genetic model envisaged to accommodate non-allelic interaction which is assumed to be absent.

Griffing (1956a) proposed a more general procedure for diallel analysis which makes provision for non-allelic interaction. In this approach mean measurement of a cross is partitioned into two major components, apart from a general mean (μ) and an environmental component, (i) the contribution of the parents, the general combining ability (*g.c.a.*) effect analogous to main effect of factorial designs, and (ii) the excess over and above the sum of the two *g.c.a* effects, called the specific combining ability (*s.c.a.*) effect, analogous to an interaction effect of a factorial design.

This approach to diallel analysis operates under sole assumption that parents of the diallel cross are inbred lines, a major advantage of this assumption is that when hybrids and parents are raised in plots (usually one row or a few rows) in the field, genetic uniformity will be maintained so that the quantitative characters can be measured on a random sample of plants from a plot. Like the Hayman's (1954) approach, Griffing's (1956a) model is not based on single diallelic gene model. The singular advantage of the model proposed by Griffing (1956a) is that the estimates of the variances due to *g.c.a.* and *s.c.a* provide an apt diagnosis of the predominant role of additive or non-allelic interaction effects of genes. The *g.c.a.* and *s.c.a.* effects help to locate the parents and crosses that are responsible in bringing about a particular type of gene action.

Arunachalam (1976) is of the opinion that combining ability analysis of Griffing (1956a) has several advantages over that of Hayman's (1954) approach. A few of these advantages are:

(i) It is not restricted to one gene and operates with limited feasible assumptions. It is, therefore, more realistic to the plant breeding problems.

(ii) The *g.c.a.* and *s.c.a.* effects and their variances are very effective genetic parameters of direct utility to decide the next phase of the breeding programme.

(iii) It enables a plant breeder to decide, for example, about hybrid or pure line breeding, the choice of parents for construction of synthetics, the selection of suitable F_1s for a multiple crossing or a composite breeding programme and the possibility of employing appropriate selection techniques like modified mass selection, recurrent selection and reciprocal recurrent selection, etc.

In this chapter, therefore, Griffing's (1956a) approach to diallel analysis is described.

In a strict sense diallel mating of p inbred lines results in p^2 progeny families. These p^2 families are made up of p inbred lines, one set of $\frac{p(p-1)}{2}$ F_1s and one set of $\frac{p(p-1)}{2}$ reciprocal F_1s. Depending upon which of the progeny families are included for analysis, four methods of diallel analysis have been proposed. These methods are:

Method 1—Comprising of all the p^2 progeny families,

Method 2—This method includes p parents and $\frac{p(p-1)}{2}$ F_1s, *i.e.* $\frac{p(p+1)}{2}$ families.

Method 3— $\frac{p(p-1)}{2}$ F_1s, and $\frac{p(p-1)}{2}$ reciprocal F_1s, *i.e.* $p(p-1)$ families are included as experimental material in this method.

and Method 4—Only one set of F_1s, *i.e.* $\frac{p(p-1)}{2}$ progeny families constitute the experimental material.

The experimental material developed according to any one of these four methods could be planted in any of the suitable experimental designs. However, we will restrict ourselves to only one design, *viz.*, the randomised block design, because it is commonly used and is applicable to this type of study.

In randomised block design we assume that there are '*a*' varieties (*i.e.* genotypes developed by the diallel crossing method), each of which is assigned at random to each of the b blocks and that there are c individuals in each of the ab plots. Thus the mathematical model for *ijkl*th observation could be expressed as:

$$Y_{ijkl} = \mu + v_{ij} + b_k + (bv)_{ijk} + e_{ijkl}$$

Where μ is the population mean effect, v_{ij} is the effect of *ij*th genotype, b_k is the effect of *k*th block, $(bv)_{ijk}$ is the interaction of *ij*th genotype with *k*th block, e_{ijkl} is the environmental effect peculiar to *ijkl*th observation. In this linear model, double subscript notation is used for variety (*i.e.* genotype) effect because it is desired to denote genotypic means in the combining ability analysis as Y_{ij}, where Y_{ii} is the mean of *i*th inbred and Y_{ij} is the mean of F_1 obtained by crossing *i*th and *j*th inbred lines. In the combining ability analysis, which does not include reciprocals, variety effect V_{ij} is expressed in terms of general and specific combining ability effects as:

$$v_{ij} = g_i + g_j + s_{ij}$$

When reciprocal cross is included, variety effect could be expressed as:

$$v_{ij} = g_i + g_j + s_{ij} + r_{ij}$$

In these expressions g_i and g_j refer to the general combining ability effects (abbreviated as *g.c.a*) of *i*th and *j*th lines, respectively, s_{ij} is the specific combining ability effect of *ij*th cross (usually expressed as *s.c.a.*) and r_{ij} is the reciprocal effect associated with *ij*th cross.

According to Sprague and Tatum (1942) the term specific combining ability is used to designate those cases in which certain combinations do relatively better or worse than would be expected on the basis of average performance of lines involved. This definition makes the concept of *s.c.a.* effects quite clear. If the mean of a cross is expressed as deviation from population mean, the mean performance of the *ij*th cross would be equal to the value conferred by *i*th and *j*th lines, *i.e.*, g_i and g_j, upon this cross, in the absence of other agencies which influence the expression of character. In other words, it implies additivity between *g.c.a* effects of *i*th and *j*th lines. However, if the performance of *ij*th cross is superior or inferior than expected on the basis of *g.c.a.* effects of *i*th and *j*th parent, non-additivity is suggested. This may be due to the dominance deviations and/or non-allelic interaction deviations. Hence $\sigma^2_{s.c.a.}$ is a measure of non-additive genetic variance. Griffing (1956b) has shown relationship between various heritable variance components and $\sigma^2_{g.c.a}$ and $\sigma^2_{s.c.a.}$. Thus,

$$2\sigma^2_{g.c.a.} = \sigma^2_A + \frac{1}{2}\sigma^2_{AA} \ldots\ldots\ldots$$

$$\sigma^2_{s.c.a.} = \sigma^2_D + \frac{1}{2}\sigma^2_{AA} + \sigma^2_{AD} + \sigma^2_{DD} \ldots\ldots\ldots$$

and $$\sigma^2_G = \sigma^2_A + \sigma^2_D + \sigma^2_{AA} + \sigma^2_{AD} + \sigma^2_{DD} \ldots\ldots\ldots$$

Griffing (1956a) gave due consideration to the sampling nature of experimental material. The parental lines employed for diallel mating or the progeny families resulting from diallel mating could be regarded as a random sample from some population about which inferences are to be drawn. Alternatively the experimental material or the parental lines could be considered as the entire population about which inferences are to be made. Based on Eisenhart's (1947) proposition, Griffing (1956a) suggested two models for combining ability analysis of the experimental progenies developed by different methods presented above. In model I, variety and block effects are regarded as constants. On the other hand, in

TABLE 7.1: Format for ANOVA when diallel progeny (= a genotypes) are planted in b blocks having c plants in each of the ab plots

Source	df	MS	Expectations of mean squares Model I (Fixed effect)	Model II (Random effect)
Replications	$(b-1)$	M_b	$\sigma_e^2 + ac\frac{1}{(b-1)}\sum_k b_k^2$	$\sigma_e^2 + c\sigma_{bv}^2 + ac\sigma_b^2$
Genotypes	$(a-1)$	M_v	$\sigma_e^2 + bc\frac{1}{(a-1)}\sum_i v_i^2$	$\sigma_e^2 + c\sigma_{bv}^2 + bc\sigma_v^2$
Genotypes × Replications	$(a-1)\ (b-1)$	M_{bv}	$\sigma_e^2 + c\frac{1}{(a-1)(b-1)}\sum_i\sum_j\sum_k (bv)_{ijk}^2$	$\sigma_e^2 + c\sigma_{bv}^2$
Error	$ab(c-1)$	M_e	σ_e^2	σ_e^2

model II, both variety and block effects are assumed to be random variables. If the 'a' genotypes produced by diallel mating, according to any one of the four methods proposed by Griffing (1956a) are planted in a randomised block design with b blocks, such that there are c plants per plot of each progeny family within each block, the format for analysis of variance will be as shown in Table 7.1 depending upon the model chosen for analysis.

In model I, the experimental material is regarded as the population about which inferences are to be drawn. The objective is to compare combining ability effects of parents, when parents themselves are used as testers, and also to identify high performing combinations. The aim is, therefore, to estimate combining ability effects of parents and their crosses and to compute appropriate standard errors for differences between the effects. For testing purposes, we assume that e_{ijkl} are normally, independently distributed with mean zero ($\mu_e = 0$) and variance, σ_e^2. On the other hand, in model II, it is assumed that we are dealing with random samples from some parent population, and the inferences are not to be drawn about individual lines in the sample but about the parameters in the parent population. The object of this model is to estimate genetic and environmental components of complex population variance. It is assumed that all the effects in this model except the μ, are normally, independently distributed with mean zero (*i.e.* $\mu_b = 0$, $\mu_g = 0$, $\mu_s = 0$ and $\mu_r = 0$) and variance σ_θ^2, where θ refers to *b* or *g* or *s* or *r*. Variance components are estimated by translating the observed mean squares to their expected values. Standard errors for estimates of variance components are calculated from variances of appropriate mean squares.

A question is frequently asked regarding the number of parents to be employed to obtain reliable estimates of components of variance from diallel mating design. Pederson's (1971) simulation studies revealed that where a random mating population is being surveyed, which has no structure-artificial or natural-imposed on it, and a sample of individuals are taken for direct involvement without prior inbreeding, using method 4, reliable estimates of heritability and degree of dominance could be obtained by establishing several replicated diallels of a minimum size of 8 to 10 parents or more. From the practical point of view, his studies indicated that 3 to 5 diallels of size 8 × 8 (each replicated 2 to 3 times) are necessary to provide reliable estimates of individual heritability. To produce reliable results with a single diallel, it would involve 17-19 parents with a total plant number generally twice that of parallel diallels.

Since each of the four methods advocated by Griffing (1956a) involve different experimental material, there are four methods of analyses. Thus there are four methods of analyses for model I and four for model II. Presently only four methods of analyses will be described for model I.

7.2 Method 1, Model I

Experimental material for this method comprises of p^2 progeny families produced by mating *p* inbred lines in all possible ways. For the sake of explanation let us suppose that $p = 3$. Then diallel mating will result in 9 progeny families as shown below:

$$\begin{matrix} Y_{11} & Y_{12} & Y_{13} \\ Y_{21} & Y_{22} & Y_{23} \\ Y_{31} & Y_{32} & Y_{33} \end{matrix}$$

Where Y_{11} is the mean of progeny obtained by mating of inbred line 1 with inbred line 1, Y_{12} is the mean of progeny obtained by mating of inbred line 1 with 2, and Y_{21} denotes the mean of progeny obtained by mating of inbred line 2 with 1. Here the expression $\overline{Y_{ij}}$ has been simplified to Y_{ij}.

We will come across some notations, while dealing with calculations of sum of squares and combining ability effects. Thus, for this method

$$Y_{i.} = \sum_j y_{ij} = y_{i1} + y_{i2} + y_{i3}$$

Where $y_{i.}$ is total of *i*th inbred line over rest of the inbred lines.

$$Y_{.j} = \sum_i y_{ij} = y_{1j} + y_{2j} + y_{3j},$$

and finally

$$Y_{..} = \sum_i \sum_j y_{ij} = y_{11}+y_{12}+y_{13}+y_{21}+y_{22}+y_{23}+y_{31}+y_{32}+y_{33}$$

$Y_{..}$ is total of all the progeny families, which comprise of the experimental material of method 1.

Linear mathematical model for combining ability analysis for method 1, model 1 is:

$$Y_{ij} = \mu + g_i + g_j + r_{ij} + s_{ij} + \frac{1}{bc} \sum_k \sum_l e_{ijkl},$$

where μ is the population mean, g_i and g_j are the general combining ability (*g.c.a.*) effects of *i*th and *j*th inbred lines, respectively, r_{ij} is the reciprocal effect, such that $r_{ij} = -r_{ji}$, s_{ij} is the specific combining ability effect (*s.c.a.*) of *ij*th cross such that $s_{ij} = s_{ji}$ and e_{ijkl} is the environmental effect associated with *ijkl*th individual observation. Restrictions are imposed on combining ability effects, such that $\sum_i g_i = 0$ and $\sum_i s_{ij} = 0$ (for each *j*). Format for analysis of variance is presented in Table 7.2.

Me' is obtained as *Me/r*, where *Me* is the error mean square from ANOVA for randomised block design. Since the combining ability analysis is based on means of each of the genotypes over *r* replications, error mean square of *r.b.d.* is divided by number of replications to make it comparable with other mean squares. Various sum of squares are obtained as:

$$S_g = \frac{1}{2p} \sum_i \left(y_{i.} + y_{.i}\right)^2 - \frac{2}{p^2} Y_{..}^2$$

$$S_s = \frac{1}{2} \sum_i \sum_j y_{ij} (y_{ij} + y_{ji}) - \frac{1}{2p} \sum_i (Y_{i.} + Y_{.i})^2 + \frac{1}{p^2} Y_{..}^2$$

and $$S_r = \frac{1}{2} \sum_i \sum_{<j} (y_{ij} - y_{ji})^2$$

TABLE 7.2 : ANOVA for method 1 (Griffing, 1956a)

Source	df	SS	MS	Expectation of mean squares: Model I	Expectation of mean squares: Model II
General combining ability	$(p-1)$	S_g	M_g	$\sigma^2 + 2p\left(\frac{1}{p-1}\right)\sum_i g_i^2$	$\sigma^2 + \frac{2(p-1)}{p}\sigma_s^2 + 2p\sigma_g^2$
Specific combining ability	$\frac{p(p-1)}{2}$	Ss	Ms	$\sigma^2 + \left(\frac{2}{p(p-1)}\right)\sum_i\sum_j s_{ij}^2$	$\sigma^2 + \frac{2(p^2-p+1)}{p^2}\sigma_s^2$
Reciprocal effects	$\frac{p(p-1)}{2}$	Sr	Mr	$\sigma^2 + 2\left(\frac{2}{p(p-1)}\right)\sum_i \sum_{<j} r_{ij}^2$	$\sigma^2 + 2\sigma_r^2$
Error	m		Me'	σ^2	σ^2

Appropriate F tests are shown below :

$$F_{g.c.a.} = Mg/Me',\ F_{s.c.a.} = Ms/Me' \text{ and } Fr = Mr/Me'$$

The value obtained for ratio Mg/Me' is referred to the F table for $(p-1)$ and m degrees of freedom. If the mean square for *g.c.a.* is found to be significant, we infer that there are significant differences among the *g.c.a.* effects. It also suggests that additive genetic variance is an important component of heritable variance for this attribute. Significance of mean square for specific combining ability indicates that significant differences exists among the *s.c.a.* effects and that non-additive genetic variance is responsible for the inheritance of the character being studied. If the value calculated for ratio Mr/Me' is greater than the table value of F for $\frac{p(p-1)}{2}$ and error degrees of freedom, we conclude that reciprocal effects are involved in the inheritance of character. While choosing a cross, in addition to its *s.c.a.* effect, we should take into consideration the reciprocal effects if later are significant. It is most important to note that when model I is adopted, components of variances such as $\sigma_s^2, \sigma_g^2, \sigma_r^2$ should not be calculated from the mean squares.

The next step would be to estimate combining ability effects. Thus

$\hat{g}_i$, the estimate of general combining ability effect (*g.c.a.*) of *i*th parent may be found as:

$$\hat{g}_i = \frac{1}{2p}(Y_{i.} + Y_{.i}) - \frac{1}{p^2}Y_{..}$$

Estimate of specific combining ability effect of *ij*th cross is computed as :

$$\hat{s}_{ij} = \frac{1}{2}(y_{ij} + y_{ji}) - \frac{1}{2p}(Y_{i.} + Y_{.i} + Y_{j.} + Y_{.j}) + \frac{1}{p^2}Y_{..}$$

And lastly, the estimate of reciprocal effect for the *ij*th cross may be got as:

$$\hat{r}_{ij} = \frac{1}{2}(y_{ij} - y_{ji}).$$

To test the significance of these estimates, standard errors are calculated as:

$$S.E._{\hat{g}_i} = \left(\frac{p-1}{2p^2}\hat{\sigma}^2\right)^{\frac{1}{2}}$$

$$S.E.(\hat{g}_i - \hat{g}_j) = \left(\frac{1}{p}\hat{\sigma}^2\right)^{\frac{1}{2}}$$

$$S.E._{\hat{s}_{ij}} = \left[\frac{1}{2p^2}(p^2 - 2p + 2)\hat{\sigma}^2\right]^{\frac{1}{2}}$$

$$S.E._{(\hat{s}_{ij} - \hat{s}_{ik})} = \left(\frac{(p-1)}{p}\hat{\sigma}^2\right)^{\frac{1}{2}}$$

$$S.E._{(\hat{s}_{ij} - \hat{s}_{kl})} = \left[\frac{(p-2)}{p}\hat{\sigma}^2\right]^{\frac{1}{2}}$$

$$S.E._{\hat{r}_{ij}} = \left(\frac{1}{2}\hat{\sigma}^2\right)^{\frac{1}{2}}$$

$$S.E._{(\hat{r}_{ij}-\hat{r}_{kl})} = (\hat{\sigma}^2)^{\frac{1}{2}}$$

How to use these standard errors for valid inferences? Let us see. Initially we begin with testing of *g.c.a.* effects. Reader should note, however, that general combining ability effects are calculated only when mean square for general combining ability is found to be significant. Same thing is applied to other effects as well. We wish to test whether estimate of g_i deviates significantly from zero or not. It is tested with the help of '*t*' test shown below:

$$t = \frac{g_i - 0}{S.E._{gi}}$$

The calculated value of ratio is referred to the 't' table for error degrees of freedom. When the degrees of freedom are larger than 30, we can take the table value of '*t*' as 1.96 and 2.578 at 5 and 1 per cent levels, respectively. Calculated value of g_i is compared with ($1.96 \times S.E._{gi}$) and ($2.58 \times S.E._{gi}$). If the estimated value of g_i is larger than ($1.96 \times S.E._{gi}$) inference can be drawn that the estimate of *g.c.a.* effect is significantly different from zero at 5 per cent level. Likewise when the estimate of g_i is larger than ($2.58 \times S.E._{gi}$), the value of *g.c.a.* effect is regarded as significantly different from zero at 1 per cent level. Compare all the *g.c.a.* effects for their significance with these values, *i.e.* ($1.96 \times S.E._{gi}$) and ($2.58 \times S.E._{gi}$).

The next operation is comparison of estimates of *g.c.a.* effects amongst themselves. Suppose for example, we notice that general combining ability effects of three parents are significant and positive. We shall be interested to know as to which of the parent is significantly superior among these three, in terms of their *g.c.a.* effects. Hence a '*t*' test is applied as:

$$t = \frac{\hat{g}_i - \hat{g}_j}{S.E._{\hat{g}_i - \hat{g}_j}}$$

A short cut method would be to compare the difference between two significant *g.c.a.* effects (in same direction) with $1.96 \times S.E._{(gi-gj)}$. If the difference between two *g.c.a.* effects is greater than $S.E._{(gi-gj)} \times 1.96$, we conclude that the *g.c.a.* effects of *i*th and *j*th inbred lines are significantly different from each other at 5 per cent level. When the difference is significant, we infer that parent with larger *g.c.a.* effect is a better combiner for the character being investigated. Parental lines with significant *g.c.a.* effects in desired direction should be chosen for hybridization.

Using $S.E._{(\hat{s}_{ij})}$, test the significance of all the specific combining ability effects. Procedure described for general combining ability effects is adopted for *s.c.a.* effects also. *S.c.a.* effects of two kinds of crosses may be significant, *viz.* crosses involving one parent in common such as 1×2, 1×4, 1×6, and crosses having no parent is common, such as 1×2, 3×4, 5×6, etc. After testing the significance of individual *s.c.a.* effects, we wish to identify crosses with superior *s.c.a.* effects. For this purpose we initially compare difference between two specific combining ability effects having one common parent, with $1.96 \times S.E._{(s_{ij}-s_{ik})}$. If the difference between two *s.c.a.* effects is larger than $1.96 \times S.E._{(s_{ij}-s_{ik})}$, we conclude that *s.c.a.* effects of two crosses having one parent in common are significantly different from each other at 5 per cent level. Subsequent to identification of superior crosses on the basis of their *s.c.a.* effects having one parent in common, we compare the differences between the specific combining ability effects of two crosses having no parent in common with a value $S.E._{(s_{ij}-s_{kl})} \times 1.96$. If the difference between two specific combining ability effects is greater than $S.E._{(s_{ij}-s_{kl})} \times 1.96$ we infer that the *s.c.a.* effects are significantly different from each other at 5 per cent level. Cross-combination having larger *s.c.a.* effect is then regarded as superior specific combination. This procedure is repeated for other *s.c.a.* effects. In this way breeders can eliminate poor crosses and choose the best.

Significance of reciprocal effects is tested as:

$$t = \frac{\hat{r}_{ij} - 0}{S.E._{\hat{r}_{ij}}}$$

After testing the significance of all reciprocal effects, two reciprocal effects are compared at a time. Thus, if difference between two reciprocal effects exceeds $S.E.(r_{ij}-r_{kl}) \times 1.96$, we infer that the two reciprocal effects are significantly different from each other and the cross with larger value or of r_{ij} is significantly superior.

7.2.1. Worked Example

Seven inbred lines of sorghum were crossed in a diallel fashion resulting in 49 progeny families. These families comprised of 21 F_1s, 21 reciprocal F_1s and 7 parental genotypes. The 49 genotypes were raised in a randomised block design with two replications. Observations were recorded on grain yield/plant (g). Data are presented in Table 7.3.

Analysis of data proceeds along conventional lines to detect significant differences among the 49 genotypes for grain yield/plant (g). Only if we observe that there are significant differences among the genotypes, we proceed for combining ability analysis. The steps are given below:

Correction factor $= \dfrac{(5785.226)^2}{49 \times 2 = 98}$

$= 341518.77419$

Total sum of squares $= (40.136^2 + 50.002^2 + ... + 45.760^2) - CF$

$= 374836.74773 - 341518.77419$

$= 33317.97354$

Genotype sum of squares $= \dfrac{1}{2}(84.89^2 + 93.282^2 + ... + 89.620^2) - CF$

$= \dfrac{1}{2}(737930.38083) - CF$

$= 27446.41623$

Replication sum of squares $= \dfrac{1}{49}(2880.965^2 + 2904.261^2) - CF$

$= 5.5378$

Error sum of squares $= 33317.97354 - (27446.41623 + 5.5378)$

$= 5866.01951$

The analysis of variance is set up as shown in Table 7.4.

TABLE 7.3: Grain yield/plant (g) of 49 genotypes obtained by 7 × 7 diallel mating.

Sl.No.	Crosses	Replication 1	Replication 2	Total	Average
1.	1 × 1	40.136	44.754	84.890	42.445
2.	2 × 2	50.002	43.280	93.282	46.641
3.	3 × 3	32.530	17.842	50.372	25.186
4.	4 × 4	21.728	13.398	35.126	17.563

(Contd.)

TABLE 7.3 : *Contd..*

Sl.No.	Crosses	Replication I	Replication 2	Total	Average
5.	5 × 5	50.002	26.324	76.326	38.163
6.	6 × 6	38.776	35.098	73.874	36.937
7.	7 × 7	33.134	26.012	59.146	29.573
8.	1 × 2	112.420	69.152	181.572	90.786
9.	1 × 3	78.828	89.560	168.388	84.194
10.	1 × 4	51.956	60.276	112.232	56.116
11.	1 × 5	79.260	62.474	141.734	70.867
12.	1 × 6	63.214	66.046	129.260	64.630
13.	1 × 7	66.928	59.522	126.450	63.225
14.	2 × 3	64.772	68.090	132.862	66.431
15.	2 × 4	69.772	66.174	135.946	67.973
16.	2 × 5	59.372	78.075	137.447	68.723
17.	2 × 6	53.334	63.860	117.194	58.597
18.	2 × 7	62.884	61.885	124.769	62.385
19.	3 × 4	43.720	56.798	100.518	50.259
20.	3 × 5	55.874	58.016	113.890	56.945
21.	3 × 6	66.974	71.296	138.270	69.135
22.	3 × 7	58.042	67.376	125.418	62.709
23.	4 × 5	49.610	35.084	84.694	42.347
24.	4 × 6	52.226	44.908	97.134	48.567
25.	4 × 7	55.284	46.752	102.036	51.018
26.	5 × 6	52.364	47.014	99.378	49.689
27.	5 × 7	38.820	48.192	87.012	43.506
28.	6 × 7	48.146	41.112	89.258	44.629
29.	2 × 1	66.042	100.290	166.332	83.166
30.	3 × 1	74.444	61.668	136.112	68.056
31.	4 × 1	64.940	67.008	131.948	65.974
32.	5 × 1	97.252	70.182	167.434	83.717
33.	6 × 1	38.349	49.890	88.239	44.120
34.	7 × 1	76.602	74.218	150.820	75.410
35.	3 × 2	77.370	53.980	131.350	65.675
36.	4 × 2	75.218	91.900	167.118	83.559
37.	5 × 2	69.492	117.996	187.488	93.744
38.	6 × 2	65.078	83.664	148.742	74.371
39.	7 × 2	78.620	90.978	169.598	84.799
40.	4 × 3	43.530	73.330	116.860	58.430
41.	5 × 3	52.765	55.970	108.735	54.368
42.	6 × 3	78.770	72.032	150.802	75.401
43.	7 × 3	65.967	68.274	134.241	67.121
44.	5 × 4	55.140	49.362	104.502	52.251
45.	6 × 4	59.080	46.885	105.965	52.983
46.	7 × 4	50.654	54.796	105.450	52.725
47.	6 × 5	52.246	55.718	107.964	53.982
48.	7 × 5	45.438	51.990	97.428	48.714
49.	7 × 6	43.860	45.760	89.620	44.810
Total		2880.965	2904.261	5785.226	

The F test for genotypes revealed significant differences among the 49 genotypes for grain yield/plant. Hence, we can carry out combining ability analysis. From the mean values of genotypes over two replications set up a diallel table (Table 7.5).

TABLE 7.4 : ANOVA for grain yield of sorghum in a 7 × 7 diallel

Source	*df*	*SS*	*MS*
Replications	1	5.5378	5.5378
Genotypes	48	27446.4162	571.8003**
Error	48	5866.0195	122.2087

** Significant at 1 per cent level

Various sums of squares are obtained from the values provided in Table 7.5. Thus, sum of squares for general combining ability is computed from the table given below:

Array	$Y_{i\cdot}$	$Y_{\cdot i}$	$(Y_{i\cdot} + Y_{\cdot i})$
1.	472.263	462.888	935.151
2.	453.916	539.575	993.491
3.	397.965	431.130	829.095
4.	367.458	349.870	717.328
5.	415.438	379.741	795.179
6.	382.423	372.365	754.788
7.	403.151	357.045	760.196

$$S.S._{g.c.a.} = \frac{1}{2 \times 7}(935.151^2 + 993.491^2 + ... + 760.196^2) - \frac{2}{49}(2892.614)^2$$

$$= \frac{1}{14}(4843402.2638) - \frac{2}{49}(8367215.753)$$

$$= 345957.3045 - 341519.01033$$

$$= 4438.2941.$$

Sum of squares for specific combining ability is obtained as:

$$\frac{1}{2}\sum_i \sum_j y_{ij}(y_{ij} + y_{ji}) - \frac{1}{2p}\sum_i (Y_{i.} + Y_{.j})^2 + \frac{1}{p^2}Y_{..}^2$$

TABLE 7.5: Diallel table for grain yield, Method 1 (Griffing, 1956a)

Sl. No.	PARENTS							TOTAL
	1	2	3	4	5	6	7	$y_{i.}$
1.	42.445	90.786	84.194	56.116	70.867	64.630	63.225	472.263
2.	83.166	46.641	66.431	67.973	68.723	58.597	62.385	453.916
3.	68.056	65.675	25.186	50.259	56.945	69.135	62.709	397.965
4.	65.974	83.559	58.430	17.563	42.347	48.567	51.018	367.458
5.	83.717	93.744	54.368	52.251	38.163	49.689	43.506	415.438
6.	44.120	74.371	75.401	52.983	53.982	36.937	44.629	382.423
7.	75.410	84.799	67.120	52.725	48.714	44.810	29.573	403.151
Total $y_{.j}$	462.888	539.575	431.130	349.870	379.741	372.365	357.045	

$Y_{..} = 2892\ 614$

Therefore, we need terms $y_{ij}(y_{ij}+y_{ji})$ for parents, F_1s and reciprocal F_1s. Thus for parents it is found as:

y_{ij}	$(y_{ij}+y_{ji})$	$y_{ij}(y_{ij}+y_{ji})$
42.445	(42.445 × 2)	3603.1560
46.641	(46.641 × 2)	4350.7657
25.186	(25.186 × 2)	1268.6691
17.563	(17.563 × 2)	616.9179
38.163	(38.163 × 2)	2912.8291
36.937	(36.937 × 2)	2728.6839
29.573	(29.573 × 2)	1749.1246
		Total 17230.1463

Therefore, $y_{ij}(y_{ij}+y_{ji})$ for parents is 17230.1463.

For F_1s, $y_{ij}(y_{ij}+y_{ji})$ is got as:

y_{ij}	$(y_{ij}+y_{ji})$	yij	$(y_{ij}+y_{ji})$
90.786	(90.786 + 83.166)	50.259	(50.259 + 58.43)
84.194	(84.194 + 68.056)	56.945	(56.945 + 54.368)
56.116	(56.116 + 65.974)	69.135	(69.135 + 75.401)
70.867	(70.867 + 83.717)	62.709	(62.709 + 67.120)
64.630	(64.630 + 44.120)	42.347	(42.347 + 52.251)
63.225	(63.225 + 75.410)	48.567	(48.567 + 52.983)
66.431	(66.431 + 65.675)	51.018	(51.018 + 52.725)
67.973	(67.973 + 83.559)	49.689	(49.689 + 53.982)
68.723	(68.723 + 93.744)	43.506	(43.506 + 48.714)
58.597	(58.597 + 74.371)	44.629	(44.629 + 44.810)
62.385	(62.385 + 84.799)		

$Y_{ij}(Y_{ij}+Y_{ji})$ for F_1s is 166746.5454

In the similar fashion we get $y_{ij}(y_{ij}+y_{ji})$ for reciprocal F_1s as:

y_{ij}	$(y_{ij}+y_{ji})$	yij	$(y_{ij}+y_{ji})$
83.166	(83.166 + 90.786)	58.430	(58.430 + 50.259)
68.056	(68.056 + 84.194)	54.368	(54.368 + 56.945)
65.974	(65.974 + 56.116)	75.401	(75.401 + 69.135)
83.717	(83.717 + 70.867)	67.120	(67.120 + 62.709)
44.120	(44.120 + 64.630)	52.251	(52.251 + 42.347)
75.410	(75.410 + 63.225)	52.983	(52.983 + 48.567)
65.675	(65.675 + 66.431)	52.725	(52.725 + 51.018)

(Contd.)

y_{ij}	$(y_{ij} + y_{ji})$	y_{ij}	$(y_{ij} + y_{ji})$
83.559	(83.559 + 67.973)	53.982	(53.982 + 49.689)
93.744	(93.744 + 68.723)	48.714	(48.714 + 43.506)
74.371	(74.371 + 58.597)	44.810	(44.810 + 44.629)
84.799	(84.799 + 62.385)		

$y_{ij}\,(y_{ij} + y_{ji})$ for reciprocal F_1s is 181919.7502

Thus $\sum_i \sum_j y_{ij}\,(y_{ij} + y_{ji}) = 17230.1463 + 166746.5454 + 181919.7502$

$= 365896.4419.$

The sum of squares for specific combining ability is, therefore,

$$\frac{1}{2}(365896.4419) - (345957.3045) + \frac{1}{49}(2892.614)^2$$
$$= 7750.4216.$$

Sum of squares of reciprocal effects is calculated as:

$$\frac{1}{2}\sum_i \sum_j (y_{ji} - y_{ji})^2$$

We, therefore, calculate $\frac{1}{2}\sum_i \sum_i (y_{ij} - y_{ji})^2$ as shown below:

$(Y_{ij} - Y_{ji})^2$	$(Y_{ij} - Y_{ji})^2$
$(90.786 - 83.166)^2$	$(62.385 - 84.799)^2$
$(84.194 - 68.056)^2$	$(50.259 - 58.430)^2$
$(56.166 - 65.974)^2$	$(56.945 - 54.368)^2$
$(70.867 - 83.717)^2$	$(69.135 - 75.401)^2$
$(64.630 - 44.120)^2$	$(62.709 - 67.120)^2$
$(63.225 - 75.410)^2$	$(42.347 - 52.251)^2$
$(66.431 - 65.675)^2$	$(48.567 - 52.983)^2$
$(67.973 - 83.559)^2$	$(51.018 - 52.725)^2$
$(68.723 - 93.744)^2$	$(49.689 - 53.982)^2$
$(58.597 - 74.371)^2$	$(43.506 - 48.714)^2$
	$(44.629 - 44.810)^2$

Thus $\sum_i \sum_i (y_{ij} - y_{ji})^2 = 3068.9041$

Therefore *S.S.* for reciprocal effect $= \frac{1}{2}(3068.9041)$

$= 1534.4520$

Now set up analysis of variance table for combining ability (Table 7.6).

TABLE 7.6: Analysis of variance for grain yield, Griffing's (1956a) model I, method I

Source	*df*	*SS*	*MS*	*F*
G.C.A.	6	4438.2941	739.7156**	12.105
S.C.A	21	7750.4216	369.067**	6.03
Reciprocal effects	21	1534.4520	73.0691	1.19
Error	48	–	61.1043	

** Significant at 1 per cent level.

In this table, error mean square (Me') is obtained as:

$$\frac{122.2087}{r = 2} = 61.1043,$$

where 122.2087 is the error mean square for 48 degrees of freedom from the analysis of original data (Table 7.4), r is the number of replications.

Results of combining ability analysis reveal that mean squares for general combining ability and specific combining ability are significant. This suggests significant differences among the general combining ability effects of 7 parents and *s.c.a.* effects of 21 crosses. The results also indicate role of additive genetic and non-additive genetic variance in the inheritance of this character. Mean square for reciprocal effects are non-significant. Since the mean squares for general and specific combining ability are significant, we proceed to compute the estimates of *g.c.a.* effects of parental lines and *s.c.a.* effects of $\frac{p(p-1)}{2}$ crosses.

Estimates of general combining ability effects are calculated in method 1 as:

$$\frac{1}{2p}(Y_{i\cdot} + Y_{\cdot i}) - \frac{1}{p^2} Y_{\cdot\cdot}$$

For example, g_1 the estimate of *g.c.a.* effect of 1st parent is got as:

$$\frac{1}{2 \times 7}(935.151) - \frac{1}{49} 2892.614$$

$$= 66.7965 - 59.0329$$

$$= 7.7636^{**}$$

G.c.a. effects of other parents, computed likewise, are presented below:

g_2	11.9307**	g_5	-2.2344
g_3	0.1881	g_6	-5.1194**
g_4	-7.7951**	g_7	-4.7331*

Standard errors required for testing *g.c.a.* effects, and difference between *g.c.a.* effects are calculated as:

$$S.E._{g_i} = \left(\frac{p-1}{2p^2}\sigma^2\right)^{\frac{1}{2}}$$

$$= \left(\frac{6}{2\times 49}61.1043\right)^{\frac{1}{2}}$$

$$= 1.9341.$$

and $$S.E._{(g_i - g_j)} = \left(\frac{1}{p}\sigma^2\right)^{\frac{1}{2}}$$

$$= \left(\frac{1}{7}61.1043\right)^{\frac{1}{2}}$$

$$= 2.9545.$$

The '*t*' test for significance of *g.c.a.* effects would be:

$$t = \frac{g_i - 0}{S.E._{gi}}$$

For example, significance of the *g.c.a.* effect of parent 1, is tested as:

$$\frac{7.7636}{1.9341} = 4.014$$

This value is highly significant (at 1 % level). Hence, we put two asterisks on 7.7636, However, as pointed out earlier, estimates of general combining ability effects exceeding 1.9341 × 1.96 = 3.7908 are regarded as significant at 5 per cent level and those greater than 1.9341 × 2.58 = 4.989 are considered as significant at 1 per cent level. Thus, we can say with confidence that 1 and 2 are desirable parents for grain yield. On the other hand, parents 4, 6 and 7 have significant but negative general combining ability effects, which suggest that they are poor combiners with respect to grain yield. We will be interested to find out which of the two combiners with positive effects, *viz.* 1 and 2, is most desirable. The '*t*' test to discriminate between these lines is then:

$$t = \frac{g_i - g_j}{S.E._{(g_i - g_j)}}$$

$$= \frac{11.9307 - 7.7636}{2.9545} = 1.41$$

This '*t*' suggests that although the *g.c.a.* effect of 2nd parent is larger in magnitude than parent 1, the two *g.c.a.* effects are non-significant. In other words, the two *g.c.a.* effects are *at par*. Therefore, we can choose either or both these parents for hybridisation programme.

If we compare the observed yields of parents 1 and 2, *i.e. per se* performance (Table 7.3), with their *g.c.a.* effects, it appears that there is a close agreement between their *per se* performance and general combining ability effects.

Estimate of the specific combining ability effect of *ij*th cross is calculated as:

$$s_{ij} = \frac{1}{2}(y_{ij} + y_{ji}) - \frac{1}{2p}(Y_{i.} + Y_{.i} + Y_{j.} + Y_{.j}) + \frac{1}{p^2} Y_{..}$$

For example, estimate of *s.c.a.* effect of cross 1 × 2 is obtained as:

$$\frac{1}{2}(90.786 + 83.166) - \frac{1}{14}(472.263 + 462.888 + 453.916 + 539.575) + \frac{1}{49} 2892.614$$

$$= 88.976 - 137.7601 + 59.0329$$

$$= 8.2488.$$

Specific combining ability effects for other crosses are calculated in similar manner (Table 7.7).

Standard errors required to test significance of specific combining ability effects and differences between *s.c.a.* effects are obtained as:

$$S.E._{s_{ij}} = \left(\frac{p^2 - 2p + 2}{2p^2}\sigma^2\right)^{\frac{1}{2}}$$

$$= \left(\frac{49 - 14 + 2}{49 \times 2} 61.1043\right)^{\frac{1}{2}}$$

$$= 4.8031$$

$$S.E._{(s_{ij}-s_{ik})} = \left(\frac{p-1}{p}\sigma^2\right)^{\frac{1}{2}}$$

$$= \left(\frac{6}{7}61.1043\right)^{\frac{1}{2}}$$

$$= 7.237$$

and
$$S.E._{(s_{ij}-s_{kl})} = \left(\frac{p-2}{p}\sigma^2\right)^{\frac{1}{2}}$$

$$= \left(\frac{5}{7}61.1043\right)^{\frac{1}{2}}$$

$$= 6.606.$$

TABLE 7.7 : Estimates of combining ability effects for grain yield of sorghum. Griffing's (1956a) method 1, model I

Inbreds	1	2	3	4	5	6	7
1.	7.763**	8.248	9.140	2.043	12.729**	−7.302	7.254
2.		11.930**	−5.098	12.597**	12.504**	0.639	7.361
3.			0.188	2.918	−1.330	18.166**	10.426*
4.				−7.795**	−1.704	4.656	5.366
5.					−2.234	0.156	−5.955
6.						−5.119**	−4.460
7.							−4.733*

Diagonal entries are *g.c.a.* effects and off-diagonal entries represent *s.c.a.* effects.

*, ** Significant at 5 and 1 per cent levels, respectively.

As a first step, we test the significance of estimates of twenty one *s.c.a.* effects. Values of those *s.c.a.* effects which are greater than 1.96 × 4.8031 = 9.414 are regarded as significant at 5 per cent and those exceeding 2.58 × 4.8031 = 12.392, as significant at 1 per cent. Put one asterisk on *s.c.a.* effects if significant at 5 per cent and two if significant at 1 per cent level.

Results presented in Table 7.7 suggest that *s.c.a.* effects of crosses 1 × 5, 2 × 4, 2 × 5, 3 × 6 and 3 × 7 are significantly different from zero.

Among these crosses, *s.c.a.* effects of 3 × 6, 2 × 4, 2 × 5, 1 × 5 and 3 × 7 are positive. These crosses could, therefore, be regarded as superior cross combinations. On the other hand, actual grain yields recorded for crosses (*per se* performance) point to 1 × 2 and 1 × 3 as superior (Table 7.3). Thus crosses found to be superior on the basis of their *per se* performance and those identified as superior on the basis of their *s.c.a.* effects are not in agreement. It is interesting to note that *s.c.a.* effect of cross 1 × 2, which involves both the parents with significant and positive *g.c.a.* effects, is not significant. Most of the crosses identified as desirable, on the basis of their *s.c.a.* effects have at least one parent with significant and positive *g.c.a.* effect.

A word regarding the choice of crosses is necessary. On the basis of simulation studies, Curnow (1980) concluded that crosses should be selected on the basis of general combining ability effects of constituent parents, unless variance due to specific combining ability exceeds twice the variance of general combining ability. When σ_s^2 is greater that $2\sigma_g^2$, selection should be based on performance of individual cross.

Although the mean square for reciprocal effects is non-significant, reciprocal effect for cross 2 × 1 will be calculated as an illustration. Thus $r_{ij} = ½\,(y_{ij} - y_{ji})$. For example, estimate of r_{12} is:

$$\frac{1}{2}(90.786 - 83.166)$$
$$= 3.81$$

Significance of the reciprocal effects is tested in a manner similar to that demonstrated for general and specific combining ability effects.

7.3. Method 2, Model I

As described earlier, the experimental material for this method comprises of $\frac{p(p-1)}{2}$ F_1s and p inbred lines. This set of progeny families is also known as half-diallel (Singh, 1981). If 3 inbred lines are crossed in a half-diallel fashion, it will result in six progeny families as shown below:

$$\begin{matrix} Y_{11} & Y_{12} & Y_{13} \\ & Y_{22} & Y_{23} \\ & & Y_{33} \end{matrix}$$

where Y_{11}, Y_{22}, Y_{33} represent the genotypes of three inbreds lines and Y_{12}, Y_{13}, Y_{23} are the hybrid combinations. Certain notations, to be used to estimate sum of squares and combining ability effects have meaning as shown below:

$$Y_{i.} = \sum_j Y_{ij} = y_{i1} + y_{i2} + y_{i3}$$

such that $y_{ij} = y_{ji}$. We need not consider for this method $Y_{.j}$

$$Y_{..} = \sum_{i \le j}\sum y_{ij} = y_{11} + y_{12} + y_{13} + y_{22} + y_{23} + y_{33}.$$

The symbol $\sum_{i \le j}\sum$ implies that i is equal to and less than j but not greater than j (because reciprocals are excluded). Thus, in the present case $i = j = y_{11}, y_{22}, y_{33} ...$ and $i < j = y_{12}, y_{13}, y_{23}$, but not y_{21}, y_{31}, y_{32}.

A linear mathematical model for an observation made on ijth genotype could be expressed as:

$$Y_{ij} = \mu + g_i + g_j + s_{ij} + \frac{1}{bc}\sum_k\sum_l e_{ijkl},$$

where μ is population mean, g_i and g_j are general combining ability effects of ith and jth parent, respectively, s_{ij} is the specific combining ability effect such that $s_{ij} = s_{ji}$. e_{ijkl} is the environmental effect associated with $ijkl$th observation. Restrictions imposed are $\sum_i g_i = 0$ and $\sum_j s_{ij} + s_{ii} = 0$ (for each i). Appropriate structure for the analysis of variance is presented in Table 7.8.

Me' = error mean square from *r.b.d./r*

Sum of squares for general (*Sg*) and specific combining ability (*Ss*) effects are found as:

$$Sg = \frac{1}{p+2}\left[\sum_i (Y_i + Y_{ii})^2 - \frac{4}{p}Y^2_{..}\right]$$

and $$Ss = \sum_{i \le j}\sum y_{ij}^2 - \frac{1}{p+2}\sum_i (Y_i + y_{ii})^2 + \frac{2}{(p+1)(p+2)}Y^2_{..}$$

It is important to keep in mind that while computing sum of squares for specific combining ability, we need a term $\sum_{i \le j}\sum y_{ij}^2$, where the squares are to be obtained for parental entries as well as for F_1s. The diagonal elements of diallel table are parental genotypes, and the off-diagonal entries to the right are values of F_1s. Off-diagonal entries to the left are mirror

TABLE 7.8: ANOVA for Griffing's (1956a) diallel analysis, method 2.

Source	*df*	*SS*	*MS*	Expectation mean square: Model I	Model II
General combining ability	$p-1$	*Sg*	*Mg*	$\sigma^2+(p+2)\left(\frac{1}{p-1}\right)\sum_i g_i^2$	$\sigma^2+\sigma^2_s+(p+2)\sigma^2_g$
Specific combining ability	$\frac{p(p-1)}{2}$	*Ss*	*MS*	$\sigma^2+\frac{2}{p(p-1)}\sum_i\sum_j s_{ij}^2$	$\sigma^2+\sigma_s^2$
Error	*m*		*Me'*	σ^2	σ^2

images of right hand side of the diagonal, which are entered in the diallel table for convenience of computational purposes. Hence these values should not be used to calculate sum of squares of *s.c.a.* *F* tests are shown below:

$$Fg = Mg/Me' \text{ for } (p-1) \text{ and } m \text{ degrees of freedom,}$$

$$\text{and} \quad Fs = Ms/Me' \text{ for } \frac{p(p-1)}{2} \text{ and } m \text{ degrees of freedom.}$$

Significance of mean square for general combining ability suggests significant differences among the *g.c.a.* effects of *p* inbred lines. It also implies that additive component of heritable variance is responsible for variation observed for the character. However, reader should note that when model I is adopted, mean square for *g.c.a.* should not be employed to calculate $\sigma^2_{g.c.a.}$ because the object of this model is not to calculate variance component. When mean square for specific combining ability is significant, inference is made that significant differences exist among the $\frac{p(p-1)}{2}$ *s.c.a.* effects. Although the estimate of $\sigma^2_{s.c.a.}$ is not calculated, we can conclude that non-additive variance is an important component for the inheritance of the character being investigated.

When mean square for general combining ability is significant, we proceed to find the estimates of *g.c.a.* effects of inbred parents. Thus $\hat{g}_i$, the estimate of *g.c.a.* effect of *i*th inbred line is got as:

$$\hat{g}_i = \frac{1}{p+2}\left[(Y_{i.}+y_{ii}) - \frac{2}{p}Y_{..}\right]$$

Standard errors required to test significance of *g.c.a* effects and difference between *g.c.a.* effects are got as:

$$S.E._{gi} = \left(\frac{p-1}{p(p+2)}\sigma^2\right)^{\frac{1}{2}} \text{ and } S.E._{(g_i-g_j)} = \left(\frac{2}{p+2}\sigma^2\right)^{\frac{1}{2}}$$

Estimates of specific combining ability effects are calculated when mean square for specific combining ability is significant. One point should be made clear. Several times, *g.c.a.* and/or *s.c.a.* effects are calculated, though the mean squares for these components are non-significant. It is meaningless. Non-significance of mean square for *g.c.a.* suggests that there are non-significant differences among the *g.c.a* effects of p parents. In other words *g.c.a.* effects of all the parental / inbred lines are comparable. Hence, it is a wasteful effort to estimate *g.c.a.* effects. Similarly non-significance of mean square for *s.c.a.* implies that there are non-significant differences among the specific combining ability effects of $\frac{p(p-1)}{2}$ cross-combinations. Hence, *s.c.a.* effects need not be calculated.

Estimate of s_{ij}, the specific combining ability effect of *ij*th cross is computed as:

$$\hat{s}_{ij} = y_{ij} - \frac{1}{p+2}[Y_{i.} + y_{ii} + Y_{j.} + y_{jj}] + \frac{2}{(p+1)(P+2)}Y_{..}$$

Various standard errors required to test the significance of *s.c.a.* effects and differences between *s.c.a.*, effects are calculated as:

$$S.E._{s_{ij}} = \left(\frac{p^2+p+2}{(p+1)(p+2)}\sigma^2\right)^{\frac{1}{2}}$$

$$S.E._{(s_{ij}-s_{ik})} = \left(\frac{2(p+1)}{p+2}\sigma^2\right)^{\frac{1}{2}}$$

and $$S.E._{(s_{ij}-s_{kl})} = \left(\frac{2p}{p+2}\sigma^2\right)^{\frac{1}{2}}$$

7.3.1. *Worked Example*

Seven parents were crossed in a half-diallel fashion so that 28 progeny families, comprising of 21 crosses and 7 parental genotypes, were obtained. The 28 progeny families were grown in a randomised block design with 2 replications. Observations were recorded on grain yield / plant (Table 7.9).

TABLE 7.9: Grain yield/plant (g) of 28 progeny families (Method 2)

Sl. No.	Cross	Replication 1	Replication 2	Total	Mean
1.	1 × 1	40.136	44.754	84.890	42.445
2.	2 × 2	50.002	43.280	93.282	46.641
3.	3 × 3	32.530	17.842	50.372	25.186
4.	4 × 4	21.728	13.398	35.126	17.563
5.	5 × 5	50.002	26.324	76.326	38.163
6.	6 × 6	38.776	35.098	73.874	36.937
7.	7 × 7	33.134	26.012	59.146	29.575
8.	1 × 2	112.420	69.152	181.572	90.786
9.	1 × 3	78.828	89.560	168.388	84.194
10.	1 × 4	51.956	60.276	112.232	56.116
11.	1 × 5	79.260	62.474	141.734	70.867
12.	1 × 6	63.214	66.046	129.260	64.630
13.	1 × 7	66.928	59.522	126.450	63.225
14.	2 × 3	64.772	68.090	132.862	66.431
15.	2 × 4	69.772	66.174	135.946	67.973
16.	2 × 5	59.372	78.075	137.447	68.723
17.	2 × 6	53.334	63.860	117.194	58.597
18.	2 × 7	62.884	61.885	124.769	62.385
19.	3 × 4	43.720	56.798	100.518	50.259
20.	3 × 5	55.874	58.016	113.890	56.945
21.	3 × 6	66.974	71.296	138.270	69.135
22.	3 × 7	58.042	67.376	125.418	62.709
23.	4 × 5	49.610	35.084	84.694	42.347
24.	4 × 6	52.226	44.908	97.134	48.567
25.	4 × 7	55.284	46.752	102.036	51.018
26.	5 × 6	52.364	47.014	99.378	49.689
27.	5 × 7	38.820	48.192	87.012	43.506
28.	6 × 7	48.146	41.112	89.258	44.629
	Total	1550.108	1468.370	3018.478	

Initially the data presented in Table 7.9 are analysed according to the procedure recommended for randomised block design in order to detect significant differences among $\frac{p(p+1)}{2}$ genotypes.

$$\text{Correction factor} = \frac{(3018.478)^2}{56}$$

$$= 162700.1685$$

$$\text{Total } s.s. = (40.136^2 + 50.002^2 + \ldots + 41.112^2) - CF$$

$$= 180248.5327 - 162700.1685$$
$$= 17548.3642$$

$$\text{Genotypes } s.s. = \frac{1}{2}(84.89^2 + 93.282^2 + ... + 89.258^2) - CF$$
$$= \frac{1}{2}(355849.109) - CF$$
$$= 15224.386$$

$$\text{Replications } s.s. = \frac{1}{28}(1550.108^2 + 1468.37^2) - CF$$
$$= 119.3053$$

$$\text{Error } s.s. = 17548.3642 - (15224.386 + 119.3035)$$
$$= 2204.6726.$$

Now set up an analysis of variance table (Table 7.10).

TABLE 7.10: ANOVA for grain yield/plant. Method 2, Model I

Source	*df*	*SS*	*MS*	*F*
Replications	1	119.3053	119.3053	1.46
Gonotypes	27	15224.386	563.8661**	6.90
Error	27	2204.6726	81.6545	

Results of the analysis reveal that there are highly significant differences among 28 genotypes for grain yield. Therefore, combining ability analysis can be carried out. A diallel table is set up from the mean values of 28 genotypes over two replications (Table 7.11).

$$\text{Grand total } (Y..) = \text{Total of } F_1s + \text{total of parents}$$
$$= 1272.731 + 236.510$$
$$= 1509.241.$$

In order to calculate sum of squares for general combining ability, we need $\sum_i (Y_{i.} + y_{ii})^2$. It is obtained as shown below:

Array	y_{ii}	$Y_{i.}$	$(y_{ii} + Y_{i.})$
1.	42.445	472.263	514.708
2.	46.641	461.536	508.177
3.	25.186	414.859	440.045
4.	17.563	333.843	351.406
5.	38.163	370.240	408.403
6.	36.937	372.184	409.121
7.	29.575	357.047	386.622

TABLE 7.11: Diallel Table for grain yield/plant (Method 2 of Griffing, 1956a)

	INBRED PARENTS							Array total
	1	2	3	4	5	6	7	$(Y_{i.})$
1.	42.445	90.786	84.194	56.116	70.867	64.630	63.225	472.263
2.	90.786	46.641	66.431	67.973	68.723	58.597	62.385	461.536
3.	84.194	66.431	25.186	50.259	56.945	69.135	62.709	414.859
4.	56.116	67.973	50.259	17.563	42.347	48.567	51.018	333.843
5.	70.867	68.723	56.945	42.347	38.163	49 689	43.506	370.240
6.	64.630	58.597	69.135	48.567	49.689	36.937	44.629	372.184
7.	63.225	62.385	62.709	51.018	43.506	44.629	29.575	357.047
$Y_{.j}$	472.263	461.536	414.859	333.843	370.240	372.184	357.047	

Thus $\sum_i (Y_{i.} + y_{ii})^2 = 1323943.5413.$

The sum of squares for *g.c.a.* is, therefore,

$$\frac{1}{p+2}\left[\sum_i (Y_{i.} + y_{ii})^2 - \frac{4}{p} Y^2_{..}\right]$$

$$= \frac{1}{9}\left[1323943.5413 - \frac{4}{7} 1509.241^2\right]$$

$$= 2482.0826.$$

Sum of squares for specific combining ability is found as:

$$\sum_i \sum_{\leq i} y_{ij}^2 - \frac{1}{p+2} \sum_i (Y_{i.} + y_{ii})^2 + \frac{2}{(p+1)(p+2)} Y^2_{..}$$

We, therefore, calculate $\sum_i \sum_{\leq j} y_{ij}^2$ as:

$(42.445^2 + 90.786^2 + 84.194^2 + 56.116^2 + 70.867^2 + 64.630^2 + 63.225^2$
$+ 46.641^2 + 66.431^2 + 67.973^2 + 68.723^2 + 58.597^2 + 62.385^2$
$+ 25.186^2 + 50.259^2 + 56.945^2 + 69.135^2 + 62.709^2$
$+ 17.563^2 + 42.347^2 + 48.567^2 + 51.018^2$
$+ 38.163^2 + 49.689^2 + 43.506^2$
$+ 36.937^2 + 44.629^2$
$+ 29.575^2)$
$= 88962.382$

Hence, *s.s.* for specific combining ability is obtained as:

$$88962.382 - \frac{1}{9}(1323943.5413) + \frac{2}{72} 1509.241^2$$

$$= 5130.0067$$

The error mean square fcr combining ability analysis is got as:

$$\frac{81.6545}{2} = 40.8272.$$

Analysis of variance for combining ability is now set up (Table 7.12).

TABLE 7.12: ANOVA for combining ability. Method 2 Model I (Griffing, 1956a)

Source	*df*	*SS*	*MS*	*F*
General combining ability	6	2482.0826	413.6804**	10.13
Specific combining ability	21	5130.0067	244.2860**	5.98
Error	27	—	40.8272	

Results of analysis revealed significance of mean squares for *g.c.a* and *s.c.a.* This suggests significant differences among the *g.c.a.* effects and also the *s.c.a.* effects. Inference could also be made that additive and non-additive components of heritable variance are involved in the inheritance.

Here one thing needs clarification. When mean squares for *g.c.a.* and *s.c.a.* are significant, scientists are tempted to conclude relative predominance of either additive genetic variance or non-additive variance on the basis of face value of mean squares corresponding to *g.c.a.* and *s.c.a.*, respectively. For example, when mean square for *g.c.a.* is larger than *s.c.a.*, conclusion is made that $\sigma^2_{g.c.a.}$ or σ^2_A is predominant cause of variation. This is erroneous. Although in the present example we assumed model I, let us calculate the estimates of $\sigma^2_{g.c.a.}$ and $\sigma^2_{s.c.a.}$, following Griffing (1956a) from mean squares. Thus,

$$\hat{\sigma}^2_{g.c.a.} = \frac{1}{p+2}[Mg - Ms]$$

$$= \frac{1}{9}(413.6804 - 244.286)$$

$$= 18.8216$$

and $$\hat{\sigma}^2_{s.c.a.} = Ms - Me'$$

$$= 244.2860 - 40.8272$$

$$= 203.4588.$$

Significance of sampling variance is tested in usual way. For this test, variance of estimate is required. According to Comstock and Moll (1963) if all the contributing factors are normally distributed, variance of a mean square is calculated as:

$$V(M) = \frac{2(EM)^2}{f}$$

Where *EM* is expectation mean square and *f* refers to the degrees of freedom associated with mean square .

Variance of any estimate can be written as a function of variance of mean squares contributing to the estimate.

The steps involved are:

(i) Write down the function of a mean square that provides estimate of variance component,

(ii) Multiply variance of each mean square by square of its coefficients in function.

(iii) Sum of these products is the sampling variance of whole function.

Thus, function of variance attributable to general combining ability is (Table 7.8)

$$\frac{Mg - Ms}{(p+2)}$$

$$\therefore\ V(M) = \frac{1}{(p+2)^2}\left[\frac{2(Mg)^2}{(p-1)} + \frac{2(Ms)^2}{p(p-1)/2}\right]$$

$$= \frac{1}{(9)^2}\left[\frac{2(413.6804)^2}{6} + \frac{2(244.2860)^2}{21}\right]$$

$$= 774.4101$$

$$\therefore\ SE\sigma_g^2 = \sqrt{774.4101}$$

$$= 27.828$$

Likewise variance for σ_s^2 is calculated. The estimates of σ_g^2 and σ_s^2 along with their standard errors are thus:

$$\sigma_g^2 = 18.8216 \pm 27.828$$

$$\sigma_s^2 = 203.4588 \pm 76.202$$

This shows that estimate of σ_g^2 is non significant but σ_s^2 is significant. Thus variance attributable to *s.c.a.* is important for variation observed for grain yield/plant. Hence, if at all inference is to be made regarding the importance of additive or non-additive components of heritable variances, it should be based on estimates of $\sigma_{g.c.a.}^2$ and $\sigma_{s.c.a.}^2$.

When the mean squares for *g.c.a.* and *s.c.a.* are significant estimates of general and specific combining ability are calculated.

Estimate of general combining ability effect ($\hat{g}_i$) of *i*th parent is got as:

$$\hat{g}_i = \frac{1}{p+2}\left[(Y_{i.} + y_{ii}) - \frac{2}{p}Y_{..}\right]$$

For example, *g.c.a.* effect of parent 1 may be computed as:

$$\hat{g}_1 = \frac{1}{9}\left[514.708 - \frac{2}{7}1509.241\right]$$

$$= \frac{1}{9}\ [514.708 - 431.211]$$

$$= 9.2774^{**}$$

Estimates of general combining ability effects of other parents calculated in similar manner are presented below:

$\hat{g}_2 = 8.5517^{**}$ $\quad\quad$ $\hat{g}_5 = -2.5342$

$\hat{g}_3 = 0.9815$ $\quad\quad$ $\hat{g}_6 = -2.4544$

$\hat{g}_4 = -8.8672^{**}$ $\quad\quad$ $\hat{g}_7 = -4.9543^{*}$

Standard errors, required to test significance of general combining ability effects and differences between *g.c.a.* effects, are calculated as:

$$S.E._{\hat{g}_i} = \left(\frac{p-1}{p(p+2)}\sigma^2\right)^{\frac{1}{2}}$$

$$= \left(\frac{6}{63}40.8272\right)^{\frac{1}{2}}$$

$$= 1.9718$$

and $$S.E._{(\hat{g}_i - \hat{g}_j)} = \left(\frac{2}{p+2}\sigma^2\right)^{\frac{1}{2}}$$

$$= \left[\frac{2}{9}40.8272\right]^{\frac{1}{2}}$$

$$= 3.012$$

Significance of *g.c.a.* effect is tested by '*t*' test as:

$$t = \frac{g_i - 0}{S.E._{gi}}$$

For example, significance of *g.c.a.* effect of parent 1 is tested as:

$$\frac{9.2774}{1.9718} = 4.705$$

This value is highly significant. Alternatively, we regard the estimate of *g.c.a.* effect as significant, if the *g.c.a.* effect is greater than $S.E._{gi} \times 1.96$. Thus, the *g.c.a.* effects are significant at 5 per cent if their values exceed 3.864. We find that although the *g.c.a.* effects of parents 1, 2, 4 and 7 are significant, only two parents are desirable combiners, *viz.*, 1 and 2, because their *g.c.a.* effects are positive. Parents 4 and 7 are unsatisfactory. If the difference between *g.c.a.* effects of parents 1 and 2 is greater than $1.96 \times S.E._{(g_i - g_j)}$, *i.e.* 5.903, we can conclude that the two *g.c.a.* effects are significantly different from each other. Since the difference is 0.7257, we infer that both the parents are equally desirable.

Estimates of specific combining ability effects are computed as:

$$\hat{s}_{ij} = y_{ij} - \frac{1}{p+2}(Y_{i.} + y_{ii} + y_{jj}) + \frac{2}{(p+1)(p+2)} Y_{..}$$

For example, s_{12}, the estimate of *s.c.a.* effect of cross 1 × 2 is got as:

$$s_{12} = 90.786 - \frac{1}{9}[514.708 + 508.177] + \frac{2}{72} 1509.241$$
$$= 19.055^*$$

Specific combining ability effects of rest of the crosses are arrived at in a similar manner (Table 7.13).

TABLE 7.13: General and specific combining ability effects (Method 2. Model I) for grain yield

	1	2	3	4	5	6	7
1.	9.2774**	19.055**	20.0336**	1.8044	10.2224	3.9056	5.0005
2.		8.5517**	2.9963	14.3870*	8.8040	-1.4017	4.8861
3.			0.9815	4.2433	4.5963	16.7065**	12.7804*
4.				-8.8672**	-0.1259	5.9873	10.9381
5.					-2.5342	0.7763	-2.9068
6.						-2.4544	-1.8635
7.							-4.9543*

Diagonal entries are *g.c.a.* effects, and off-diagonal entries *s.c.a.* effects.

*, ** Significant at 5 and 1 per cent levels, respectively.

Three standard errors, which are necessary in connection with testing the significance of *s.c.a.* effects, and differences between various *s.c.a.* effects are calculated as:

$$S.E._{\hat{s}_{ii}} = \left(\frac{p^2 + p + 2}{(p+1)(p+2)} \sigma^2 \right)^{\frac{1}{2}}$$

$$= \left(\frac{58}{72} 40.8272 \right)^{\frac{1}{2}}$$

$$= 5.7348$$

$$S.E._{(\hat{s}_{ij} - s_{ik})} = \left(\frac{2(p+1)}{p+2} \sigma^2 \right)^{\frac{1}{2}}$$

$$= \left[\frac{16}{9} 40.8272 \right]^{\frac{1}{2}}$$

$$= 8.5194$$

and $$S.E._{(\hat{s}_{ij} - s_{kl})} = \left(\frac{2p}{p+2} \sigma^2 \right)^{\frac{1}{2}}$$

$$= \left[\frac{14}{9} 40.8272 \right]^{\frac{1}{2}}$$

$$= 7.9692.$$

Significance of *s.c.a.* effect is tested by '*t*' test. Thus,

$$t = \frac{s_{ij} - 0}{S.E._{sij}}$$

Alternatively those *s.c.a.* effects which exceed the values 11.2402, ($S.E._{sij} \times 1.96$) and 14.795, ($S.E._{sij} \times 2.58$) could be regarded as significant at 5 and 1 per cent levels, respectively. Estimates of *s.c.a.* effects of crosses 1 × 2, 1 × 3, 2 × 4, 3 × 6 and 3 × 7 are significant. All the significant *s.c.a.* effects are positive in direction. Therefore, all these crosses are regarded as desirable. Next step is to test the significance of difference between *s.c.a.* effects of two crosses, which include one common parent. This '*t*' test is performed as shown below for crosses 1 × 2 and 1 × 3:

$$t = \frac{20.0336 - 19.055}{8.5194}$$

$= 0.1148.$

This ratio is non-significant when the value is referred to the '*t*' table. Both the crosses are, therefore, equally desirable. Alternatively, if the difference between *s.c.a.* effects of two crosses having one parent in common is greater than $8.5194 \times 1.96 = 16.698$, *s.c.a.* effects are regarded as significantly different at 5 per cent level. In the present example, crosses 1×2 and 1×3, 3×6 and 3×7 are *at par* with each other. In order to test the significance of difference between *s.c.a.* effects of two crosses, having no parent in common, standard error of difference, *i.e.* $S.E._{sij-skl}$, is required. For the present example, *s.c.a.* effects of two such crosses will be significantly different, if the difference between *s.c.a.* effects exceeds $7.9692 \times 1.96 = 15.6196$.

From the analysis it appears that parental lines 1 and 2 are desirable combiners. Reference to the Table 7.11 shows that the *per se* performance of these lines is superior than other lines. There is thus a close agreement between parental lines selected on the basis of *per se* performance and their *g.c.a.* effects. This is true with respect to the poor combiner parental line 4 as well.

There is a close agreement between crosses selected on the basis of their *s.c.a.* effects and *per se* performance. Cross combination 1×2 has both the parents which are desirable combiners. Hence selection from the segregating generations of this cross is excepted to lead to substantial genetic improvement.

7.4 Method 3, Model I

Unlike methods 1 and 2, experimental material for this method comprises of $\frac{p(p-1)}{2}$ $F_{1}s$ and $\frac{p(p-1)}{2}$ reciprocal F_1s. In other words, $p\,(p-1)$ progeny families constitute the experimental material for this method. Hence this method is known as "modified diallel" (Griffing, 1956b). When random samples are drawn from the population of inbred lines, "modified diallel" analysis is expected to provide unbiased estimates of population parameters (Griffing, 1956b).

Suppose 3 inbred lines are chosen to develop experimental material for this method. Diallel mating, according to method 3, will result in progeny families shown below:

$$\begin{matrix} 0 & Y_{12} & Y_{13} \\ Y_{21} & 0 & Y_{23} \\ Y_{31} & Y_{32} & 0 \end{matrix}$$

While calculating sum of squares and combining ability effects some notations are used. Meanings of these notations are given below:

$$Y_{i.} = \sum_{j \neq i} y_{ij}\text{, e.g. } Y_{2.} = y_{21} + y_{23}$$

$$Y_{.j} = \sum_{i \neq j} y_{ij}\text{, e.g. } Y_{.2} = y_{12} + y_{32}$$

and $$Y_{..} = \sum_{i \neq j}\sum y_{ij} = y_{12} + y_{13} + y_{21} + y_{23} + y_{31} + y_{32}$$

Among these notations, signs $i \neq j$ or $j \neq i$ indicate that i is not equal to j and j not equal to i, respectively and remind that parental genotypes do not form a part of the experimental material.

Observation recorded on ijth genotype could be linearly expressed as:

$$Y_{ij} = \mu + g_i + g_j + r_{ij} + s_{ij} + \frac{1}{bc}\sum_k\sum_l e_{ij}kl.$$

Where μ is the population mean, g_i and g_j are the *g.c.a.* effects of ith and jth parent, respectively, s_{ij} is the specific combining ability effect such that $s_{ij} = s_{ji}$, and r_{ij} is the reciprocal effect such that $r_{ij} = -r_{ji}$. e_{ijkl} is the error effect peculiar to $ijkl$th observation.

Restrictions imposed on combining ability effects are $\sum_i g_i = 0$, and $\sum_{i \neq j} s_{ij} = 0$ (for each j). Format for analysis of variance is given in Table 7.14, along with expectation mean squares. Construction of this analysis was provided by Yates (1947) and detailed derivation of the expectation mean squares for random effects model was given Kempthorne (1952).

TABLE 7.14: Format for combining ability analysis method 3

Source	*df*	*SS*	*MS*	Expectation mean squares	
				Model I	Model II
General combining ability	$(p-1)$	*Sg*	*Mg*	$\sigma^2 + 2(p-2)\left(\frac{1}{p-1}\right)\sum_i g_i^2$	$\sigma^2 + 2\sigma_s^2 + 2(p-2)\sigma_g^2$
Specific combining ability	$\frac{p(p-3)}{2}$	*Ss*	*Ms*	$\sigma^2 + 2\frac{2}{p(p-3)}\sum_{i<j}\sum s_{ij}^2$	$\sigma^2 + 2\sigma_s^2$
Reciprocal effects	$\frac{p(p-1)}{2}$	*Sr*	*Mr*	$\sigma^2 + 2\frac{2}{p(p-1)}\sum_{i<j}\sum r_{ij}^2$	$\sigma^2 + 2\sigma_r^2$
Error	*m*		*Me'*	σ^2	σ^2

In this method also, *Me'* is found as:

$$\frac{Me}{bc}$$

where *Me* is the error mean square from original analysis (*r.b.d.*), *b* is the number of replications and *c* the number of plant/plot. The three sums of squares are calculated as:

$$Sg = \frac{1}{2(p-2)}\sum_i (Y_{i.} + Y_{.i})^2 - \frac{2}{p(p-2)}Y_{..}^2$$

$$Ss = \frac{1}{2}\sum_i\sum_j (y_{ij} + y_{ji})^2 - \frac{1}{2(p-2)}\sum_i (Y_{i.} + y_{.i})^2 + \frac{1}{(p-1)(p-2)}Y_{..}^2$$

$$\text{and } Sr = \frac{1}{2}\sum_{i<j}\sum (y_{ij} - y_{ji})^2$$

Significance of various mean squares is tested by *F* tests. For mean squares of general combining ability, specific combining ability and reciprocal effects, *Me'* is used as denominator. Only when mean squares for *g.c.a.*, *s.c.a.* and reciprocal effects are significant we proceed to calculate the estimates of general and specific combining ability effects, as well as the reciprocal effects.

Estimate of general combining ability effect for the *i*th parent ($\hat{g}_i$)

is found as:

$$\hat{g}_i = \frac{1}{2p(p-2)}[p(Y_{i.} + y_{.i}) - 2Y_{..}]$$

Significance of *g.c.a.* effects is tested by means of '*t*' test. Standard error required to test this significance is got as:

$$S.E._{\hat{g}_i} = \left(\frac{p-1}{2p(p-2)}\sigma^2\right)^{\frac{1}{2}}$$

Standard error to test significance of difference between *g.c.a.* effects is calculated as:

$$S.E.(\hat{g}_i - \hat{g}_j) = \left(\frac{1}{p-2}\sigma^2\right)^{\frac{1}{2}}$$

For $\frac{p(p-1)}{2}$ F_1s, estimates of specific combining ability effects are found as:

$$\hat{S}_{ij} = \frac{1}{2}(y_{ij} + y_{ji}) - \frac{1}{2(p-2)} \cdot (Y_{i.} + Y_{.i} + Y_{j.} + Y_{.j}) + \frac{1}{(p-1)(p-2)} Y_{..}$$

Standard error required to test the significance of estimates of *s.c.a.* effects ($S.E._{sij}$) is got as:

$$S.E._{\hat{s}_{ij}} = \left(\frac{p-3}{2(p-1)}\sigma^2\right)^{\frac{1}{2}}$$

Other standard errors needed in connection with testing the significance of differences between *s.c.a.* effects are found as:

$$S.E._{(\hat{s}_{ij} - \hat{s}_{ik})} = \left(\frac{p-3}{p-2}\sigma^2\right)^{\frac{1}{2}}$$

$$S.E._{(\hat{s}_{ij} - \hat{s}_{kl})} = \left(\frac{p-4}{p-2}\sigma^2\right)^{\frac{1}{2}}$$

Estimate of the reciprocal effect of *ij*th cross, $\hat{r}_{ij}$, is got as:

$$\hat{r}_{ij} = \frac{1}{2}(y_{ij} - y_{ji})$$

Standard error required to test the significance of reciprocal effects, $S.E._{\hat{r}_{ij}}$ is calculated as:

$$\left(\frac{1}{2}\sigma^2\right)^{\frac{1}{2}}$$

7.4.1 *Worked Example*

Seven inbred lines of sorghum were crossed to produce 21 F_1s and 21 reciprocal F_1s, which were raised in a randomised block design with two replications. Grain yield/plant was recorded in each replication on 42 crosses (Table 7.15).

Data are subjected initially to the analysis of variance according to the method suggested for randomised block design. Various sum of squares are calculated as:

$$\text{Correction factor} = \frac{(5312.21)^2}{84}$$

$$= 335947.3224$$

$$\text{Total sum of squares} = (112.42^2 + 78.828^2 + \ldots + 45.76^2) - CF$$

$$= 357118.3332 - 335947.3224$$

$$= 21171.0108$$

$$\text{Genotype s.s.} = \tfrac{1}{2}(181.572^2 + 168.388^2 + \ldots + 89.62^2) - CF$$

$$= 15787.7213$$

$$\text{Replication sum of squares} = 81.8065$$

$$\text{Error sum of squares} = 21171.0108 - (15787.7213 + 81.8065)$$

$$= 5301.483$$

Analysis of variance table is presented in Table 7.16.

Genotype mean square is found to be highly significant suggesting significant genetic differences among the 42 cross combinations.

Combining ability analysis is now taken up on mean values of 42 crosses over two replications (Table 7.17).

TABLE 7.15: Grain yield/plant (g) of p (p – 1) genotypes of sorghum (Method 3)

Sl. No.	Cross	Replication I	Replication 2	Total	Mean
1.	1 × 2	112.420	69.152	181.572	90.786
2	1 × 3	78.828	89.560	168.388	84 194
3	1 × 4	51.956	60.276	112.232	56.116
4.	1 × 5	79.260	62.474	141.734	70.867
5.	1 × 6	63.214	66.046	129.260	64.630
6.	1 × 7	66.928	59.522	126.450	63.225
7.	2 × 3	64.772	68.090	132.862	66.431
8.	2 × 4	69.772	66.174	135.946	67.973
9.	2 × 5	59.372	78.075	137.447	68.723
10	2 × 6.	53.334	63.860	117.194	58.597
11.	2 × 7	62.884	61.885	124.769	62.385
12.	3 × 4	43.720	56.798	100.518	50.259
13.	3 × 5	55.874	58.016	113.890	56.945
14.	3 × 6	66.974	71.296	138.270	69.135
15.	3 × 7	58.042	67.376	125.418	62.709
16.	4 × 5	49.610	35.084	84.694	42.347
17.	4 × 6	52.226	44.908	97.134	48.567
18.	4 × 7	55.284	46.752	102.036	51.018
19.	5 × 6	52.364	47.014	99.378	49.689
20.	5 × 7	38.820	48.192	87.012	43.506
21.	6 × 7	48.146	41.112	89.258	44.629
22.	2 × 1	66.042	100.290	166.332	83.166
23.	3 × 1	74.444	61.668	136.112	68.056
24.	4 × 1	64.940	67.008	131.948	65.974
25.	5 × 1	97.252	70.182	167.434	83.717
26.	6 × 1	38.349	49.890	88.239	44.120
27.	7 × 1	76.602	74.218	150.820	75.410
28.	3 × 2	77.370	53.980	131 350	65.675
29.	4 × 2	75.218	91.900	167.118	83.559
30.	5 × 2	69.492	117.996	187.488	93.744
31.	6 × 2	65.078	83.664	148.742	74.371
32.	7 × 2	78.620	90.978	169.598	84.799
33.	4 × 3	43.530	73.330	116.860	58.430
34.	5 × 3	52.765	55.970	108.735	54.368
35.	6 × 3	78.770	72.032	150.802	75.401
36.	7 × 3	65.967	68.274	134.241	67.121
37.	5 × 4	55.140	49.362	104.502	52.251
38.	6 × 4	59.080	46.885	105.965	52.983
39.	7 × 4	50.654	54.796	105.450	52.725
40.	6 × 5	52.246	55.718	107.964	53.982
41.	7 × 5	45.438	51.990	97.428	48.714
42.	7 × 6	43.860	45.760	89.620	44.810
	Total	2614.657	2697.553	5312.210	

TABLE 7.16 : Analysis of variance for grain yield/plant (Method 3)

Source	*df*	*SS*	*MS*	*F*
Replications	1	81.8065	81.8065	
Genotypes	41	15787.7213	385.0663**	2.97
Error	41	5301.483	129.3044	

**Significant at 1 percent level.

From the marginal totals of Table 7.17, sum of squares for general combining ability is calculated as shown below:

Arrays	$Y_{i.}$	$Y_{.i}$	$(Y_{i.} + Y_{.i})$
1.	429.818	420.443	850.261
2.	407.275	492.934	900.209
3.	372.779	405.945	778.724
4.	349.895	332.307	682.202
5.	377.275	341.578	718.853
6.	345.486	335.428	680.914
7.	373.579	327.472	701.051

Therefore $\sum_i (Y_{i.} + Y_{.i})^2 = 4076996.6643$

$$S.S._g = \frac{1}{2(p-2)} \sum_i (Y_{i.} + Y_{.i})^2 - \frac{2}{p(p-2)} Y_{..}^2$$

$$= \frac{1}{10}(4076996.6643) - \frac{2}{35} 2656.107^2$$

$$= 407699.6664 - 403137.3940$$

$$= 4562.2724.$$

TABLE 7.17: Diallel table for grain yield (Method 3)

	PARENTS							Array total
	1	2	3	4	5	6	7	$Y_{i.}$
1.	–	90.786	84.194	56.116	70.867	64.630	63.225	429.818
2.	83.166	–	66.431	67.973	68.723	58.597	62.385	407.275
3.	68.056	65.675	–	50.259	56.945	69.135	62.709	372.779
4.	65.974	83.559	58.430	–	42.347	48.567	51.018	349.895
5	83.717	93.744	54.368	52.251	–	49.689	43.506	377.275
6	44.120	74.371	75.401	52.983	53.982	–	44.629	345.486
7	75.410	84.799	67.121	52.725	48.714	44.810	–	373.579
Array total Y	420.443	492.934	405.945	332.307	341.578	335.428	327.472	
								Grand total 2656.107

Sum of squares for specific combining ability requires a quantity $\sum_{i<j}\sum (y_{ij}+y_{ji})^2$, which is calculated as:

y_{ij}	y_{ji}	$(y_{ij}+y_{ji})$
90.786	83.166	173.952
84.194	68.056	152.250
56.116	65.974	122.090
70.867	83.717	154.585
64.630	44.120	108.750
63.225	75.410	138.635
66.431	65.675	132.106
67.973	83.559	151.532
68.723	93.744	162.467
58.597	74.371	132.968
62.385	84.799	147.184
50.259	58.430	108.689
56.945	54.368	111.313
69.135	75.401	144.536
62.709	67.121	129.830
42.347	52.251	94.598
48.567	52.983	101.550
51.018	52.725	103.743
49.689	53.982	103.671
43.506	48.714	92.220
44.629	44.810	89.439

$$\sum_{i<j}\sum (y_{ij}+y_{ji})^2 = 348666.5553$$

S.s. for specific combining ability is, therefore, got as:

$$\frac{1}{2}(348666.5553) - \frac{1}{10}(4076996.6643) + \frac{1}{30}\,2656.107^2$$

$= 1797.091$

Finally, we calculate the sum of squares for reciprocal effects as:

$$\frac{1}{2}\sum_i\sum_j (y_{ij}-y_{ji})^2.$$

Value of $\sum_i\sum_j (y_{ij}-y_{ji})^2$ is got from the following table:

y_{ij}	y_{ji}	$y_{ij} - y_{ji}$	y_{ij}	y_{ji}	$y_{ij} - y_{ji}$
90.786	83.166	7.620	62.385	84.799	-22.414
84.194	68.056	16.138	50.259	58.430	-8.171
56.116	65.974	-9.858	56.945	54.368	2.577
70.867	83.717	-12.850	69.135	75.401	-6.266
64.630	44.120	20.510	62.709	67.121	-4.412
63.225	75.410	-12.185	42.347	52.251	-9.904
66.431	65.675	0.756	48.567	52.983	-4.416
67.973	83.559	-15.586	51.018	52.725	-1.707
68.723	93.744	-25.021	49.689	53.982	-4.293
58.597	74.371	-15.774	43.506	48.714	-5.208
			44.629	44.810	-0.181

Hence, *s.s.* for reciprocal effects is:

$$\frac{1}{2}(3068.9129)$$
$$= 1534.4564$$

Analysis of variance table is now set up (Table 7.18).

TABLE 7.18: Combining ability analysis for grain yield (Method 3, Model I)

Source	*df*	*SS*	*MS*	*F*
General combining ability	6	4562.2724	760.3787**	11.76
Specific combining ability	14	1797.091	128.3636*	1.98
Reciprocal effects	21	1534.4564	73.0693	1.13
Error	41		64.6522	

*, ** Significant at 5 and 1 per cent levels, respectively.

Mean squares for *g.c.a.* and *s.c.a.* are significant (Table 7.18). Hence we can conclude that there are significant differences among the general combining ability effects of seven parents and *s.c.a.* effects of 21 crosses. Since the mean square for reciprocal effects is non-significant there is no indication of maternal inheritance.

Significance of mean square for general combining ability suggests that additive genetic variance is responsible for variation observed for yield in this material. Non-additive variance is also involved in the inheritance of this trait.

Estimates of general combining ability effects are now calculated. For example $\hat{g}_1$, the estimate of *g.c.a.* effect of parent 1, is got as:

$$\hat{g}_1 = \frac{1}{2p(p-2)}[Y_i.+y_{.i})-2Y..]$$

$$= \frac{1}{70}\ [7(850.261) - 2\ (2656.107)]$$
$$= 9.1373$$

Estimates of *g.c.a.* effects of rest of the parents are obtained in similar fashion (Table 7.19). Standard errors which are required to test the significance of *g.c.a.* effects and differences between two *g.c.a.* effects are calculated as:

$$S.E._{\hat{g}_i} = \left(\frac{p-1}{2p(p-2)}\sigma^2\right)^{\frac{1}{2}}$$

$$= \left(\frac{6}{70}64.6522\right)^{\frac{1}{2}}$$

$$=2.354$$

and $$S.E._{(\hat{g}_i - \hat{g}_j)} = \left(\frac{1}{p-2}\sigma^2\right)^{\frac{1}{2}}$$

$$= \left(\frac{1}{5}64.6522\right)^{\frac{1}{2}}$$

$$= 3.5988$$

Significance of *g.c.a.* effect is tested by means of '*t*' test. Alternatively, if *g.c.a.* effects exceed value 2.354 × 1.96 = 4.613 and 2.354 × 2.58 = 6.073, we infer that the *g.c.a.* effects are significant at 5 and 1 per cent levels, respectively. Although *g.c.a.* effects of all the parents, except 3 and 5 are significant, direction is desirable only for parents 1 and 2. Other parents have negative general combining ability effects and, therefore, appear undesirable. Which of the parents having significant and positive *g.c.a.* effect is more desirable? Answer is provided by a '*t*' test involving a ratio of difference of *g.c.a.* effects to the standard error of differences of *g.c.a.* effects. Thus,

$$t = \frac{14.1321 - 9.1373}{3.5958} = 1.38$$

Since the '*t*' test is non-significant both the parents could be regarded as equally desirable for hybridisation.

Let us calculate the specific combining ability effects. *S.c.a.* effect of cross 1 × 2 is found as:

$$s_{12} = \frac{1}{2}(Y_{12} + Y_{21}) - \frac{1}{2(p-2)}(Y_1.+Y._1+Y_2.+Y._2) + \frac{1}{(p-1)(p-2)}Y..$$

$$= \frac{1}{2}(173.952) - \frac{1}{10}(850.261 + 900.209) + \frac{1}{30}2656.107$$

$$= 86.976 - 175.047 + 88.5369$$

$$= 0.4659$$

Estimates of specific combining ability effects of rest of the crosses are obtained in a like manner (Table 7.19). Standard errors required to test the significance of *s.c.a.* effects and differences between various *s.c.a.* effects are found as:

$$S.E._{\hat{s}_{ij}} = \left(\frac{p-3}{2(p-1)}\sigma^2\right)^{\frac{1}{2}}$$

$$= \left(\frac{4}{12}64.6533\right)^{\frac{1}{2}}$$

$$= 4.6422$$

$$S.E._{(\hat{S}_{ij}-\hat{S}_{ik})} = \left(\frac{p-3}{p-2}\sigma^2\right)^{\frac{1}{2}}$$

$$= \left(\frac{4}{5}64.6522\right)^{\frac{1}{2}}$$

$$= 7.1917$$

and lastly $$S.E._{(\hat{s}_{ij}-\hat{s}_{kl})} = \left(\frac{p-4}{p-2}\sigma^2\right)^{\frac{1}{2}}$$

$$= \left(\frac{3}{5}64.6522\right)^{\frac{1}{2}}$$

$$= 6.2282.$$

TABLE 7.19: General and specific combining ability effects for grain yield (Method 3)

	PARENTS						
	1	2	3	4	5	6	7
1.	9.137**	0.4659	1.7634	-3.6644	8.9175	-10.2056*	2.7232
2.		14.1321**	-13.3034**	6.0618	7.8642	-3.0914	2.0029
3.			1.9836	-3.2112	-5.5643	14.8440**	5.4744
4.				-7.6685**	-4.2696	3.0003	2.0831
5.					-4.0034	0.3957	-7.3435
6.						-7.7973**	-4.9401
7.							-5.7836*

Diagonal entries are *g.c.a.* effects and off-diagonal entries are *s.c.a.* effects.
*, ** Significant at 5 and 1 per cent levels, respectively.

Significance of *s.c.a.* effects is tested with the help of a '*t*' test. Alternatively, if the specific combining ability effects exceed values $4.6422 \times 1.96 = 9.0987$ and $4.6422 \times 2.58 = 11.9768$, we infer that the *s.c.a.* effects are significant at 5 and 1 per cent levels, respectively. From Table 7.19 it appears that *s.c.a.* effects of only three crosses are significant, *viz.*, 3 × 6, 2 × 3 and 1 × 6. The *s.c.a.* effects of 2 × 3 and 1 × 6 are negative and, therefore, these crosses are unsatisfactory. Solitary cross, 3 × 6 with significant and positive *s.c.a.* effect has one parent with *g.c.a.* effect which is significant but undesirable in direction. On the basis of *per se* performance, crosses 5 × 2 and 1 × 2 appear superior. This shows that there is no agreement between crosses selected on the basis of their *s.c.a.* effects and *per se* performance. Cross 1 × 2 involves parents both of which have been identified as superior combiners.

Since the mean square for reciprocal effects is non-significant, estimates of reciprocal effects need not be calculated. Only one reciprocal effect will be calculated in order to describe the procedure. Thus

$\hat{r}_{ij} = \frac{1}{2}(y_{ij} - y_{ji})$. For example, $\hat{r}_{12}$ is found as:

$$\frac{1}{2}(90.786 - 83.166)$$

$$= 3.81$$

7.5 Method 4, Model I

Since the experimental material for this method comprises of

$\frac{p(p-1)}{2}$ F_1s only, this method is also a "modified diallel". This method could be chosen for genetic investigation when maternal inheritance is not suspected.

If p is equal to 3, diallel mating according to this method will result in 3 progeny families as shown below:

$$\begin{matrix} 0 & Y_{12} & Y_{13} \\ 0 & 0 & Y_{23} \\ 0 & 0 & 0 \end{matrix}$$

Notations used for estimation of the sums of squares and combining ability effects for this method are:

$$Y_{i.} = \sum_{j \neq i} y_{ij}$$

where $y_{ij} = y_{ji}$. For example $Y_{3.} = Y_{13} + Y_{23}$, and $Y_{2.} = Y_{12} + Y_{23}$. We need not consider $Y_{.j}$

and $Y_{..} = \sum_{i<} \sum_{j} y_{ij} = Y_{12} + Y_{13} + Y_{23}$

Linear model for the observation recorded on *ij*th genotype could be expressed as:

$$Y_{ij} = \mu + g_i + g_j + s_{ij} + \frac{1}{bc} \sum_k \sum_l e_{ijkl}$$

Where μ is the population mean, g_i is the general combining ability effect of *i*th parent, g_j is the *g.c.a.* effect of *j*th parent, s_{ij} is the specific combining ability of *ij*th cross and e_{ijkl} is error effect peculiar to the *ijkl*th observation.

Restrictions imposed on the combining ability effects are $\sum_i g_i = 0$,

and $\sum_{i \neq j} s_{ij} = 0$ (for each j).

Analysis of variance was originally given by Sprague and Tatum (1942). Structure for ANOVA of this method is given in Table 7.20.

Like the other methods Me', the error mean square for combining ability analysis, is found as:

$$\frac{Me}{bc}$$

Sum of squares for general combining ability (Sg) is calculated as:

$$Sg = \frac{1}{p-2} \sum_i Y_{i.}^2 - \frac{4}{p(p-2)} Y_{..}^2$$

TABLE 7.20: ANOVA for combining ability analysis (Method 4)

Source	df	SS	MS	Expectation mean squares: Model I	Model II
General combining ability	$(p-1)$	Sg	Mg	$\sigma^2 + (p-2)\left(\frac{1}{p-1}\right)\sum_i g_i^2$	$\sigma^2 + \sigma_s^2 + (p-2)\sigma_g^2$
Specific combining ability	$\frac{p(p-3)}{2}$	Ss	Ms	$\sigma^2 + \frac{2}{p(p-3)}\sum\sum_{i<j} s_{ij}^2$	$\sigma^2 + \sigma_s^2$
Error	m		Me'	σ^2	σ^2

And sum of squares for specific combining ability (Ss) is computed as:

$$Ss = \sum\sum_{i<j} y_{ij}^2 - \frac{1}{p-2}\sum_i Y_{i.}^2 + \frac{2}{(p-1)(p-2)} Y_{..}^2$$

Mean square for error should be used as denominator to test the significance of general and specific combining ability. Thus,

$$Fg = \frac{Mg}{Me'} \text{ for } (p-1) \text{ and } m \text{ degrees of freedom, and}$$

$$F_s = \frac{Ms}{Me'} \text{ for } \frac{p(p-3)}{2} \text{ and } m \text{ degrees of freedom.}$$

Significance of mean square for general combining ability suggests that there are significant differences among the general combining ability effects of p inbred parents. Since variance of *g.c.a.* effects measures the additive variance, conclusion may also be drawn that additive genetic variance is responsible for expression of the character being investigated. When mean square for specific combining ability is significant, we infer that there are significant difference among the *s.c.a.* effects of crosses. Significance of mean square for *s.c.a.* implies that non-additive genetic variance is responsible for the inheritance of attribute being studied. If both the mean squares are significant, additive as well as non-additive gene effects govern the expression of character. Calculate the *g.c.a.* effects of the p inbred parents, only when mean square for *g.c.a.* is found to be significant. Likewise *s.c.a.* effects are calculated only when mean square for specific combining ability is significant. Estimate of general combining ability effect of ith inbred line is obtained as:

$$\hat{g}_i = \frac{1}{p(p-2)}[pY_{i.} - 2Y_{..}]$$

Estimate of specific combining ability effect of *ij*th cross may be got as:

$$\hat{s}_{ij} = y_{ij} - \frac{1}{p-2}[Y_{i.} + Y_{j.}] + \frac{2}{(p-1)(p-2)}Y_{..}$$

We require standard errors to test the significance of *g.c.a.* effects of *p* parents and also standard error of difference of *g.c.a.* effects to test the significance of difference between general combining ability effects. Thus

$$S.E._{\hat{g}_i} = \left(\frac{p-1}{p(p-2)}\sigma^2\right)^{\frac{1}{2}}$$

and $$S.E._{(\hat{g}_i - \hat{g}_j)} = \left(\frac{2}{p-2}\sigma^2\right)^{\frac{1}{2}}$$

Standard error required to test the significance of specific combining ability effects is computed as:

$$S.E._{\hat{s}_{ij}} = \left(\frac{(p-3)}{p-1}\sigma^2\right)^{\frac{1}{2}}$$

Standard errors are also required to test significance of differences between *s.c.a.* effects. Estimates of these standard errors are obtained as:

$$S.E._{(\hat{s}_{ij} - \hat{s}_{ir})} = \left(\frac{2(p-3)}{p-2}\sigma^2\right)^{\frac{1}{2}}$$

$$S.E._{(\hat{s}_{ij} - \hat{s}_{kl})} = \left(\frac{2(p-4)}{p-2}\sigma^2\right)^{\frac{1}{2}}$$

7.5.1 *Worked Example*

Experimental material, comprising of 21 F_1s, was generated by crossing 7 inbred lines of sorghum. These twenty-one F_1s were raised in randomised block design with 2 replications. Observations were recorded on grain yield/plant (Table 7.21).

The data presented in Table 7.21 are subjected to analysis of variance to detect genetic differences. Various sums of squares are calculated as:

$$\text{Correction factor} = \frac{(2545.462)^2}{42}$$
$$= 154270.876$$

$$\text{Total sum of squares} = (112.420^2 + 78.828^2 + ... + 41.112^2) - CF$$
$$= 162530.1182 - 154270.876$$
$$= 8259.2422$$

$$\text{Genotype sum of squares} = \frac{1}{2}(181.572^2 + 168.388^2 + ... + 89.258^2) - CF$$
$$= \frac{1}{2}(321388.8156) - 154270.876$$
$$= 6423.5318$$

$$\text{Replication sum of squares} = \frac{1}{21}(1283.80^2 + 1261.662^2) - CF$$
$$= 11.6688$$

$$\text{Error sum of squares} = 1824.0416$$

TABLE 7.21 : Grain yield/plant (g) of 21 F_1 s of sorghum (Method 4)

Sl. No.	Pedigree	Replication 1	Replication 2	Total	Mean
1.	1 × 2	112.420	69.152	181.572	90.786
2.	1 × 3	78.828	89.560	168.388	84.194
3.	1 × 4	51.956	60.276	112.232	56.116
4.	1 × 5	79.260	62.474	141.734	70.867
5.	1 × 6	63.214	66.046	129.260	64.630
6.	1 × 7	66.928	59.522	126.450	63.225
7.	2 × 3	64.772	68.090	132.862	66.431
8.	2 × 4	69.772	66.174	135.946	67.973
9.	2 × 5	59.372	78.075	137.447	68.723
10.	2 × 6	53.334	63.860	117.194	58.597
11.	2 × 7	62.884	61.885	124.769	62.385
12.	3 × 4	43.720	56.798	100.518	50.259
13.	3 × 5	55.874	58.016	113.890	56.945
14.	3 × 6	66.974	71.296	138.270	69.135
15.	3 × 7	58.042	67.376	125.418	62.709
16.	4 × 5	49.610	35.084	84.694	42.347
17.	4 × 6	52.226	44.908	97.134	48.567
18.	4 × 7	55.284	46.752	102.036	51.018
19.	5 × 6	52.364	47.014	99.378	49.689
20.	5 × 7	38.820	48.192	87.012	43.506
21.	6 × 7	48.146	41.112	89.258	44.629
	Total	1283.800	1261.662	2545.462	

These sum of squares are entered in the analysis of variance table (Table 7.22).

TABLE 7.22 : ANOVA for grain yield/plant (g) in sorghum (Method 4)

Source	*df*	*SS*	*MS*	*F*
Replications	1	11.6688	11.6688	
Genotypes	20	6423.5318	321.1765**	3.52
Error	20	1824.0416	91.2020	

** Significant at 1 per cent level.

Because significant differences have been observed for genotypes we proceed for combining ability analysis. From the mean values given in Table 7.21, a diallel table is prepared (Table 7.23).

Sum of squares for general combining ability is calculated from Table 7.23. Thus :

$$Sg = \frac{1}{p-2}\sum_i Y_{i.}^2 - \frac{4}{p(p-2)}Y_{..}^2$$

$$\frac{1}{5}(429.818^2 + 414.895^2 + ... + 327.472^2) - \frac{4}{35}(1272.731)^2$$

$$= 187732.611 - 185125.0512$$

$$= 2607.5598$$

Sum of squares for specific combining ability is got as:

$$Ss = \sum_{i<}\sum_{j} y_{ij}^2 - \frac{1}{p-2}\sum_i Y_i^2 + \frac{2}{(p-1)(p-2)}Y_{..}^2$$

Where $\sum_{i<}\sum_{j} Y_{ij}^2$ is found as:

$90.786^2 + 84.194^2 + 56.116^2 + 70.867^2 + 64.630^2 + 63.225^2$
$+ 66.431^2 + 67.973^2 + 68.723^2 + 58.597^2 + 62.385^2$
$+ 50.259^2 + 56.945^2 + 69.135^2 + 62.709^2$
$+ 42.347^2 + 48.567^2 + 51.018^2 + 49.689^2$
$+ 43.506^2$
$+ 44.629^2$
$= 80347.1976$

TABLE 7.23: Diallel table for combining ability analysis of grain yield, Method 4

Inbred parents	Inbred Parents							Total $Y_{i.}$).
	1	2	3	4	5	6	7	
1.	–	90.786	84.194	56.116	70.867	64.630	63.225	429.818
2.	90.786	–	66.431	67.973	68.723	58.597	62.385	414.895
3.	84.194	66.431	–	50.259	56.945	69.135	62.709	389.673
4.	56.116	67.973	50.259	–	42.347	48.567	51.018	316.280
5.	70.867	68.723	56.945	42.347	–	49.689	43.506	332.077
6.	64.630	58.597	69.135	48.567	49.689	–	44.629	335.247
7.	63.225	62.385	62.709	51.018	43.506	44.629	–	327.472

Grand total ($Y_{..}$) = 1272.731

Hence sum of squares for specific combining ability is:

$$80347.1976 - 187732.611 + \frac{2}{30}(1272.731)^2$$

$$= 604.1998$$

These sum of squares are entered in the analysis of variance in Table 7.24.

The error mean square Me' is got as:

$$\frac{91.202}{2} = 45.601$$

Where 91.202 is the error mean square from analysis of variance for original data (Table 7.22).

Mean square for general combining ability is highly significant. This significance suggests significant differences among the *g.c.a.* effects of seven inbred lines of sorghum. On the contrary, mean square for *s.c.a* effects is non-significant which implies that all the *s.c.a.* effects are statistically *at par*. Only source of variability for grain yield in the present material is attributable due to *g.c.a.*

TABLE 7.24: Combining ability analysis for grain yield (Method 4)

Source	*df*	*SS*	*MS*	*F*
General combining ability	6	2607.5598	434.5933	9.53
Specific combining ability	14	604.1998	43.1571	0.94
Error	20	–	45.6010	–

Estimate of general combining ability effect of *i*th line is calculated as:

$$\hat{g}_i = \frac{1}{p(p-2)}[pY_{i.} - 2Y_{..}]$$

For example, estimate of *g.c.a.* effect of parent 1 is got as:

$$\hat{g}_1 = \frac{1}{35}[7(429.818) - 2(1272.731)]$$

$$= \frac{1}{35}(3008.726 - 2545.462)$$

$$= 13.2361^{**}$$

Likewise estimates of *g.c.a* effects of rest of the genotypes are obtained, which are listed below:

$\hat{g}_2 = 10.2515^{**}$ $\hat{g}_5 = -6.312^{*}$

$\hat{g}_3 = 5.2071$ $\hat{g}_6 = -5.678^{*}$

$\hat{g}_4 = -9.4714^{**}$ $\hat{g}_7 = -7.233^{**}$

Standard errors required to test the significance of *g.c.a.* effects of parents and differences of *g.c.a.* effects are obtained as:

$$S.E._{\hat{g}i} = \left(\frac{p-1}{p(p-2)}\sigma^2\right)^{\frac{1}{2}}$$

$$= \left(\frac{6}{35}45.601\right)^{\frac{1}{2}}$$

$$= 2.7959$$

and $$S.E._{(\hat{g}_i - \hat{g}_j)} = \left(\frac{2}{p-2}\sigma^2\right)^{\frac{1}{2}}$$

$$= \left(\frac{2}{5}45.601\right)^{\frac{1}{2}}$$

$$= 4.2708$$

Those *g.c.a* effects which are greater than 2.7959 × 1.96 = 5.4799 and 2.7959 × 2.58 = 7.2134 are regarded as significantly different from zero at 5 and 1 per cent levels, respectively. We put one asterisk on estimate of *g.c.a.* effects to denote significance at 5 per cent and two asterisks at 1 per cent level.

The *g.c.a.* effects of parents, 1, 2, 4, 5, 6 and 7 are significant. Nevertheless, *g.c.a.* effects of genotypes 1 and 2 are positive in direction. Therefore, these two parents could be considered as desirable combiners. Rest of the parents are unsatisfactory. If the difference between *g.c.a* effects of two parents exceeds 1.96 × 4.2708 = 8.3707, genotype with large value of *g.c.a.* effect is considered as significantly superior combiner. In the present example, *g.c.a* effects of genotypes 1 and 2 are statistically *at par* and, therefore, both these genotypes are considered as equally desirable.

Although the component of variance due to specific combining ability is non-significant, estimate of *s.c.a.* effect of cross 1×2 will be calculated for demonstration. Thus,

$$\hat{S}_{ij} = y_{ij} - \frac{1}{p-2}(Y_{i.} + Y_{j.}) + \frac{2}{(p-1)(p-2)} Y_{..}$$

$$\hat{S}_{12} = 90.786 - \frac{1}{5}(429.818 + 414.895) + \frac{2}{30} 1272.731$$

$$= 90.786 - 168.9426 + 84.8487$$

$$= 6.6921$$

The three standard errors required for testing the *s.c.a.* effects and diferences of *s.c.a.* effects are found as:

$$S.E._{\hat{s}ij} = \left(\frac{p-3}{p-1} \sigma^2 \right)^{\frac{1}{2}}$$

$$= \left(\frac{4}{6} 45.601 \right)^{\frac{1}{2}}$$

$$= 5.5136$$

$$S.E._{(\hat{s}_{ij} - S_{ik})} = \left(\frac{2(p-3)}{p-2} \sigma^2 \right)^{\frac{1}{2}}$$

$$= \left(\frac{8}{5} 45.601 \right)^{\frac{1}{2}}$$

$$= 8.5417$$

and $S.E._{(\hat{s}_{ij} - S_{kl})} = \left(\frac{2(p-4)}{p-2} \sigma^2 \right)^{\frac{1}{2}}$

$$= \left(\frac{6}{5} 45.601 \right)^{\frac{1}{2}}$$

$$= 7.3973.$$

7.6. Combining ability analysis over environments

When several genotypes are raised in different environments (including locations or years or both) their relative rankings are not same in each of the environment. Change of the environment usually does not have similar effects on different genotypes. This aspect of genotype × environment interaction is dealt with in chapter 8. However, breeder wants to know if the general and specific combining ability effects of parents and crosses, respectively are influenced by environmental effects. To investigate this aspect, the experimental material produced by either of the methods suggested by Griffing (1956) is grown in l environments. Methods of analysis for data pooled over environments were developed by Singh (1973a, 1973b, 1979).

The data recorded on character of interest is subjected to analysis of variance at each of the location. Means (over replications) of each of the genotypes (of experimental material developed according to the method adopted) are then subjected to pooled analysis. The procedures are described for this in the standard text books of statistics. Means over replications in each of the environments are then used for combining ability analysis (in other words environments take place of replications for analysis).

Although Singh (1973a, 1973b, 1979) described analysis for both the models I and II, procedure for analysis will be described here only for model I (fixed effects model).

7.6.1 Method 1, Model I

The mathematical model used for this method is :

$$Y_{ijkl} = u + g_i + g_j + S_{ij} + r_{ij} + l_k + (gl)_{ik} + (gl)_{jk} +$$

$$(sl)_{ijk} + (rl)_{ijk} + \frac{1}{bc}\sum_m \frac{1}{bc}\sum_m\sum_n e_{ijkmr}$$

Format for ANOVA is presented in table 7.25.

TABLE 7.25 ANOVA *for Method 1, Model I over environments (Singh 1973a, 1979)*

Source	df	SS	MS	EMS
GCA (G)	$(p-1)$	SS_g	M_g	$\sigma^2 + \frac{2pl}{(p-1)}\Sigma g_i^2$
SCA (S)	$\frac{p(p-1)}{2}$	SS_s	M_s	$\sigma^2 + \frac{2l}{p(p-1)}\Sigma\Sigma s_{ij}^2$
Reciprocals (R)	$\frac{p(p-1)}{2}$	SSr	Mr	$\sigma^2 + \frac{4l}{p(p-1)}\Sigma\Sigma r_{ij}^2$
Environments (L)	$(l-1)$	SS_l	M_l	$\sigma^2 + \frac{p^2}{l-1}\Sigma l^2$
G × L	$(p-1)(l-1)$	SS_{gl}	M_{gl}	$\sigma^2 + \frac{2p}{(p-1)(l-1)}\Sigma\Sigma(gl)_{ik}^2$
S × L	$\frac{p(p-1)}{2}(l-1)$	SS_{sl}	M_{sl}	$\sigma^2 + \frac{2}{p(p-1)(l-1)}\Sigma\Sigma(sl)_{ijk}^2$
R × L	$\frac{p(p-1)}{2}(l-1)$	SS_{rl}	M_{rl}	$\sigma^2 + \frac{4}{p(p-1)(l-1)}\Sigma\Sigma\Sigma(rl)_{ijk}^2$
Error	$l(v-1)(r-1)$*		Me'	σ^2

*Where $v = p^2$

In this table value of *Me*' is obtained as pooled error mean square over locations divided by number of environments and also the replications (because mean values over replications are taken for analysis). Various sums of squares are computed as:

$$SS(g) = \frac{1}{2pl}\sum_i (Y_{i..} + Y_{.i.})^2 - \frac{2}{p^2 l} Y^2_{...}$$

$$SS(s) = \frac{1}{2l}\sum_i \sum_j (y_{ij.} + y_{ji.})y_{ij.} - \frac{1}{2pl}\sum_i (Y_{i..} + Y_{.i.})^2 + \frac{Y^2_{...}}{p^2 l}$$

$$SS_{(r)} = \frac{1}{2l}\sum_i \sum_j (y_{ij.} - y_{ji.})^2$$

$$SS_{(l)} = \frac{\sum Y^2_{..k}}{p^2} - \frac{Y^2...}{p^2 l}$$

Interaction sum of squares are calculated as:

$$SS_{(gl)} = \frac{1}{2p}\sum_k \sum_i (Y_{i.k} + Y_{.ik})^2 - \frac{1}{2pl}\sum_i (Y_{i..} + Y_{.i.})^2$$

$$\frac{-2\sum_k Y^2_{..K}}{p^2} + \frac{2Y^2..}{p^2 l}$$

Where $\sum_k \sum_i \frac{(Y_{i.k} + Y_{\bullet ik})^2}{2p}$ denotes the sum of term $\sum_i (Y_{i.} + Y_{.i})^2$ over locations and $\sum_i (Y_{i..} + Y_{.i.})^2$ is the value obtained while computing sum of squares for general combining ability effects from pooled data.

$$SS_{(sl)} = \frac{1}{2}\sum_k \sum_i \sum_j (y_{ijk} + y_{jik})\, y_{ijk} - \frac{1}{2l}\sum_k \sum_i (y_{ij.} + y_{ji.})\, y_{ij.}$$

$$-\frac{1}{2p}\sum_k \sum_i (y_{i.k} + y_{.ik})^2 + \frac{1}{2pl}\sum_i (Y_{i..} + Y_{.i.})^2$$

$$+\sum_k \frac{Y^2..k}{p^2} - \frac{Y^2...}{p^2 l}$$

In this expression $\sum_k \sum_i \sum_j (y_{ijk} + y_{jik})y_{ijk}$ denotes sum of items $\sum_i \sum_j (y_{ij} + y_{ji})y_{ij}$ over k environments, whereas $\sum_i \sum_j (y_{ij.} + y_{ji.})y_{ij.}$ is the value used to calculate sum of squares for specific combining ability effects from pooled data. $\sum_k Y^2..k$ is sum of grand total squared over k environments.

And lastly, *SS* (r_l) is got as:

$$\frac{1}{2}\sum_k\sum_i\sum_j (y_{ijk} - y_{jik})^2 - \frac{1}{2l}\sum_i\sum_j (y_{ij.} - y_{ji.})^2$$

Significance of various mean squares is tested in usual way, *i.e.* error mean square is taken as denominator for *F* tests. When the mean squares for general combining ability effects and specific combining ability effects are significant *g.c.a* and *s.c.a* effects are calculated. Thus

$$\hat{g}_i = \frac{1}{2pl}[Y_{i..} + Y_{.i.})] - \frac{Y...}{p^2 l}$$

$$\hat{S}_{ij} = \frac{1}{2l}(y_{ij.} + y_{ji.}) - \frac{1}{2pl}(Y_{i..} + Y_{.i.} + Y_{j..} + Y_{.j.}) + \frac{Y^2...}{p^2 1}$$

$$\hat{r}_{ij} = \frac{1}{2l}(y_{ij.} - y_{ji.})$$

The interaction effects of *g.c.a.*, *s.c.a* and r_{ij} with environments could also be calculated as shown below:

$$(gl)_{ik} = \frac{y_{i.k} + y_{.ik})}{2p} - \frac{(Y_{i.} + Y_{.i.})}{2p1} - \frac{Y_{..k}}{p^2} + \frac{Y_{...}}{p^2 l}$$

$$(sl)_{ijk} = \frac{1}{2}(y_{ijk} + y_{jik}) - \frac{1}{2l}(y_{ij.} + y_{ji.}) - \frac{1}{2p}(Y_{.i.k} + Y_{.ik} + Y_{j.k} + Y_{.jk})$$

$$+ \frac{1}{2pl}(Y_{i..} + Y_{.i.} + Y_{j..} + Y_{.j.}) + \frac{Y..k}{p^2} - \frac{Y...}{p^2 l}$$

and

$$(rl) = \frac{1}{2}(Y_{ijk} - Y_{jik}) - \frac{1}{2l}(y_{ij.} + y_{ji.})$$

Standard errors required to test the significance of these effects are calculated as:

$$SE_{gi} = \sqrt{\frac{p-1}{2p^2 l}\sigma^2}$$

$$SE_{(gi-gj)} = \sqrt{\frac{1}{pl}\sigma^2}$$

$$SE_{sij} = \sqrt{\frac{p^2 - 2p + 2}{2p^2 l}\sigma^2}$$

$$SE_{sij-sik}\sqrt{\frac{(p-1)}{pl}\sigma^2}$$

$$SE_{sij-skl}=\sqrt{\frac{(p-2)}{pl}\sigma^2}$$

$$SE_{rij}=\sqrt{\frac{1}{2l}\sigma^2}$$

where σ^2 represents error mean square.

Singh (1973 a, b, 1979) has also given formulae for calculating values of interaction of *g.c.a* effects of each of the parent and interaction of *s.c.a.* effects of crosses with environments. Reader may refer to these papers for more details.

7.6.2. *Method 2, Model I*

The format for analysis of variance is presented in table 7.26.

TABLE 7.26 : ANOVA for Method 2,Model I over environments (Singh, 1973b, 1979)

Source	*df*	*SS*	*MS*	*EMS*
GCA (*G*)	$(p-1)$	*SSg*	*Mg*	$\sigma^2+\frac{(p+2)l}{(p-1)}\sum_i g_i^2$
SCA (S)	$\frac{p(p-1)}{2}$	*SSs*	*Ms*	$\sigma^2+\frac{2l}{p(p-1)}\sum_{i\le j}\sum s_{ij}^2$
Environments (L)	$(l-1)$	*SSl*	M_l	$\sigma^2+\frac{p(p+1)}{2(l-1)}\sum l_k^2$
G × L	$(p-l)(l-1)$	*SSgl*	*Mgl*	$\sigma^2+\frac{p+2}{(p-1)(l-1)}\sum_k\sum_i (gl)_{ik}^2$
S × L	$\frac{p(p-1)}{2}(l-1)$	*SSsl*	*Msl*	$\sigma^2+\frac{2}{p(p-1)(l-1)}\sum_k\sum_{i\le j}\sum (Sl)_{ijk}^2$
Error	$l(v-1)(r-1)$*	-	*Me'*	σ^2

* Where $v=\frac{p(p+1)}{2}$

Various sums of squares are calculated as shown below:

$$SS_g = \frac{1}{(p+2)l}\sum_i (Y_{i..} + Y_{ii.})^2 - \frac{4Y^2_{...}}{p(p+2)l}$$

$$SS_s = \frac{1}{l}\sum_{i\leq}\sum_j y^2_{ij.} - \frac{1}{(p+2)l}\sum_i (Yi.. + yii.)^2 + \frac{2\Psi^2_{...}}{(\pi+1)(\pi+2)\lambda}$$

$$SSl = \frac{2\sum_k Y^2_{..k}}{p(p+1)} - \frac{2Y^2...}{p(p+1)l}$$

$$SS_{gl} = \frac{1}{(p+2)}\sum_k\sum_i (Y_{i.k} + y_{i.i.k})^2 - \frac{4\sum_k Y^2_{..k}}{p(p+2)} - \frac{1}{(p+2)l}\sum_i (y_{i..} + y_{ii.})^2$$

$$+ \frac{4Y^2_{...}}{p(p+2)l}$$

In this expression $\sum_k\sum_i (Y_{i.k} + y_{iik})^2$ is the sum over environments of the item $\sum_i (Y_{i.} + y_{ii})^2$, and $\frac{4\sum Y^2_{..k}}{p(p+2)}$ is sum of the items $\frac{4Y^2_{..}}{p(p+2)}$ over environments. As shown by Singh (1979) sums of squares for interaction of *g.c.a.* or *s.c.a.* effects with environments could be obtained as:

$$SS\,(A \times l) = \sum_{l=1}^{k} SS_l\,(A) - SS\,(A),$$

Where $SS(A)$ is the sums of squares for factor A (in this case either *g.c.a* or *s.c.a.*) calculated from the total of means over k environments and $\sum_{l=1}^{k} SS_l(A)$ is the total of sums of squares of A factor at each of the environments. And hence the $SS(sl)$ is computed as:

$$\sum_k \sum_{i\le} \sum_j y^2_{ijk} - \frac{1}{p+2} \sum_k \sum_i (Y_{i.k} + y_{iik})^2 + \frac{2\sum_\kappa \Psi^2_{..\kappa}}{(\pi+1)(\pi+2)}$$

$$-\sum_{i\le}\sum_j \frac{y^2_{ij.}}{l} + \frac{1}{(p+2)l}\sum_i (Y_{i..} + y_{ii.})^2 - \frac{2Y^2_{...}}{(p+1)(p+2)l}$$

Significance of various mean squares is then tested in usual fashion, *i.e.* F test using error mean square as denominator. When the mean squares for general and specific combining ability effects are significant, estimates of *g.c.a.* and *s.c.a* are calculated and tested for significance. The *g.c.a.* (g_i) and *s.c.a* (s_{ij}) effects are got as:

$$\hat{g}_i = \frac{1}{(p+2)l} [(Y_{i..} + y_{ii.}) - \frac{2}{p} Y_{...}]$$

$$\acute{s}_{ij} = \frac{1}{l} y_{ij.} - \frac{1}{(p+2)l} (Y_{i..} + y_{ii.} + Y_{j..} + y_{jj.}) + \frac{2\Psi_{...}}{(\pi+1)(\pi+2)\lambda}$$

We can also calculate interaction of *g.c.a.* and *s.c.a.* when these two kinds of effects manifest interaction with environments. Thus:

$$(gl)_{ik} = \frac{1}{p+2} [(Y_{i.k} + y_{iik}) - \frac{2Y_{..k}}{p}] - \frac{1}{(p+2)l} [(Y_{i..} + y_{ii.}) - \frac{2}{p} Y_{...}]$$

$$(Sl)_{ijk} = y_{ijk} - \frac{1}{p+2} (Y_{i.k} + y_{iik} + Y_{j.k} + y_{jjk}) + \frac{2Y_{..k}}{(p+1)(p+2)}$$

$$\frac{y_{ij.}}{l} + \frac{1}{(p+2)l} (y_{i..} + y_{ii.} + y_{j..} + y_{jj.})$$

$$-\frac{2Y_{...}}{(p+1)(p+2)l}$$

Various standard errors required to test the significance of the estimates of *g.c.a* and *s.c.a* effects are estimated as:

$$SE_{gi} = \sqrt{\frac{(p-1)}{p(p+2)l}\sigma^2}$$

$$SE_{gi-gj} = \sqrt{\frac{2}{(p+2)l}\sigma^2}$$

$$SE_{sij} = \sqrt{\frac{p^2+p+2}{(p+1)(p+2)l}\sigma^2}$$

$$SE_{sij-sik} = \sqrt{\frac{2(p+1)}{(p+2)l}\sigma^2}$$

$$SE_{sij-skl} = \sqrt{\frac{2p}{(p+2)l}\sigma^2}$$

7.6.2.1. *Worked Example*

Data was provided by Dr. P.N. Gadewadikar. Seven varieties of cotton were crossed in diallel fashion, according to method 2 of Griffing (1956). The 21 F_1s and 7 parental lines were planted in randomized block design with 3 replications each in 3 environments, *viz,* Indore two dates of sowings (E_1 = 14 July, E_2 = 29 July) and Khandwa (E_3). Observations were recorded on 3 plants/plot on ginning per cent after harvesting. The mean ginning per cent over replications for 3 enviroments is presented in table 7.27. Results of combining ability analyses for this character in each environment are shown in table 7.28.

TABLE 7.27: Mean ginning % of 28 genotypes of cotton (over 3 replications) in 3 environments

S.No.	Genotypes	E_1	E_2	E_3	Total
1.	Khandwa 2	39.17	39.67	34.67	113.51
2.	Vikram	33.33	31.26	32.67	97.26
3.	GS 23	33.67	34.50	33.07	101.24
4.	Bikaneri Nerma	34.17	35.33	31.93	101.43
5.	Reba B 50	32.00	33.20	33.83	99.03
6.	Okra 100	31.80	30.73	32.23	94.76
7.	Cocker 315	35.34	34.53	30.30	100.17
8.	Khandwa 2 × Vikram	34.00	34.83	34.33	103.16
9.	Khandwa 2 × GS 23	35.00	36.83	35.70	107.53
10.	Khandwa 2 × BN	36.33	35.50	33.73	105.56
11.	Khandwa 2 × Reba	36.67	36.17	31.23	104.07
12.	Khandwa 2 × Okra	37.67	38.17	34.43	110.27
13.	Khandwa 2 × Cocker	36.83	37.50	32.23	106.56
14.	Vikram × GS 23	31.67	33.17	31.30	96.14
15.	Vikram × BN	32.77	32.43	32.40	97.60
16.	Vikram × Reba	32.33	35.00	32.60	99.93
17.	Vikram × Okra	33.33	34.50	34.00	101.83
18.	Vikram × Cocker	34.17	32.67	33.97	100.81
19.	GS 23 × BN	33.17	33.67	34.80	101.64
20.	GS 23 × Reba	32.50	33.33	35.10	100.93
21.	GS 23 × Okra	33.50	33.67	33.47	100.64
22.	GS 23 × Cocker	34.83	34.50	35.07	104.40
23.	BN × Reba	34.67	36.00	33.23	103.90
24.	BN × Okra	36.33	33.90	33.20	103.43
25.	BN × Cocker	34.00	31.47	33.63	99.10
26.	Reba × Okra	36.33	34.50	36.80	107.63
27.	Reba × Cocker	35.33	33.67	36.67	105.67
28.	Okra × Cocker	35.17	35.50	35.40	106.07

TABLE 7.28: ANOVA for combining ability in 3 environments (Griffing's 1956 Method 2, Model I)

Source	*df*	Mean squares		
		E_1	E_2	E_3
GCA	6	10.814**	12.00**	1.507
SCA	21	1.407	1.878*	2.812**
Error	54	0.851	0.872	0.852
$Y_{..}$		966.08	966.20	941.99
$\sum_i (Y_{i.} + y_{ii})^2$		533904.3	534101.23	507135.75
$\sum\sum_{i \le j} y_{ij}^2$		33426.958	33452.294	31758.987

From the diallel table 7.29, sums of squares for general and specific combining ability and interaction of *GCA* and *SCA* with environments are calculated as shown below:

TABLE 7.29: Diallel table for ginning % of cotton (over 3 environments)

	Khandwa2	Vikram	GS23	Bika-neri Nerma	Reba B 50	Okra 100	Cocker 315
Khandwa 2	113.51	103.16	107.53	105.56	104.07	110.27	106.56
Vikram	103.16	97.26	96.14	97.60	99.93	101.83	100.81
GS 23	107.53	96.14	101.24	101.64	100.93	100.64	104.40
Bikaneri N	105.56	97.60	101.64	101.43	103.90	103.43	99.10
Reba B 50	104.07	99.93	100.93	103.90	99.03	107.63	105.67
Okra	110.27	101.83	100.64	103.43	107.63	94.76	106.07
Cocker	106.56	100.81	104.40	99.10	105.67	106.07	100.17
Array Total $Y_{i..}$	750.66	696.73	712.52	712.66	721.16	724.63	722.78

The experimental material for method 2 as described by Griffing (1956) is F_1s and parents *i.e.* $p + p\,(p-1)/2 = p\,(p+1)/2$. The grand total therefore equals 707.40 + 2166.87 = 2874.27.

TABLE 7.30: $Y_{i..} + Y_{ii.}$ for seven arrays (over 3 environments)

Array	$y_{i..}$	$y_{ii.}$	$Y_{i..} + y_{ii.}$
1	750.66	113.51	864.17
2	696.73	97.26	793.99
3	712.52	101.24	813.76
4	712.66	101.43	814.09
5	721.16	99.03	820.19
6	724.63	94.76	819.39
7	722.78	100.17	822.95

From the table 7.30 we compute the value $\sum_i (Y_{i..} + y_{ii.})^2$ required for estimation of sum of squares for general combining ability. This is found to be 4723516.10.

$$SS_g = \frac{1}{(p+2)l}\sum_i (Y_{i..} + Y_{ii.})^2 - \frac{4}{p(p+2)l} Y^2...$$

$$= \frac{1}{27}(4723516.1) - \frac{4}{189}(2874.27)^2$$

$$= 174945.04 - 174845.04$$

$$= 100.00$$

$$SS_s = \frac{1}{l}\sum_{i\leq}\sum_j y_{ij.}^2 - \frac{1}{(p+2)l}\sum_i (Y_{i..} + y_{ii.})^2 + \frac{2}{(p+1)(p+2)l} Y^2...$$

$$= \frac{295541.7}{3} - \frac{1}{27}(4723516.1) + \frac{2}{216}(2874.27)^2$$

$$= 63.5632$$

As shown in section 7.3.1, $\sum_{i\leq}\sum_j y_{ij.}^2$ is obtained by squaring the mean values of 21 F_1s and 7 parents and adding together.

$$SS_l = \frac{2\Sigma Y_{..k}^2}{P(p+1)} - \frac{2Y^2...}{p(p+1)l}$$

$$= \frac{2(966.08^2 + 966.20^2 + 941.99^2)}{56} - \frac{2(2874.27)^2}{168}$$

$$= 13.8862$$

Interaction sum of squares of general and specific combining ability effects are got as:

$$SS_{gl} = \frac{1}{p+2}\sum_k\sum_i (Y_{i.k} + y_{iik})^2 - \frac{4\sum_k Y_{..k}^2}{p(p+2)}$$

$$- \frac{1}{(p+2)l}\sum_i (Y_{i..} + Y_{ii.})^2 + \frac{4Y_{...}^2}{p(p+2)l}$$

$$= \frac{1}{9}(533904.30 + 534101.23 + 507135.75) -$$

$$\frac{4}{63}(966.08^2+966.20^2+941.99^2)-\frac{1}{27}(4723516.1)+$$

$$\frac{4}{189}(2874.27)^2=45.97$$

$$SS_{sl}=\sum_k\sum_{i\leq}\sum_j y_{ijk}^2-\frac{1}{(p+2)}\sum_k\sum_i(Y_{i.k}+y_{iik})^2+\frac{2\sum_K \Psi_{..K}^2}{(\pi+1)(\pi+2)}$$

$$-\sum_{i\leq}\sum_j\frac{y_{ij.}^2}{l}+\frac{1}{(p+2)l}\sum_i(Y_{i..}+y_{ii.})^2-\frac{2Y^2...}{(p+1)(p+2)l}$$

$$=(33426.956+33452.294+31758.987)-\frac{1}{9}(1575141.30)$$

$$+\frac{2}{72}(966.08^2+966.20^2+941.99^2)-\frac{1}{3}(295541.70)$$

$$+\frac{1}{27}(4723516.1)-\frac{2}{216}(2874.27)^2$$

$$=64.480$$

The analysis of variance is then set up as in table 7.31. The error mean square is calculated as mean over 3 environments. It is clear from

TABLE 7.31: ANOVA for pooled combining ability (Singh 1973b)

Source	*df*	*SS*	*MS*	*F*
GCA(*G*)	6	100.00	16.667**	19.4
SCA (*S*)	21	63.563	3.026*	3.5
Environments (L)	2	13.886	6.943**	8.0
G × L	12	45.970	3.830**	4.5
S × L	42	64.480	1.535**	1.8
Error	168	–	0.858	

this table that there are significant differences among the *g.c.a.* and *s.c.a.* effects of parents and F_1s, respectively as revealed by significance of items *GCA* and *SCA* in table 7.31. Significance of $G \times L$ and $S \times L$ point out that the *g.c.a.* and *s.c.a.* effects also exhibit interaction with environments (in the present case locations). Hence choice of parents and F_1s should be based on combiners and F_1 combinations which show least interaction with environments. Singh (1973 *b*) has given least square estimates to calculate interaction of *g.c.a.* with environments (g_l) and *s.c.a.* effects with environments (s_l).

Since the mean squares for *GCA* and *SCA* are significant, estimates of *g.c.a.* effects of 7 parents and *s.c.a.* effects of 21 F_1s are calculated (Table 7.32). The estimate of g_1 is got as:

$$g_1 = \frac{1}{(p+2)l}\left[\sum_i (Y_{i..} + y_{ii.}) - \frac{2Y...}{p}\right]$$

$$= \frac{1}{27}\left[864.17 - \frac{2}{7}2874.27\right]$$

$$= 1.5907^{**}$$

Estimate of S_{12} is calculated as:

$$\frac{y_{ij.}}{l} - \frac{(Y_{i..} + y_{ii.} + Y_{j..} + y_{jj.})}{(p+2)l} + \frac{2Y...}{(p+1)(p+2)l}$$

$$S_{12} = \frac{103.16}{3} - \frac{1}{27}(864.17 + 793.99) + \frac{2}{216}2874.27$$

$$= -0.4130$$

Estimates of various standard errors are calculated as:

$$SE_{gi} = \sqrt{\frac{p-1}{p(p+2)l}\sigma^2} = \sqrt{\frac{6}{189}0.858}$$

$$= 0.165$$

$$SE_{gi-gj} = \sqrt{\frac{2}{(p+2)l}\sigma^2} = \sqrt{\frac{6}{186}0.858}$$

$$= 0.252$$

$$SE_{sij} = \sqrt{\frac{p^2+p+2}{(p+1)(p+2)l}\sigma^2} = \sqrt{\frac{58}{216}0.858}$$

$$= 0.4799$$

$$SE_{sij-sik} = \sqrt{\frac{2(p+1)}{(p+2)l}\sigma^2} = \sqrt{\frac{16}{27}0.858}$$

$$= 0.713$$

$$SE_{sij} - s_{kl} = \sqrt{\frac{2p}{(p+2)l}\sigma^2} = \sqrt{\frac{14}{27}0.858}$$

$$= 0.666$$

TABLE 7.32 : Estimates of *g.c.a.* and *s.c.a.* effects of cotton over 3 environments (Singh, 1973 b)

	Khandwa2	Vikram	*GS* 23	Bika-neri Nerma	Reba B 50	Okra 100	Cocker 315
Khandwa	1.591**	−0.413	0.311	−0.357	−1.080*	1.016*	−0.352
Vikram		−1.008**	−0.886	−0.411	0.139	0.802	0.330
GS 23			−0.276	0.202	−0.259	−0.326	0.794
Bikaneri *N*				−0.264	0.718	0.591	−0.984*
Reba B 50					−0.038	1.765**	0.979*
Okra 100						−0.068	1.142*
Cocker 315							0.064

Diagonal entries are *g.c.a.* effects. *, ** significant at 5 and 1 per cent levels, respectively.

The estimates of interaction of *g.c.a.* effects of genotype 1, *i.e.* Khandwa 2, could be calculated in the 3 environments as:

$$(gl)_{ik} = \frac{1}{p+2}\left[\,(Y_{i.k}+y_{iik}) - \frac{2Y_{..k}}{p}\,\right] - \frac{1}{(p+2)l}\left[\,(Y_{i..}+y_{ii.}) - \frac{2Y_{...}}{p}\,\right]$$

$$g_{11} = \frac{1}{9}\left[294.84 - \frac{2\times966.08}{7}\right] - \frac{1}{27}\left[864.17 - \frac{2\times2874.27}{7}\right]$$
$$= 0.4993$$

$$g_{12} = \frac{1}{9}\left[298.34 - \frac{2\times966.20}{7}\right] - \frac{1}{27}\left[864.17 - \frac{2\times2874.27}{7}\right]$$
$$= 0.8851, \text{ and}$$

$$g_{13} = \frac{1}{9}\left[270.99 - \frac{2\times941.99}{7}\right] - \frac{1}{27}\left[864.17 - \frac{2\times2874.27}{7}\right]$$
$$= -1.3851$$

Where 294.84, 298.34 and 270.99 are values of $(Y_{i.} + y_{ii})$ in environments 1, 2 and 3 respectively and 966.08, 966.20 and 941.99 are values of $Y..$ in these 3 environments. 864.17 and 2874.27 are the values of $(Y_{i..} + y_{ii.})$ and $Y...$, from pooled data, respectively.

Similarly the interaction of *s.c.a.* effects are obtained as:

$$(Sl)_{12k} = y_{ijk} - \frac{1}{p+2}(Y_{i.k} + y_{iik} + Y_{j.k} + y_{jjk}) + \frac{2Y..k}{(p+1)(p+2)}$$
$$- \frac{y_{ij.}}{l} + \frac{1}{(p+2)l}(Y_{i..} + y_{ii.} + Y_{j..} + y_{jj.}) - \frac{2Y...}{(p+1)(p+2)l}$$

$$S_{12.1} = 34.0 - \frac{1}{9}(294.84+264.93) + \frac{2\times966.08}{72} - \frac{103.16}{3}$$
$$+ \frac{1}{27}(864.17 + 793.99) - \frac{2\times2874.27}{216}$$
$$= -0.9481$$

$$S_{12.2} = 34.83 - \frac{1}{9}(298.34+265.12) + \frac{966.20\times2}{72}$$
$$- \frac{103.16}{3} + \frac{1}{27}(864.17+793.99) - \frac{2\times2874.27}{216}$$
$$= -0.5247$$

$$S_{12.3} = 34.33 - \frac{1}{9}(270.99 + 263.94) + \frac{2\times941.99}{72}$$
$$- \frac{103.16}{3} + \frac{1}{27}(864.17 + 793.99) - \frac{2\times2874.27}{216}$$
$$= 1.472$$

The interaction of *g.c.a.* with environments shows that Khandwa 2 is a desirable general combiner in E_1 and E_2 but undesirable in E_3. Likewise, specific combination Khandwa 2 × Vikram has desirable specific combining ability in E_3 but not in E_1 and E_2.

7.6.3 *Method 3, Model I*

Mathematical model used to derive estimates of parameters and expectation mean squares is:

$$Y_{ijk} = u_i + g_i + g_j + S_{ij} + r_{ij} + l_k + (gl)_{ik} + (gl)_{jk}$$

$$+ (Sl)_{ijk} + (rl)_{ijk} + \frac{1}{bc}\sum_m \sum_r eijkmr$$

The format for ANOVA, alongwith expectation mean squares is presented in table 7.33.

TABLE 7.33 : ANOVA for method 3 (Model I) over environments (Singh, 1973b, 1979)

Source	*df*	*SS*	*MS*	*EMS*
GCA (*G*)	$(p-1)$	SSg	Mg	$\sigma^2 + \frac{2(p-2)l}{(p-1)}\sum_i g_i^2$
SCA (*S*)	$\frac{p(p-3)}{2}$	SSs	Ms	$\sigma^2 + \frac{4l}{p(p-3)}\sum_{i\le}\sum_j s_{ij}^2$
Reciprocal effects (*R*)	$\frac{p(p-1)}{2}$	SSr	Mr	$\sigma^2 + \frac{4l}{p(p-1)}\sum_{i\le}\sum_j r_{ij}^2$
Environments	$(l-1)$	SS_l	M_l	$\sigma^2 + \frac{p(p-1)}{l-1}\sum_k l_k^2$
G × L	$(p-1)(l-1)$	$SS(g_l)$	Mg_l	$\sigma^2 + \frac{2(p-2)}{(p-1)(l-1)}\sum\sum(gl)_{ik}^2$
S × L	$\frac{p(p-3)}{2}(l-1)$	$SS(sl)$	Msl	$\sigma2 + \frac{4}{p(p-3)(l-1)}\sum\sum(Sl)_{ijk}^2$

R × L	$\frac{p(p-1)}{2}(l-1)$	SS_{rl}	M_{rl}	$\sigma^2 + \frac{4}{p(p-1)(l-1)}\sum\sum\sum(rl)^2_{ijk}$	
Error	$l(v-1)(r-1)$		m	σ^2	

* $v = p(p-1)$

Various sums of squares are obtained as:

$$SSg = \frac{1}{(p-2)l}\left[\frac{\sum_i (Y_{i..} + Y_{.i.}}{2} - \frac{2Y^2_{...}}{p}\right]$$

$$SS_s = \frac{\sum_i\sum_j (y_{ij.} + y_{ji.})^2}{2l} - \frac{\sum_i (Y_{i..} + Y_{.i.})^2}{2(p-2)l} + \frac{Y^2...}{(p-1)(p-2)l}$$

$$SS_r = \frac{1}{2l}\sum_i\sum_j (y_{ij.} - y_{ji.})^2$$

$$SS_{gl} = \frac{1}{(p-2)}\left[\frac{\sum_k\sum_i (Y_{i.k} + Y_{.ik})^2}{2} - \frac{2\sum_k Y^2_{..k}}{p}\right] - \frac{1}{(p-2)l}\left[\sum_i \frac{(Y_{i..} + Y_{.i.})^2}{2} - \frac{2Y^2_{...}}{p}\right]$$

$$SS_{sl} = \frac{1}{2}\sum_k\sum_i\sum_j (y_{ijk} + y_{jik})^2 - \frac{1}{2(p-2)}\sum_k\sum_i (Y_{i.k} + Y_{.ik})^2 + \frac{\sum_k Y^2_{..k}}{(p-1)(p-2)} - \frac{1}{2l}\sum_i\sum_j (y_{ij.} + y_{ji.})^2 + \frac{1}{2(p-2)l}\sum_i (Y_{i..} + Y_{.i.})^2 - \frac{Y^2...}{(p-1)(p-2)l}$$

$$SS_{(rl)} = \frac{1}{2}\sum_k\sum_i\sum_j (y_{ijk} - y_{jik})^2 - \frac{1}{2l}\sum_i\sum_j (y_{ij.} - y_{ji.})^2$$

Significance of various mean squares is then tested in customary fashion applying the '*F*' test. When the *GCA*, *SCA* and reciprocal effects are significant, general combining ability effects, specific combining ability effects and reciprocal effects are calculated as shown below. Their significance is tested using standard errors for '*t*' test. Thus:

$$\hat{g}_i = \frac{1}{2p(p-2)l}[p(Y_{i..} + Y_{.i.}) - 2Y...]$$

$$\hat{S}_{ij} = \frac{1}{2l}(y_{ij.} + y_{ji.}) - \frac{1}{2(p-2)l}(Y_{i..} + Y_{.i.} + Y_{j..} + Y_{.j.}) + \frac{Y...}{(p-1)(p-2)l}$$

$$\hat{r}_{ij} = \frac{1}{2l}(y_{ij.} - y_{ji.})$$

$$(gl)_{ik} = \frac{1}{2p(p-2)}[p(Y_{i.k} + Y_{.ik}) - 2Y_{..k}]$$

$$-\frac{1}{2p(p-2)l}[p(Y_{i..} + Y_{.i.}) - 2Y...]$$

$$(sl)_{ijk} = \frac{1}{2}(y_{ijk} + y_{jik}) - \frac{1}{2(p-2)}(Y_{i.k} + Y_{.ik} + Y_{j.k} + Y_{.jk})$$

$$+\frac{Y_{..k}}{(p-1)(p-2)} - \frac{1}{2l}(y_{ij} + y_{ji.}) + \frac{1}{2(p-2)l}(Y_{i..} + Y_{.i.} + Y_{j..} + Y_{.j.})$$

$$-\frac{Y...}{(p-1)(p-2)l}$$

$$(rl)_{ijk} = \frac{1}{2}(y_{ijk} - y_{jik}) - \frac{1}{2l}(y_{ij.} - y_{ji.})$$

The standard errors are calculated as:

$$SE_{gi} = \sqrt{\frac{p-1}{2p(p-2)l}\sigma^2}$$

$$SE_{(gi-gj)} = \sqrt{\frac{1}{(p-2)l}\sigma^2}$$

$$SE_{sij} = \sqrt{\frac{(p-3)}{2(p-1)l}\sigma^2}$$

$$SE_{sij-sik} = \sqrt{\frac{(p-3)}{(p-2)l}\sigma^2}$$

$$SE_{sij-s_{kl}} = \sqrt{\frac{p-4}{(p-2)l}\sigma^2}$$

$$SE_{rij} = \sqrt{\frac{1}{2l}\sigma^2}$$

7.6.4 *Method 4 Model I*

Procedure in the analysis of data obtained from the experimental material developed according to this method which is grown in l environments is not much different than the procedures shown for earlier analyses. The mathematical model is

$$Y_{ijk} = u + g_i + g_j + s_{ij} + l_k + (gl)_{jk} + (gl)_{ik} + (sl)_{ijk} + \frac{1}{bc}\Sigma\Sigma\, eijkmr$$

Format for analysis of variance would be as shown in table 7.34.

TABLE 7.34 : ANOVA for combining ability over environments for method 4 (Singh 1973b, 1979) Model I

Source	df	SS	MS	EMS
$GCA(G)$	$(p-1)$	SSg	Mg	$\sigma^2 + \frac{(p-2)l}{(p-1)}\sum_i g_i^2$
$SCA\ (S)$	$\frac{p(p-3)}{2}$	SSs	Ms	$\sigma^2 + \frac{2l}{p(p-3)}\sum_i\sum_j s_{ij}^2$
Environments (L)	$(l-1)$	SS_l	Ml	$\sigma^2 + \frac{p(p-1)}{2}\sum_k l_k^2$
G × L	$(p-1)\ (l-1)$	SS_{gl}	M_{gl}	$\sigma^2 + \frac{(p-2)}{(p-1)(l-1)}\sum_k\sum_i (gl)_{ik}^2$
S × L	$(l-1)\frac{(p-3)p}{2}$	SSs_l	M_{sl}	$\sigma^2 + \frac{2}{p(p-3)(l-1)}\sum_k\sum_i\sum_j (sl)_{ijk}^2$
Error	$1(v-1)\ (r-1)-$		Me'	σ^2

Various sums of squares are calculated as per Singh (1973b, 1979) as shown below:

$$SS_g = \frac{1}{(p-2)l}\left[\sum_i Y_{i..}^2 - \frac{4Y_{...}^2}{p}\right]$$

$$SS_s = \frac{1}{l}\sum_i \sum_{<j} y_{ij.}^2 - \frac{1}{(p-2)l}\sum_i Y_{i..}^2 + \frac{2Y_{...}^2}{(p-1)9p-2)l}$$

$$SS_{(l)} = \frac{1}{p(p-1)}\left[2\sum_k Y_{..k}^2 - \frac{2Y_{...}^2}{l}\right]$$

$$SS_{(gl)} = \frac{1}{p-2}\left[\sum_k \sum_i Y_{i.k}^2 - \frac{4\sum_k Y_{..k}^2}{p} - \frac{\sum_i Y_{i..}^2}{l} + \frac{4Y_{...}^2}{pl}\right]$$

$$SS_{S1} = \sum_k \sum_i \sum_j y_{ijk}^2 - \frac{1}{p-2}\sum_k \sum_i (Y_{i.k}^2) + \frac{2\sum_k Y_{..k}^2}{(p-1)9p-2)}$$

$$-\frac{1}{l}\sum_i \sum_{<j} y_{ij.}^2 + \frac{1}{(p-2)l}\sum_i Y_{i..}^2 - \frac{2Y_{...}^2}{(p-1)(p-2)l}$$

When the mean squares for *GCA* and *SCA* are found to be significant, estimates of general and specific combining ability effects are computed. Thus estimates of g_i and S_{ij} could be obtained as:

$$\hat{g}_i = \frac{1}{p(p-2)l}\left[p(Y_{i..}) - 2Y...\right]$$

$$\hat{S}_{ij} = \frac{1}{l}y_{ij.} - \frac{1}{(p-2)l}(Y_{i..} + Y_{j..}) + \frac{2Y...}{(p-1)(p-\cdot 2)l}$$

And the interaction of general and specific combining ability effects according to Singh (1973b, 1979) are calculated as:

$$(gl)_{ik} = \frac{1}{p(p-2)}[p(Y_{i.k}) - 2Y_{..k}] - \frac{1}{p(p-2)l}[p(Y_{i..}) - 2Y...]$$

$$(sl)_{ijk} = y_{ijk} - \frac{1}{(p-2)}(Y_{i.k} + Y_{j.k}) + \frac{2Y..k}{(p-1)(p-2)}$$

$$-\frac{1}{l}y_{ij.} + \frac{1}{(p-2)l}(Y_{i..} + Y_{j..}) - \frac{2Y...}{(p-1)(p-2)l}$$

Estimates of various standard errors are got as:

$$SE_{gi} = \sqrt{\frac{p-1}{p(p-2)l}\sigma^2}$$

$$SE_{(gi-gj)} = \sqrt{\frac{2}{(p-2)l}\cdot\sigma^2}$$

$$SE_{sij} = \sqrt{\frac{p-3}{(p-1)l}\sigma^2}$$

$$SE_{(sij-sik)} = \sqrt{\frac{2(p-3)}{(p-2)l}\sigma^2}$$

$$SE_{(sij-skl)} = \sqrt{\frac{2(p-4)}{(p-2)l}\sigma^2}$$

8

GENOTYPE-ENVIRONMENT INTERACTION AND STABILITY PARAMETERS

8.1 Genotype-Environment Interaction

We know that the phenotype of an individual is determined by the effects of its genotype and environment surrounding it. The effects of genotype and environment on phenotype may not be always independent. The phenotypic response to change in environment is not same for all genotypes, the consequences of variation in phenotype depend upon the environment. Very often breeders encounter situations where the relative rankings of varieties change from location to location and/or from year to year. The interplay in the effect of genetic and non-genetic on development is termed as 'genotype-environment interaction' (Comstock and Moll, 1963).

Genotype-environment interactions are of major consequence to the breeders in the process of evolution of improved varieties. When varieties are grown at several locations for testing their performance, their relative rankings usually do not remain same. This causes difficulty in demonstrating significant superiority of any variety. Genotype-environment interaction is present whether varieties are pure lines, single-crosses, double-crosses, top-crosses, S_1 lines or any other material with which breeder is working. Stratification of the environment has been recommended to reduce the genotype-environment interaction. The geographical region for which a breeder is working may be large and hence heterogeneous with respect to environment. This region could be so subdivided that the environment within each sub-region is relatively homogeneous. This stratification is usually based on such macro-environmental differences as temperature gradients, rainfall distribution and soil types, *etc.* However, even with this refinement of technique, interaction of genotypes with environment in a given sub-region remains too large.

Genotype and environment may exhibit their interaction in several ways (Mather and Jinks, 1971). Environment may cause change in the genetic constitution of a population by pressure of selection (such as differential fertility and/or viability) it exercises on the population. In the long run it may lead to evolutionary changes. But in the short run also, pressure of selection from environment may alter the genetic constitution of segregating material that the genetic theory leads us to expect. In other words, differential fertility and/or viability of various genotypes may change the genetic constitution of segregating material.

Permanent changes in the genetic material can also be induced by environmental agencies. These changes may be of two kinds. One is the familiar mutagenic effect of the radiations and various chemicals. Other effect of environment on the genotype is known as "conditioning" (Durrant, 1958). It was observed by Durrant (1958) that certain varieties of flax plants when grown in soil carrying combinations of nitrogenous, phosphatic and potassic fertilizers reflected the effect of their treatments not only in their own growth but also transmitted them to their progeny. This kind of change was transmitted equally efficiently by the pollen and egg.

Genotype and environment may interact and produce differences among the individuals within a family. The interactions may appear in two ways, *viz.* as non-heritable variation of a character displayed by individuals within a family, changing with genotype, and as difference in the mean expressions of two or more genotypes grown in two or more environments. The non-heritable variance of individuals or families may reflect differences of mircro-environment in which different members of a family are grown or in which different parts of given organism develop.

There is a general agreement among the breeders that interaction of genotypes with environments have an important bearing on the breeding of better varieties. However, there is not much agreement regarding what should be done about it. Since genotype-environment interaction has masking effect on genotype, some breeders attempt to estimate the magnitude of this interaction variance so that precise estimate of genotypic variance could be obtained. The choice of an efficient breeding programme for the improvement of a character is determined by the relative magnitudes of components of genotypic variance. As shown in section 4.8.2, estimate of genotypic variance (σ_g^2) is biased when genotypes are not grown in adequate number of environments. This may have an adverse implication on the breeding programme. For instance, if the magnitude of σ_g^2 is overestimated the breeder is likely to waste his time and effort not justified by the real potential for improvement of segregating material being handled. The breeding procedure also varies according to the nature and relative magnitudes of components of heritable variance. If the genotypic variance is underestimated, sound breeding programmes may be abandoned prematurely or unwisely.

Although the importance of genotype-environment interaction is recognised well and these are known to be heritable (Jinks and Mather, 1955) and statistical techniques are available, main efforts of geneticists are to reduce them or to scale them out.

Some breeders feel that a direct and systematic approach is required which will throw light on the genetic systems that will result in high and stable performance.

Though the conventional statistical procedures of splitting the interaction variance into various components, *viz.*, varieties × locations, varieties × years and varieties × years × locations, yield useful information for planning and apportioning of the available resources for testing programme and handling the breeding material, yet these analyses do not pin-point the genotypes which are stable in productivity, owing to the change in ranks in different environments. Significant advances have been made in the measurement of contribution of genotypes to the genotype-environment interaction and in making predictions of performance of genotypes over environments by using regression technique originally given by Yates and Cochran (1938) and revived by Finlay and Wilkinson (1963).

Before we discuss various techniques developed to characterise stable genotypes it would be desirable to understand what geneticists mean by environment and what are the probable reasons for genotype-environment interactions.

8.2 The Environment

To a geneticist, environment is the sum total of physical, chemical and biological factors that influence the development of an organism.

Comstock and Moll (1963) classified environment into two kinds, *viz.* the macro-environment and the micro-environment. Micro-environment refers to the environment of a single plant which is made up of all the things, other than genotype of a plant, which influence its development. This includes physical and chemical attributes of the soil in which the plant grows; climatic variables (such as temperature, humidity, etc.), amount, distribution and quality of solar radiation; and the number and kinds of biological organisms (such as pathogens, insects, etc.) to which the plant is exposed. Potential number of micro-environments will be infinite, even within a given area, and the probability that the environments experienced by two plants growing in the same field at the same time are same is very small. It is this unique complex of forces in development that is called as micro-environment (of a single plant).

The environment that organisms experience in one area as compared to the other in one period of time than in another is not same. Environments that are potential or experienced within a given area and period of time are collectively known as macro-environment. A macro-environment is a population of micro-environments.

In order to distinguish among the environmental sources of variation that contribute to the genotype-environment interaction, Allard and Bradshaw (1964) coined two terms, *viz.* predictable and unpredictable environmental variations. Predictable variation includes all the permanent characters of environment such as general features of climate and soil type as well as those characters of environment that fluctuate in a systematic manner, such as the day length. It also includes those aspects of environment which are determined by man and can, therefore, be fixed more or less at will, *e.g.*, planting date, sowing density, etc.

The unpredictable variation includes fluctuations in weather, such as amount and distribution of rainfall and temperature.

8.3 Causes of Genotype-Environment Interaction

In the past, breeders were primarily interested in the "final" characters. Plant breeders have, however, recognised that higher plants are dynamic living systems in which change takes place from germination to maturity.

The pattern of change is not same from one genotype to another in the same environment or for same genotype in different environments. It is felt that efficiency of a breeding programme will improve if developmental pathways by which the final characters are reached are well understood.

Most of the characters of living organisms are determined by nuclear borne genes. The genetic material in higher organisms is DNA which is composed of nucleotides of four kinds. Metabolic processes in living organisms are catalysed by enzymes which are mainly composed of proteins. Structure and function of proteins is determined by genetic material – the genes. It is now well known that the sequence of nucleotides on DNA strands determines the sequence of amino acids on polypeptides. Any change in the sequence of nucleotides leads to a corresponding change in the sequence of amino acids in polypeptides and ultimately change in gene function. Environmental agencies, both internal and external, can lead to altered nucleotide sequence which is recognised as mutations. Mutation is reflected in altered gene function and subsequently changed phenotype. We know that bio-synthesis takes place in a stepwise fashion such that each step is governed by an enzyme whose structure/ function is determined by a particular gene. Thus there are many opportunities for environmental fluctuations to induce genotype-environment interactions at various levels of metabolism. While this provides an insight into the complex causes of genotype-environment interactions and offers more opportunities by which they could be investigated, many basic problems at the molecular level are yet unresolved. Presently what can be said is that there is a wide gap between the genetic code and the final character and, therefore, much light cannot be focused on relationships between the genotypes and the environments at molecular level. However, several attempts have been made to consider pathways above the molecular level through which final characters are reached.

Example of the pathway approach at enzyme level was provided by Sarkissian and Huffaker (1962). They studied the effect of chloramphenicol on carboxylation systems in isogenic lines of barley. Barley plants heterozygous at hooded locus exhibited better carboxylation and growth rate than the homozygotes when treated with chloramphenicol.

Schwartz (1960) investigated the genetic control of an enzyme with esterase activity in maize. This is an example of pathway approach at biochemical level to understand the cause of genotype-environment interaction. Schwartz (1960) observed that heterozygotes form "hybrid" enzymes. Karve (1980) explained stability in the performance of hybrids on a biochemical basis. He noted that polyphenol oxidase activity was greater in hybrids of safflower than their parents. According to him "isoenzyme complementation" could have been responsible for this enhanced enzyme activity. (Enzymes which catalyse one and the same reaction but are different physico-chemical entities, are known as "isoenzymes"). Since isoenzymes differ in physico-chemical properties, they also differ in their sensitivity to various external factors such as *pH* of the substrate, temperature, light, etc. which are presumably responsible for stable performance of safflower hybrids in varying environments. Langridge and Griffing (1959) and Griffing and Langridge (1963) while working with *Arabidopsis thaliana* observed that hybrids had greater mean growth as compared to their parents, especially at the higher temperature regimes. Hybrids manifested greater stability of phenotypic expression over a wide temperature range. Homozygotes ceased growth at higher temperature presumably because of deficiencies in particular enzymes which distinguish different homozygous ecological races. According to these workers, vigour and stability are the consequence of combination of alleles which condition more thermostable products in hybrids.

Lewis (1954) explained stable performance of hybrids on the basis of alternative pathways. In its simplest form let us assume that a single change from substrate to a product is governed by one gene (A). Homozygote A_1A_1 will have only one genetic pathway between the substrate and the product while the heterozygote may have one or two pathways according to the action of alleles. This will also apply to different loci A and B having duplicate effects.

Besides satisfaction that accompanies the understanding of biochemical, physiological or morphological basis of interplay between genotype-environment interaction, these basic causes are not directly useful to the breeder, whose primary responsibility is to evolve and identify superior and stable varieties. Therefore, we have to turn to analysis of genotype-environment interaction.

8.4 Significance of Genotype-Environment Interaction

What breeders can do to overcome this complication depends upon the relative importance of variance components. Moreover, breeding programmes aimed to evolve stable genotypes also depend upon whether a breeder is dealing with predictable or unpredictable environmental variation.

When a breeder is concerned with predictable environmental variation the first step that he should take is to identify the differences. There is no difficulty when differences are recognisable, for example, differences in the seasons such as varieties to be developed for *kharif* (rainy season) or *rabi* (post-rainy season) season. Sorghum is grown in Maharashtra, Karnataka and Andhra Pradesh in *kharif* as well as in *rabi* seasons. Breeders can evolve varieties suitable for both these seasons because environmental variation is defined.

Significance of mean square for genotypes$\times$locations suggests that the region for which genotypes are being bred comprises of a number of special environments. In such circumstances the geographic region could be subdivided into sub-regions which are relatively homogeneous. Varieties should be bred which are specifically adapted to these ecotypes. Implication of genotypes$\times$years interaction is very different from the genotypes$\times$locations interaction. This is so because year-to-year fluctuations cannot be predicted in advance and breeders can hardly aim their programmes to develop varieties suited to particular years. This is also not practicable.

In some situations environmental variation is predictable but it can also be corrected. For example, saline soils can be corrected by certain agronomic practices or by addition of some amendments. This is easier and quicker than evolving varieties suitable for such situations. However, breeding of varieties suitable for saline or acidic soils is a low cost input and also a relatively permanent solution to the problem.

Whereas it is relatively easier to evolve varieties specifically adapted to predictable environmental situations it is very difficult to breed for unpredictable environmental variations. The aim of a breeding programme should, therefore, be to develop genotypes that can withstand unpredictable transient environmental fluctuations. In other words, breed widely adapted genotypes. According to Allard and Bradshaw (1964) "a variety which can adjust its genotypic or phenotypic state in response to transient fluctuations in environment in such ways that it gives high and stable economic returns for place and year is termed as well buffered". Plant breeders generally agree that the new variety must show high degree of stability in performance. However, the stability with which a plant breeder is concerned does not refer to constancy of phenotype in varying environments. It implies stability in those aspects of phenotype which are important economically such as grain yield and quality. Such stability may depend upon holding some aspects of morphology and physiology in steady state but allowing others to vary. In this way the desirable varieties will show low genotype×environment interaction for agriculturally important characters, especially grain yield, but not necessarily for others. Two basic concepts of phenotypic stability are distinguished: (i) the biological concept, and (ii) the agronomical concept. The biological concept of stability is referred to the constant performance of a genotype over a wide range of environments. This idea of stability is in agreement with the concept of homeostasis widely used in genetics. On the other hand, agronomical concept of stability implies that a stable genotype should always give high yield expected at the level of productivity of the respective environments, *i.e.*, a variety with genotype × environments interaction as small as possible. Is such stability under genetic control? Is it possible to measure stability in performance? Answers to these questions will be provided in next sections.

8.5 Stability and Buffering

All the living things can make physiological adjustments which permit them to cope with fluctuations in their immediate environment. These adjustments themselves are known as adaptations. Adaptation is the property of a genotype which permits its survival under selection. An adapted genotype or population is simply one which survives the selection procedure of a breeder, that is, one which performs better than the standard under comparison. According to Simmonds (1962) adaptation has four separable aspects. These are:

(a) Specific genotypic adaptation: It is close to adaptation of the corresponding genotypes to a limited environment.
(b) General genotypic adaptation is the capacity of a genotype to produce a range of phenotypes adapted to a variety of environments.
(c) Specific population adaptation is analogous to (a) and is the aspect of specific adaptation of heterogeneous population that is attributable to interaction between components rather than to the adaptations of components themselves.

(d) General population adaptation is analogous to general genotypic adaptation and is the capacity of heterogeneous population to adapt to a variety of environments.

The aim of a breeding programme is to identify genotypes which are widely adapted. According to Frey (1964), a variety having wide or good adaptability is one which gives consistently superior performance over several environments. There are two ways by which a variety can achieve stability in performance (Allard and Hansche, 1964). Firstly, the variety can be made up of a number of genotypes each of which is adapted to a somewhat different range of environments. It is called as populational buffering. Secondly, individuals themselves may be well buffered so that each member of the population is well adapted to a range of environments. This phenomenon is known as individual buffering. Genetically homogeneous populations, such as pure line varieties or single crosses, obviously depend upon individual buffering for stability in production. On the other hand, both individual and populational buffering are open to the genetically heterogeneous populations.

8.5.1 *Individual Buffering*

There is considerable evidence to show that buffering is a property of specific genotypes. Cereal breeders usually observe that there are some varieties which perform reasonably well under favourable as well as unfavourable conditions. They also notice varieties, performance of which is erratic. According to Lerner (1954) adaptedness—the attribute of an individual to be fit in Darwinian sense to their immediate environment – is mediated by heterozygous advantage in buffering ability. This holds true for plants also. Shank and Adams (1960) for example, compared inbred lines of maize with their hybrids for six characters. Coefficient of variability was relatively larger for inbred lines than for F_1 for these characters.

Heterozygosity also plays significant role for buffering in self-pollinated crops. Good evidence has been provided by Langridge and Griffing (1959) and Griffing and Langridge (1963).

8.5.2 *Populational Buffering*

Populational buffering arises due to interaction among different cohabiting genotypes within a population, *i.e.*, it is buffering above and beyond the individual buffering of specific constituents of the population. Like the individual buffering it should be possible to measure populational buffering in terms of genotype-environment interaction. Most precise information on populational buffering in crop plants comes from comparison between pure line varieties grown singly and in mixtures. Simmonds (1962) provided evidence to show that stability in yield is commonly associated with mixtures.

Information on populational buffering in heterozygous material comes both from cross-fertilizing and inbreeding species. In maize, Sprague and Federer (1951) and Eberhart and Russell (1969) showed that double-cross hybrids were relatively more stable in performance than single-cross hybrids. Jones (1958) compared performance of single and double-cross hybrids of maize in a number of yield trials and found that coefficient of variability was smaller for double-cross hybrids (12.3%) than for single-cross hybrids (21.4%). He attributed this stability of double-cross hybrids to populational buffering and suggested that it is the stability that permits double-crosses to give high yields when averaged over several environments, although highest yield in anyone place and year may be attained by a particular single-cross.

8.6 Detection of Genotype-Environment Interaction

Interaction of genotypes with the environment contributes to the total phenotypic variation which can be isolated and tested for significance. Usual procedure for detection of interaction involves multi-environmental testing of the genotypes in replicated trials. When all the genotypes behave consistently in all the environments, interaction term is absent. Variance due to genotype-environment interaction will get confounded with σ_g^2, if the genotypes are raised in one location for only one year. When the genotypes are raised at several locations and/or for several years, appropriate interpretation of results can be made after the joint statistical analysis by combining the results of individual trials. If error mean squares of individual analyses are homogeneous, pooled analysis of experiments is simple. We can regard the replications in each environment (location or year or both) as a group of replications. Mean of each genotype over all the replications in each environment or the total over replications in the environment can be taken for pooled analysis.

This simple analysis assumes that the error variances in all the environments are similar in magnitude. It is further assumed that the interactions of various genotypes with environments are of similar magnitude. In other words, the interactions of genotypes with environments are homogeneous. The experimental material may, therefore, belong to anyone of the following classes (Panse and Sukhatme, 1967):

(i) Experimental errors homogeneous and interactions absent
(ii) Experimental errors homogeneous and interactions present
(iii) Experimental errors heterogeneous and interactions absent, and
(iv) Experimental errors heterogeneous and the interactions present.

Before the data are subjected to pooled analysis, it is essential to test for homogeneity of error variances of individual analyses.

8.6.1 *Homogeneity of Experimental Errors*

Very often it is observed that when a treatment is repeated several times the results are not in perfect agreement with each other. For example, if a variety of wheat is planted in several plots of same size at a certain fertility level, kernel yields of all the plots will not be exactly alike. Failure of repeated observations, under similar conditions, to be identical is known as the experimental error. Linear mathematical model for observation recorded on *i*th genotype grown in *j*th environment may be expressed as:

$$x_{ij} = \mu + g_i + p_j + g_{ij} + \bar{e}_{ij}$$

where μ is the overall mean, g_i, p_j represent the effects of *i*th genotype, *j*th environment, respectively and g_{ij} is the effect due to genotype × environment interaction. $\bar{e}_{ij}$ is average of the errors associated with *i*th genotype grown in r plots in *j*th environment. It is assumed here that experimental errors, e_{ij}, of individual observations are normally and independently distributed with zero mean and same variance, σ_e^2. Further it is also assumed that the interaction terms g_{ij} are normally and independently distributed with zero population means and same variance, *i.e.*, σ_g^2 and are independent of *e's*. Both these assumptions may not be satisfied. Presently, we are concerned with error variances and, therefore, let us see how homogeneity of error variances is detected.

In general, magnitudes of error variances, σ_e^2*s* may not be same in all the experiments, unless the experiments have been conducted in same way, with same amount of control over environmental conditions and the experimental material is of same variability. In experiments with crops such high degree of uniformity is seldom attainable. In such experiments, therefore, we expect the experimental error variances to change from place-to-place and/or year-to-year. Heterogeneity of σ_e^2*s* invalidates the *F* test of interaction mean square against pooled error mean square. When experimental errors are homogeneous, pooled error mean square is obtained simply as average of error mean squares over all the environments, provided the error degrees of freedom are also identical. For more details on this subject, the reader is referred to Cochran and Cox (1957). Bartlett's test of homogeneity of variances is applied to the error mean squares, S^2, in the experiments.

When an experiment is conducted in *n* environments there will be *n* error mean squares. Provided that each error mean square, *i.e.*, S^2_1, S^2_2, S^2_3,..., S^2_n is based on k_1, k_2, k_3, ..., k_n degrees of freedom, pooled error mean square ($\overline{s^2}$) is obtained as:

$$\overline{s^2} = \Sigma \frac{1}{k_i} (\Sigma k_i s_i^2)$$

A quantity χ'^2 is then computed as:

$$\left(\sum_1^n k_i\right) \log_e \overline{s^2} - \sum_1^n k_i \log_e s_i^2$$

However, when the number of degrees of freedom (*i.e.*, *k*) are equal in all the environments, expression given above reduces to

$$k\left(n.\log_e \overline{s^2} - \sum_1^n \log_e s_i^2\right)$$

For convenience logarithms are taken to the base 10 and the result is multiplied by 2.3026 to obtain a value $\log_e$. Thus, log of $\overline{s^2}$ is found from the log table and the quantity so obtained is multiplied by 2.3026. This gives $\log_e \cdot \overline{s^2}$. Log values of individual s^2 are multiplied by 2.3026 and added which yields $\Sigma \log_e s_i^2$. The quantity χ'^2 is distributed approximately as chi-square with $(n-1)$ degrees of freedom, but is slightly biased upwards. It can be corrected by dividing χ^2 by c which is got as:

$$1+\frac{1}{3(n-1)}\left[\sum_1^n \frac{1}{k_i} - \frac{1}{\Sigma k_i}\right]$$

When the k s are equal, c is got simply as:

$$1+\frac{n+1}{3nk}$$

The quantity χ'^2/c is then referred to the table of chi-square for $(n-1)$ degrees of freedom. If the value of this ratio is less than the table value of χ^2 for 5 per cent level of significance, variances are regarded as homogeneous. We then proceed further for pooled analysis.

First step involved in the detection of genotype-environment interaction is to analyse and interpret the data in each environment (location and/or year) separately. If the individual analyses indicate significant differences among the genotypes, Bartlett's test is carried out to detect homogeneity of error variances. Provided the error mean squares are homogeneous, pooled analysis of the data follows the pattern of factorial analysis. We can employ either the means of genotypes over replications in each environment or the totals over the replications for pooled analysis. Because the stability analysis, to be described in section 8.7, is performed on means, it is desirable to use the means for detection of genotype-environment interaction.

8.6.2 *Worked Example*

Eight genotypes of sorghum were grown in four environments, *viz.* E_1, E_2, E_3 and E_4. In each environment, these genotypes were planted in a randomised block design with three replications. Data were recorded on grain yield/plot in kilograms (Table 8.1). Results of the analysis of variance in each of the four environments are presented in Table 8.2. Significant differences were observed among the eight genotypes for yield in each environment. Hence, we can proceed for pooled analysis.

TABLE 8.1: Grain yield (kg) of sorghum genotypes in four environments (means over 3 replications)

Genotypes	Environments				Total
	E_1	E_2	E_3	E_4	
G_1	3.165	5.183	5.692	5.375	19.415
G_2	3.257	5.225	6.561	5.608	20.651
G_3	3.812	5.866	6.769	5.708	22.155
G_4	2.310	4.656	4.103	4.583	15.652
G_5	2.633	5.883	6.391	5.950	20.857
G_6	3.673	5.383	6.469	5.450	20.975
G_7	2.957	4.233	4.632	3.500	15.322
G_8	2.564	4.883	4.667	5.200	17.314
Total	24.371	41.312	45.284	41.374	152.241

TABLE 8.2: Analysis of variance of grain yield (kg/plot) of sorghum (mean squares)

Source	*df*	Environments			
		E_1	E_2	E_3	E_4
Replications	2	0.0279	0.0846	0.8381	0.4375
Genotypes	7	0.8529	0.9710	3.2995	2.7109
Error	14	0.1380	0.2091	0.4040	0.3619

Estimate of pooled error mean square (s^{-2}) is calculated as:

$$\frac{\sum_{1}^{n} k_i s_i^2}{\sum_{1}^{n} k_i}$$

Usually totals of genotypes over replications are used to calculate the pooled error mean square. When means (over replications) of each of the genotypes are used for analysis, estimate of pooled error mean square is calculated as:

$$\frac{\sum_{1}^{n} k_i s_i^2}{\sum_{1}^{n} k_i r},$$

where r is the number of replications in each environment. The degrees of freedom for pooled error mean square are obtained by adding the degrees of freedom for error mean square in each of the n environments. The Bartlett's test of homogeneity of variances is:

$$\chi'^2 = k\,[(n \log_e s^{-2}) - \Sigma \log_e s^2_i]$$

For Bartlett's homogeneity test we need $\log_e s^{-2}$. For this example, s^{-2} is got as:

$$\frac{14(0.1380)+14(0.2091)+14(0.4040)+14(0.3619)}{56}$$

$$=0.2782$$

The log of 0.2782 is $\bar{1}.4443$. The characteristic is negative and mantissa positive, therefore, log value is $(-1+0.4443) = -0.5557$. However, we need $\log_e$ of 0.2782, which is got as:

$$-0.5557 \times 2.3026$$
$$= -1.2795$$

A term $\sum_{1}^{n} \log_e s_i^2$ is also required. For this purpose, the log values of four error mean squares are found, which are subsequently converted to $\log_e$ values. The four $\log_e$ values are then added to get $\Sigma \log_e s^2_i$. Thus,

$\log 0.1380 = \bar{1}.1399$ or -0.8601

$\log 0.2091 = \bar{1}.3203$ or -0.6797

$\log 0.4040 = \bar{1}.6064$ or -0.3936

$\log 0.3619 = \bar{1}.5586$ or -0.4414

The $\log_e$ values are then obtained as:

$\log_e 0.1380 = -0.8601 \times 2.3026 = -1.9805$
$\log_e 0.2091 = -0.6797 \times 2.3026 = -1.5651$
$\log_e 0.4040 = -0.3936 \times 2.3026 = -0.9063$
$\log_e 0.3619 = -0.4414 \times 2.3026 = -1.0164$

The χ'^2 is calculated as:

$$k\,[(n\,.\,\log_e \bar{s}^2) - \Sigma \log_e s_i^2]$$
$$= 14\,[(4 \times -1.2795) - (-1.9805 - 1.5651 - 0.9063 - 1.0164)]$$
$$= 14\,(-5.1180 + 5.4683)$$
$$= 4.9042$$

The correction factor is computed as:

$$1 + \frac{n+1}{3nk}$$
$$= 1 + \frac{4+1}{3 \times 4 \times 14}$$
$$= 1 + \frac{5}{168}$$
$$= 1.0298$$

The chi-square is, therefore, obtained as:

$$\frac{4.9042}{1.0298} = 4.7622$$

This value is referred to the table of chi-square for $(n-1)$, *i.e.*, 3, degrees of freedom. Since the observed value of χ^2 is less than the table value at 5 per cent level of significance, we can infer that the error variances in four environments are homogeneous. Using data provided in Table 8.1, we proceed for the pooled analysis. Thus,

Correction factor

$$\frac{(152.341)^2}{8 \times 4}$$
$$= 725.24312$$

Total sum of squares $= (3.165^2 + 3.257^2 + 3.812^2 + ... + 5.200^2) - CF$

$$= 48.9409$$

$$\text{Genotype S.S.} = \frac{1}{4}(19.415^2 + 20.651^2 + \ldots + 17.314^2) - CF$$

$$= \frac{1}{4}(2948.7382) - CF$$

$$= 11.9414$$

$$\text{Environment SS} = \frac{1}{8}(24.371^2 + 41.312^2 + 45.284^2 + 41.374^2) - CF$$

$$= 757.88441 - CF$$

$$= 32.6413$$

The sum of squares for genotype-environment interaction is got as a difference. Thus

Genotype-environment *s.s.* = Total *s.s.* – Genotype *s.s.* – Environment *s.s.*

$$= 48.9409 - 11.9414 - 32.6413$$

$$= 4.3582$$

Because means of the genotypes have been employed for the pooled analysis, error mean square for pooled analysis is obtained by dividing $\overline{s^2}$ by number of replications. Thus error mean square is

$$\frac{0.2782}{3}$$

$$= 0.0927$$

The analysis of variance is now set up as shown in Table 8.3.

TABLE 8.3: Pooled analysis of variance for grain yield of sorghum

Source	*df*	*SS*	*MS*	*F*
Genotypes	7	11.9414	1.7059**	8.22
Environments	3	32.6413	10.8804**	117.37
Geno. × Env.	21	4.3582	0.2075**	2.23
Pooled Error	56	–	0.0927	

What is the appropriate denominator to test the significance of genotype × environment interaction? The null hypothesis (H_0) is that genotype × environment interaction is absent (*i.e.*, $\sigma^2_{ge} = 0$). The F test is, therefore,

$$\frac{g \times e \text{ mean square}}{\text{Pooled error mean square}}$$

Value of this ratio is referred to the F table for 21 and 56 degrees of freedom. If the observed value is larger than the table value, significance of this mean square is indicated and we reject the null hypothesis.

The next step is to detect whether there are significant differences among the genotypes. Which mean square should be used as correct denominator for the F test to test significance among the genotypes? There are two candidates, *viz.* pooled error mean square and genotype × environment interaction mean square. A glance at Table 8.4 shows that the F test for $g \times e$ interaction is a ratio M_2/M_3.

TABLE 8.4: Format for ANOVA when g genotypes are grown in e environments

Source		Expectation mean squares		
	df	Means used	Totals used	*M.S.*
Environments	$(e-1)$			
Genotypes	$(g-1)$	$\sigma_e^2 + \sigma_{ge}^2 + e\sigma_g^2$	$\sigma^2 + r\sigma_{ge}^2 + re\sigma_g^2$	M_1
Geno. × Env.	$(g-1)(e-1)$	$\sigma_e^2 + \sigma_{ge}^2$	$\sigma^2 + r\sigma_{ge}^2$	M_2
Pooled Error	m*	σ_e^2	σ^2	M_3

* Degrees of freedom pooled over environments and σ_e^2 is got as $\overline{s^2}/r$.

The null hypothesis, as pointed out earlier, is that $\sigma_{ge}^2 = 0$. If this ratio is non-significant, we accept the null hypothesis (*i.e.*, $\sigma_{ge}^2 = 0$). However, when this ratio is significant we accept alternative hypothesis (H_1) which is $\sigma_{ge}^2 \neq 0$. An appropriate denominator for genotypes should be considered in this light. When the null hypothesis is rejected and alternative hypothesis accepted, mean square for genotype × environment interaction is the appropriate denominator for *F* test of genotypes. Thus *F* test for testing the significance of genotypes would be:

$$\frac{\sigma_e^2 + \sigma_{ge}^2 + e\sigma_g^2}{\sigma_e^2 + \sigma_{ge}^2}$$

The null hypothesis for this *F* test would be $\sigma_g^2 = 0$. If this is true, the ratio will be equal to unity. When the ratio is significant, we accept the alternative hypothesis ($H_1 = \sigma_g^2 \neq 0$). If we choose pooled error mean square for this *F* test, it will be:

$$\frac{\sigma_e^2 + \sigma_{ge}^2 + e\sigma_g^2}{\sigma_e^2}$$

This very clearly shows that even if $\sigma_g^2 = 0$, the ratio will be greater than unity, because σ_{ge}^2, which is the component of genotype × environment interaction mean square is present. This *F* test, therefore, leads to a wrong inference.

In the present example, *F* test for genotype × environment interaction is:

$$\frac{0.2075}{0.0927} = 2.23$$

This value is significant. Therefore, we conclude that genotype × environment interaction is present.

If the mean square for genotype × environment interaction is found to be non-significant, mean squares for pooled error and genotype × environment interaction are pooled as:

$$\frac{n_1 s_1 + n_2 s_2}{n_1 + n_2}$$

where n_1, n_2 are the degrees of freedom for genotype × environment interaction and pooled error, respectively, and s_1, s_2 are corresponding mean squares. The degrees of freedom for the two sources are also pooled. The new mean square represents the error mean square ,which should be then used as denominator to test the significance of genotypes and environments.

Since the mean square for genotypes × environment interaction is significant in the present example, the F test for genotypes is:

$$\frac{1.7059}{0.2075} = 8.22$$

This ratio suggests that there are significant differences among the eight genotypes for grain yield.

8.7 Stability Parameters – Statistical Approach

The process of identification of stable genotypes is difficult because of genotype-environment interaction. Although the plant breeders have observed genetic differences for adaptability they have been unable to fully exploit these differences in breeding of stable genotypes. This has been largely due to the problems of defining and measuring the phenotypic stability. Various attempts were made to characterise the behaviour of genotypes in response to varying environments.

Lewis (1954) introduced a term "stability factor" to measure the phenotypic stability. It is calculated as:

$$S.F. = \frac{\overline{X}_{HE}}{\overline{X}_{LE}},$$

where $\overline{X}_{HE}$ and $\overline{X}_{LE}$ refer to the mean measurements in high-yielding and low-yielding environments, respectively. Performance of stable genotype should be same, *i.e.*, $S.F. = 1$, according to Lewis (1954). The greater the deviation of $S.F.$ from unity lesser the phenotypic stability.

Plaisted and Peterson (1959) suggested calculation of mean σ^2_{gl} in order to detect a stable genotype. When g genotypes are raised at several locations, a combined analysis of variance over all the locations is carried out for each pair of genotypes (there will be $g(g-1)/2$ pairs). Combined analysis will provide an estimate of σ^2_{gl} for each pair. Each genotype appears in $(g-1)$ analyses. Mean σ^2_{gl} is calculated from $(g-1)$ combined analyses for each genotype. A genotype with smallest σ^2_{gl} is regarded as the 'most' stable genotype. If large number of genotypes are to be evaluated, this method would call for large number of analyses and hence is not practicable.

Statistical approach of Finlay and Wilkinson (1963) has proved considerably useful to measure phenotypic stability in the performance of genotypes. They recognised an interesting fact that the components of genotype-environment interaction are linearly related to the environmental effects when the environmental effects are measured on the same scale as the genotypic effects. The procedure developed by Finlay and Wilkinson (1963) comprised of calculating for each variety a linear regression of its yield on mean yields of all the varieties at each of the locations and/or seasons. They quantified the natural environments in terms of mean yields of all the varieties at a location and/or season, which was designated as 'site means'. No attempt was made to measure the variation in moisture or nitrogen supply, radiation, temperature or any other environmental factors. For calculation of means and regressions, Finlay and Wilkinson (1963) measured the data on a logarithmic scale. In their opinion measurement of yields on logarithmic scale induced a high degree of linearity in the regressions of individual yields on site means. Logarithmic scale also induced a reasonable degree of homogeneity of experimental errors. Regression coefficients and mean performance of varieties were considered by them as a useful criterion for characterising the phenotypic stability (Table 8.5). Genotypes with b lesser than unity do not respond favourably to improved environmental conditions and hence could be regarded as specifically adapted to poor environments when their mean performance is more than average of all varieties. On the other hand, a genotype is recognised as below average in stability when b_i is > 1 and mean performance is more than the average performance.

Such genotypes tend to respond favourably to better environments but give poor yield in unfavourable environments. An ideal genotype would be one with $b_i = 0$ and mean performance above the average of all the varieties. However, this is practically difficult to achieve.

The regression analysis proposed by Finlay and Wilkinson (1963) to measure phenotypic stability was improved upon by Eberhart and Russell (1966). They introduced (in addition to two parameters proposed by Finlay and Wilkinson, 1963, $\overline{X}_i$ and b_i) one more parameter, which accounts for unpredictable irregularities in the responses of genotypes to varying environments measured as the deviation from the regression lines, to characterise a stable genotype.

TABLE 8.5. A generalised interpretation of varietal adaptation (Finlay and Wilkinson, 1963)

Mean performance ($\bar{X}_i$)	Regression Coefficient (b_i)	Nature of adaptation
Higher than the average of all varieties	1.0 (average)	Well adapted to all the environments
Lower than the average of all varieties	1.0	Poorly adapted to all the environments
Higher than the average	Greater than 1.00 (Below average)	Specifically adapted to favourable environments
Higher than the average	Lesser than 1.0 (Above average)	Specifically adapted to unfavourable (poor) environments.

In the model proposed by Eberhart and Russell (1966), sum of the mean squares attributable to environments and genotypes × environments interaction is partitioned into three components, *viz*. Environments (linear), Genotypes × environments (linear) and deviations from regression (Pooled deviation over all the genotypes). A linear model proposed by Eberhart and Russell (1966) is:

$$Y_{ij} = \mu_i + \beta_i I_j + \delta_{ij}$$

where Y_{ij} is the mean performance of *i*th variety ($i = 1, 2, ..., v$) in *j*th ($j = 1, 2, ..., n$) environment, μ_i is the mean of *i*th variety over all the environments, β_i is the regression coefficient which measures the response of *i*th variety to varying environments, δ_{ij} the deviation from regression of *i*th variety in the *j*th environment, and I_j is the environmental index of *j*th environment. The environmental index, I_j, for *j*th environment is calculated as:

$$\left[\left(\frac{\sum_i Y_{ij}}{v}\right) - \left(\frac{\sum_i \sum_j Y_{ij}}{vn}\right)\right], \sum_j I_j = 0$$

This quantification of environments differs from that of the Finlay and Wilkinson (1963) in that the means of all the varieties at a site and/or season was regarded by them as "site mean". Eberhart and Russell (1966) preferred to measure the environment as deviation of mean of all the varieties at a location from the overall mean. They recognised a need for defining environmental index which is independent of the experimental varieties but is based on environmental factors such as rainfall, temperature and soil fertility. However, our present knowledge of the relationship of these factors and yield does not permit computation of such an index. Until we can measure such factors in order to formulate a mathematical relationship with yield, average yield of the varieties in particular environment must suffice. Eberhart and Russell (1966) recommended growing of varieties in adequate number of environments, covering a full range of possible environmental conditions, so that a useful information is available regarding stability.

The estimate of stability factor b_i, is obtained for ith variety as:

$$b_i = \frac{\sum_j Y_{ij} I_j}{\sum_j I_j^2}$$

Another stability parameter is the squared deviations from this regression. Estimate of this stability parameter $\left(s_{di}^2\right)$ is obtained as:

$$S_{d_i}^2 = \left[\frac{\sum_j \delta_{ij}^2}{(n-2)}\right] - \frac{S_e^2}{r}$$

δ_{ij} is the deviation of ith variety in jth environment from regression and is got as:

$$\delta_{ij} = y_{ij} - \hat{y}_{ij}$$

where $\hat{y}_{ij}$ is expected value of ith variety in jth environment. It is predicted as $\overline{X}_i + b_i I_j$. s_e^2/r is the estimate of pooled error mean square. In practice $\sum_j \delta_{ij}^2$ is calculated as:

$$\left[\sum_j Y_{ij}^2 - \frac{Y_{i.}^2}{n}\right] - \frac{\left(\sum_j Y_{ij} I_j\right)^2}{\sum_j I_j^2}$$

This approach to the measurement of phenotypic stability is based on regression analysis. In the regression analysis, variation of dependent variable (y) can be partitioned into two components, *viz*. due to its regression on independent variable (x) and deviation from regression or residual variation. The former could be expressed as $b\,\Sigma(x-\bar{x})(y-\bar{y})$, while the latter as $\Sigma(y-\bar{y})^2 - b\,\Sigma(x-\bar{x})(y-\bar{y})$. In the present context, the regression component could be expressed as:

$$\frac{\sum_j Y_{ij} I_j}{\sum_j I_j^2} \cdot \sum_j Y_{ij} I_j = \frac{\left(\sum_j y_{ij} I_j\right)^2}{\sum_j I_j^2}$$

And, therefore, the residual variation for ith variety $\left(\sum_j \delta_{ij}^2\right)$ is obtained as shown above. This model, therefore, provides a means of partitioning the genotype-environment interaction of each variety into two parts:

(i) Variation due to the response of a variety to varying environmental indexes (sums of squares due to regression), and

(ii) deviations from regression on environmental index.

An appropriate structure for analysis of variance for stability is presented in Table 8.6.

Various sums of squares are calculated as:

(i) Genotypes sum of squares:

$$\left(\frac{1}{n}\sum_i Y_{i.}^2\right) - C.F.$$

where $\sum_i Y_{i.}^2$ is got by squaring totals of each genotype over environments and adding all the squared values.

(ii) Environments (linear) sum of squares:

This value is obtained from pooled analysis. Environments S.S. of pooled analysis is environments (linear) S.S. of the stability analysis. It is calculated as:

$$\frac{\frac{1}{v}\left(\sum_{j} Y_{.j} I_{.j}\right)^2}{\sum_{j} I_j^2}$$

TABLE 8.6: Format for analysis of variance for stability analysis (Eberhart and Russell, 1966)

Source	*df*	*SS*	*MS*
Genotypes	$(v - 1)$		M_1
Environment +	$(n - 1) + (v-1)(n-1)$		
(Genotypes × Env.)	$= v(n - 1)$		
Env. (linear)	1		
Geno. × Env. (linear)	$(v - 1)$		M_2
Pooled deviations	$v(n - 2)$		M_3
Genotype 1	$(n - 2)$		
Genotype 2	$(n - 2)$		
.	.		
.	.		
.	.		
Genotype v	$(n - 2)$		
Pooled error	$n(r - 1)(v - 1)$		M_4
Total	$(nv - 1)$		

(iii) Genotypes × environments (linear) sum of square:

$$\sum_i \left[\frac{\left(\sum_j Y_{ij} I_j \right)^2}{\sum_j I_j^2} \right] - \text{environments (linear) sum of squares}$$

(iv) Sum of squares for pooled deviations are obtained as:

$$\sum_i \sum_j \delta_{ij}^2$$

Pooled deviation sum of squares are made up of v components each with $(n - 2)$ degrees of freedom. For ith genotype $\sum_j \delta_{ij}^2$ is calculated as (described earlier also):

$$(\sum_j Y_{ij}^2 - \frac{Y_{i.}^2}{n}) - \frac{(\sum_j Y_{ij} I_j)^2}{\sum_j I_j^2}$$

The pooled deviations mean square is tested against the pooled error mean square. Thus F test is:

$$\frac{M_3}{M_4}$$

When the mean square for pooled deviations is significant but mean square for genotype × environments (linear) is non-significant, variation in the performance of genotypes is entirely unpredictable. On the other hand, significance of mean square for pooled deviations, when mean square for genotypes × environments (linear) is also significant, implies that part of the variability is unpredictable in nature.

Appropriate denominator to test the significance of mean square for genotypes is pooled deviations mean square (if it is significant), the null hypothesis (H_0) being that $\mu_1 = \mu_2 = ... = \mu_v$. $\mu_1, \mu_2 ... \mu_v$ denote the mean performances of genotypes 1, 2, ..., v, respectively. Thus,

$$F = \frac{M_1}{M_3}$$

Here we assume that deviations are homogeneous over all the varieties. If the deviations are not homogeneous, difficulty arises.

The hypothesis that there are non-significant differences among the regression coefficients is tested approximately by F test as M_2/M_3, provided that M_3 is significant.

The null hypothesis in this case being $\beta_1 = \beta_2 = \beta_3 ... = \beta_{r}$. If the mean square for genotypes × environments (linear) is found to be significant, conclusion is drawn that variation in the performance of genotypes is due to the regression of genotypes on environments and hence the performance is predictable in nature. The next step is to test the significance of b_i from zero. A 't' test is employed for this purpose. Thus,

$$t = \frac{b_i - 0}{S.E._{b_i}}$$

If b_i is significant, it's significant deviation from unity is tested as:

$$t = \frac{1 - b_i}{S.E._{b_i}}$$

Standard error of b_i is got from the component of mean square for pooled deviations corresponding to the ith genotype. Thus, for genotype i, the mean square for deviation corresponding to this genotype should be employed to calculate standard error of b_i. Thus

$$S.E._{bi} = \sqrt{\frac{\left(\sum_j \delta_{ij}^2 / n - 2\right)}{\sum_j I_j^2}}$$

Why? The answer is simple. We know that the standard error for linear regression of y on x is:

$$\left[\frac{\Sigma(y-\bar{y})^2 - b\,\Sigma(x-\bar{x})(y-\bar{y})}{(n-2)\,\Sigma(x-\bar{x})^2}\right]^{\frac{1}{2}}$$

In the regression analysis for stability, term $\sum_j \delta_{ij}^2$ is equal to $\Sigma(y-\bar{y})^2 - b\Sigma(x-\bar{x})(y-\bar{y})$ and $\delta_{ij}^2 / n - 2$ is the mean square component of pooled deviation corresponding to *i*th genotype. $\Sigma(x-\bar{x})^2$ is the sum of squares of environmental index and it is simply $\sum_j I_j^2$ (because $\sum_j I_j = 0$).

Significance of the deviation of each genotype from its regression can be tested by an appropriate F test. Thus

$$F = \frac{\left(\dfrac{\sum_j \delta_{ij}^2}{n-2}\right)}{\text{Pooled error mean square}}$$

8.7.1 *Worked Example*

In section 8.6, data were presented for grain yield of eight genotypes of sorghum grown in four environments. It was observed that genotypes manifested significant interaction with environments (Table 8.3). Data provided in Table 8.1 will be used to describe steps involved in the stability analysis.

The first stability parameter is b_i. It is got as:

$$\frac{\sum_j Y_{ij} I_j}{\sum_j I_j^2}$$

We, therefore, require estimates of environmental indices, *viz.* I_j, which is calculated as:

$$I_j = \frac{\sum_i Y_{ij}}{v} - \frac{\sum_i \sum_j Y_{ij}}{vn}$$

Grand mean, $(\sum_i \sum_j Y_{ij} / vn)$, is $152.341/32 = 4.761$. Means of E_1, E_2, E_3 and E_4 are 3.046, 5.164, 5.660 and 5.172, respectively. Therefore, the four environmental indices are found as:

$$I_1 = 3.046 - 4.761 = -1.715$$
$$I_2 = 5.164 - 4.761 = 0.403$$
$$I_3 = 5.660 - 4.761 = 0.899$$
$$I_4 = 5.172 - 4.761 = 0.411$$

It was pointed out in section 8.7 that sum of environmental indices over all the environments is zero. Thus.

$$(-1.715) + (0.403) + (0.899) + (0.411)$$
$$= -0.002$$

which is practically equal to zero.

In order to compute the regression coefficients, covariances of genotypes with environmental indices are required for each genotype, which are obtained as:

$$\begin{matrix} G_1 \\ G_2 \\ G_3 \\ G_4 \\ G_5 \\ G_6 \\ G_7 \\ G_8 \end{matrix} \underbrace{\begin{bmatrix} 3.165 & 5.183 & 5.692 & 5.375 \\ 3.257 & 5.225 & 6.561 & 5.608 \\ 3.812 & 5.866 & 6.769 & 5.708 \\ 2.310 & 4.656 & 4.103 & 4.583 \\ 2.633 & 5.883 & 6.391 & 5.950 \\ 3.673 & 5.383 & 6.469 & 5.450 \\ 2.957 & 4.233 & 4.632 & 3.500 \\ 2.564 & 4.883 & 4.667 & 5.200 \end{bmatrix}}_{Y_{ij}} \underbrace{\begin{bmatrix} -1,715 \\ \\ 0.403 \\ 0.899 \\ \\ 0.411 \end{bmatrix}}_{I_j} = \underbrace{\begin{bmatrix} 3.987 \\ 4.723 \\ 4.258 \\ 3.487 \\ 6.046 \\ 3.926 \\ 2.237 \\ 3.903 \end{bmatrix}}_{\sum_j Y_{ij} I_j}$$

Among these matrices, the first matrix comprises of the mean values of eight genotypes in four environments. Environmental indices constitute the second matrix. Multiplication of first and second matrix gives the third matrix, which comprises of covariance values of eight genotypes with four environmental indices. For example, the covariance of first genotype is obtained as:

$$\sum_j Y_{ij} I_j = 3.165 \times (-1.715) + 5.183 \times 0.403$$

$$+ 5.692 \times 0.899 + 5.375 \times 0.411$$

$$= 3.98701 \text{ or } 3.987$$

Variance of the environmental indices (ΣI_j^2) is

$$(-1.715)^2 + (0.403)^2 + (0.899)^2 + (0.411)^2$$

$$= 4.0807 \text{ or } 4.081.$$

Regression coefficient for the first genotype is then calculated as:

$$b_1 = \frac{3.987}{4.081}$$

$$= 0.97697 \text{ or } 0.977$$

Regression coefficients for other genotypes are also calculated in like manner (Table 8.7).

Now let us calculate the second parameter of stability, *viz.* S_{di}^2. It is got as:

$$\left[\frac{\sum_j \delta_{ij}^2}{(n-2)}\right] - \frac{S_e^2}{r}$$

For *i*th genotype $\sum_j \delta_{ij}^2$ is got as:

$$\Sigma(Y_i - \overline{Y}_i)^2 - b_i \sum_j Y_{ij} I_j \quad ,$$

where $\Sigma(Y_i - \overline{Y}_i)^2$ is the sum of deviations squared for *i*th genotype. For the first genotype, for example, it is found as :

$$(3.165^2 + 5.183^2 + 5.692^2 + 5.375^2) - \frac{(19.415)^2}{4}$$

$$= 3.935$$

$\therefore$ $\sum_j \delta_{ij}^2$ for 1st genotype is:

$$3.935 - 3.895 = 0.04$$

Information required to calculate $\sum_j \delta_{ij}^2$ for other genotypes is given in Table 8.7.

TABLE 8.7: Steps involved in the calculation of $\sum_j \delta_{ij}^2$ for eight genotypes of sorghum

$\Sigma(y-\bar{y})^2$	b	$\sum_j Y_{ij} I_j$	$b\sum_j Y_{ij} I_j$	$\sum_j \delta_{ij}^2 = \Sigma(Y-\bar{Y})^2 - b\Sigma Y_{ij} I_j$
1	2	3	4	5
3.935	0.977	3.987	3.895	0.040
5.789	1.157	4.723	5.465	0.324
4.631	1.043	4.258	4.441	0.190
3.607	0.854	3.487	2.978	0.629
9.036	1.482	6.046	8.960	0.076
4.030	0.962	3.926	3.777	0.253
1.677	0.548	2.237	1.226	0.451
4.295	0.956	3.903	3.731	0.564
Total	7.979		34.473	2.527

For genotype 1, S^2_d is calculated as:

$$\left(\frac{0.04}{2}\right) - 0.0927$$

$$= -0.0727$$

Deviations squared for other genotypes are also computed in similar fashion, which are presented below:

Genotypes	S_{di}^2
2	0.0693
3	0.0023
4	0.2220
5	−0.0547
6	0.0343
7	0.1330
8	0.1890

Now let us proceed to the analysis of variance for stability. The sum of squares for genotypes have been calculated (Table 8.3). Environment sum of squares, presented in Table 8.3, is the sum of squares for environments (linear). Sum of squares for genotypes × environments (linear) is obtained as:

$$\sum_i \left(b_i \sum_j Y_{ij} I_j \right) - \text{Environments (linear) s.s.}$$

Total at the end of fourth column of Table 8.7 is $\sum_i \left(b \sum_j Y_{ij} I_j \right)$ or

$\sum_i \left[\left(\sum_j Y_{ij} I_j \right)^2 \Big/ \sum_j I_j^2 \right]$. Thus, genotypes × environments (linear) s.s.

is:

$$34.473 - 32.6413 = 1.8317$$

Deviations squared from the regression for each genotype have been computed in the fifth column of Table 8.7. Sum of the eight deviations squared gives sum of squares for pooled deviations $\left(\sum_i \sum_j \delta_{ij}^2 \right)$. It is 2.527 in the present example. Pooled error mean square is also available (Table 8.3). The analysis of variance for stability is now set up as shown in Table 8.8 As a first step we test the validity of assumption that there are non-significant differences among the deviations of genotypes being evaluated from their expected performances. Thus,

1 $$F = \frac{0.1579}{0.0927}$$

$$= 1.70.$$

When referred to the F table this value is found to be non-significant. This suggests that deviations of all the genotypes, from their expected performances, are similar in magnitude, and unpredictable causes of variation are not responsible for observed genotype × environment interaction.

In order to test the validity of hypothesis that there are non-significant differences among the eight genotypes with respect to their mean grain yields ($H_0 = \mu_1 = \mu_2 ... = \mu_v$), mean square for pooled error is used as denominator (because mean square for pooled deviations is non-significant). Thus,

$$F = \frac{M_1}{M_4} = \frac{1.7059}{0.0927} = 18.40.$$

This value is highly significant when referred to the *F* table for 7 and 56 degrees of freedom, hence we accept the alternate hypothesis, H_1, that $\mu_1 \neq \mu_2 \neq \ldots \neq \mu_v$. Thus there are significant differences among the eight genotypes with respect to the average grain yield/plant. Do the regression coefficients of eight genotypes differ significantly from each other? The answer is provided by *F* test. Thus.

$$F = \frac{M_2}{M_4} = \frac{0.2616}{0.0927} = 2.82$$

References to the *F* table for 7 and 56 degrees of freedom suggests that there are significant differences among the regression coefficients of eight genotypes. Thus differential performance of varieties when grown in 4 environments is predictable in nature. Prediction can be made on the basis of linear regression equation.

TABLE 8.8: ANOVA for stability of grain yield of sorghum

Source	*df*	*SS*	*MS*		*F*
Genotypes	7	11.9415	1.7059 **	M_1	18.40
Env. + (Geno × env.)	24	36.9995	1.5416		
Env. (linear)	1	32.6413	32.6413		
Geno. × Env. (linear)	7	1.8317	0.2616 *	M_2	2.82
Pooled deviations	16	2.527	0.1579	M_3	1.70
Genotype 1	2	0.040	0.020		0.21
2	2	0.324	0.162		1.74
3	2	0.190	0.095		1.02
4	2	0.629	0.315 *		3.39
5	2	0.076	0.038		0.41
6	2	0.253	0.127		1.37
7	2	0.451	0.226		2.43
8	2	0.564	0.282		3.04
Pooled error	56	–	0.0927	M_4	

The hypothesis that regression coefficient of a given genotype does not differ from zero can be tested by a '*t*' test. For example '*t*' test for regression coefficient of the first genotype (b_1) would be:

$$t = \frac{b_1}{SE_{b_1}}$$

Standard error of b_1 is calculated as:

$$\left(\frac{\sum_j \delta_{1j}^2 / n-2}{\sum_j I_j^2} \right)^{\frac{1}{2}}$$

$$= \left(\frac{0.02}{4.081} \right)^{\frac{1}{2}}$$

$$= 0.07$$

The '*t*' test for b_1 is then

$$\frac{0.977}{0.07}$$

$$= 13.95$$

The value is significant at 1 per cent level of significance. We, therefore, place two asterisks on the *b* value. This significance suggests that the *b* value is significantly different from zero.

In the next step, we test the validity of assumption that the *b* does not differ from unity. Thus,

$$t = \frac{1.0 - 0.977}{0.07}$$

$$= 0.32$$

Value of this ratio is found to be non-significant. We, therefore, conclude that b_1 is not significantly different from unity.

Standard error of rest of the regression coefficients are given below:

Genotypes	Standard errors of b
2	0.199
3	0.152
4	0.278
5	0.096
6	0.176
7	0.235
8	0.262

The tests of significance reveal that only the regression coefficient of fifth genotype is significantly different from unity, which implies that all the genotypes being tested are average in stability, except the fifth genotype (provided we consider only the b values). Fifth genotype appears to be specifically adapted to the favourable environments (*i.e.*, below average in stability).

Significance of each $\sum_j \delta_{ij}^2 / n-2$ is tested against mean square for pooled error (only if pooled deviations mean square is significant). Significance of $\sum_j \delta_{ij}^2 / n-2$, for example, is tested as:

$$F = \frac{0.020}{0.0927}$$

$$= 0.215$$

When referred to the F table, this value is found to be non-significant. Other deviations, except the 4th, are also non-significant.

According to Eberhart and Russell (1966) a variety can be considered as stable if it meets following requirements:

(i) high mean yield ($\bar{x}$),

(ii) $b = 1$, and

(iii) s^2_d approaching zero

TABLE 8.9 : Showing $\overline{x}$, b, and S^2_d of eight genotypes

Genotype	$\overline{x}$		b	S^2_d
1	4.854		0.977**	−0.072
2	5.163		1.157**	0.069
3	5.387		1.043**	0.002
4	3.913		0.854**	0.222*
5	5.214		1.482**	−0.054
6	5.244		0.962**	0.034
7	3.830		0.548**	0.133
8	4.328		0.956**	0.189
$\overline{\overline{x}}$	4.741	$\overline{b}$	0.997	

*, ** Significantly different from zero at 1 and 5 per cent level, respectively.

It appears from Table 8.9 that genotype 3 has mean yield higher than the overall mean, $b = 1.043$ and $s^2d = 0.002$. This genotype could be regarded as stable and widely adapted. On the other hand, genotype 5 is specifically adapted to favourable environments because its regression is significantly more than unity ($b = 1.482$), mean yield is higher than the average and s^2d is nearly zero. Genotypes 2 and 6 are also desirable.

Performance of genotypes in different environments could be presented in a graphical form. The abscissa (X axis) is marked with environmental indices and the ordinate (Y axis) with yield levels. Expected yield of a variety is plotted against corresponding environmental indices. Join these points which gives regression line for a genotype. In this way regression lines for all the genotypes being investigated are plotted. Expected yield of ith genotype in jth environment is calculated as:

$$\hat{Y}_{ij} = \overline{X}_i + b_i I_j$$

For example, the expected yields of first genotype in four environments are obtained as:

$$\text{Environment } 1 = 4.854 + 0.977\,(-1.715) = 3.178$$
$$\text{Environment } 2 = 4.854 + 0.977\,(0.403) = 5.247$$
$$\text{Environment } 3 = 4.854 + 0.977\,(0.899) = 5.732$$
$$\text{Environment } 4 = 4.854 + 0.977\,(0.411) = 5.255$$

Expected yields of other genotypes are computed in similar fashion.

Figure 8.1 shows that the first environmental index is negative and has a large value. Hence it is the most unfavourable environment. Environment 3 appears to be the most favourable one, followed by environments 4 and 2 in that order. Genotype 3 has not only given better performance in favourable environments but also in poorest environment. On the other hand, yield levels of genotype 5 have increased with the improvement in environment.

A scatter graph of the stability is also sometimes plotted. On a graph paper the abscissa is marked with yield levels and the ordinate with regression coefficients. Observed yield of given genotype is then plotted against it's b value. The two vertical lines on this graph respresent the values $\overline{x} \pm \sigma$ and the horizontal ones denote the values $\overline{b} \pm \sigma_b$. It will be apparent from the graph (Fig. 8.2) that although the points for genotypes 2, 3, 5 and 6 fall near the line for $\overline{x} + \sigma$, genotypes 3, 6 and 2 appear desirable because the point for genotype 5 is far away from the lines $\overline{b} + \sigma_b$.

8.8 Stability Parameters—Genetical Approach

In the earlier section a statistical approach to stability analysis was described. The components in this analysis have not been related to the parameters in a biometrical genetical model. The other approach is based on fitting models which specify the contribution of genetic, environmental and genotype-environmental interaction effects to generation means and variances (Mather and Jones, 1958; Jones and Mather, 1958; Bucio Alanis, 1966; Bucio Alanis and Hill, 1966).

The analysis of Eberhart and Russell (1966) is applicable to any number and kinds of strains grown in any number of environments. Bucio Alanis (1966) and Bucio Alanis and Hill (1966) developed an alternative analysis which was appropriate only for a pair of inbred lines and generations derived from an initial cross between them. This analysis, however, leads to more informative conclusions and can be employed to predict the performance across generations as well as across environments. However, the most important conclusion to emerge from analysis of the data is same for both kinds of analyses, *viz.* that genotype-environmental interactions are linear functions of environmental effects. This conclusion also applies to the interactions of environment with additive and dominance effects of genes.

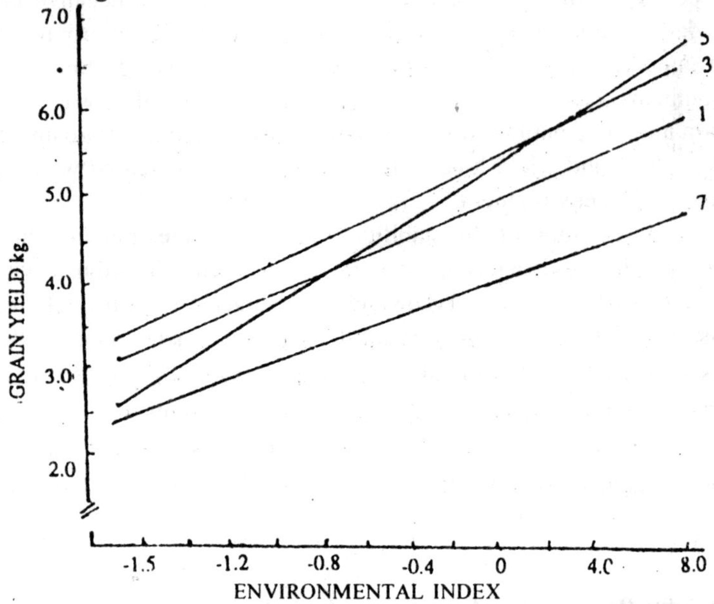

FIG. 8.1: *Stability performance of genotypes. Linear regression of grain yield on environmental indices are plotted on this graph. In this figure, lines for only four genotypes have been shown. Other lines have not been drawn.*

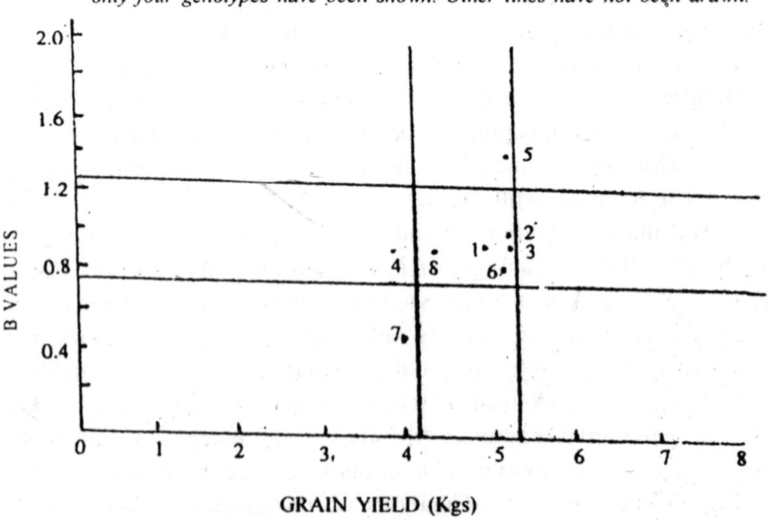

FIG. 8.2: *Stability of genotypes*

To explain the basic concepts involved in this approach let us begin with a simple situation of single locus with two alleles, *A* and *a*. With respect to this locus there will be two inbred lines *AA* and *aa*. If these inbred lines are grown in two environments *X* and *Y*, three parameters are required to describe differences among the four phenotypes (Table 8.10). Following Mather and Jinks (1971) these could be described by three parameters *d*, *e* and gd_1.

TABLE 8.10: Showing phenotypes of two genotypes grown in two environments

		Genotypes		Mean
		AA	*aa*	
Environ-ments	*X*	$d + e_1 + gd_1$	$-d + e_1 - gd_1$	e_1
	Y	$d - e_1 - gd_1$	$-d - e_1 + gd_1$	$-e_1$
Mean		*d*	$-d$	0

Where *d* measures the difference between two genotypes expressed as deviation from the overall mean (m). In the present case $m = 0$. e_1 represents the difference between two environments. It is measured as deviation of means of two genotypes *AA* and *aa* from overall mean. Parameter gd_1 measures the interaction of genetical and environmental components *d* and e_1.

We can now generalise the situation to consider several loci affecting a given character. In this case *d* is replaced by [*d*]. Estimates of parameters [*d*], e_1 and gd_1 could be obtained in several ways. However, simple procedure would be:

$$\hat{m} = \frac{1}{4}(AAX + aaX + AAY + aaY)$$

$$[\hat{d}] = \frac{1}{4}(AAX + AAY - aaX - aaY)$$

$$\hat{e}_1 = \frac{1}{4}(AAX + aaX - AAY - aaY), \text{ and}$$

$$\hat{g}d_1 = \frac{1}{4}(AAX - aaX - AAY + aaY)$$

where AAX, aaX, AAY and aaY denote the mean performance of AA and aa genotypes in X and Y environments, respectively.

8.8.1 *Worked Example*

Two inbred lines of sorghum, *viz.* 2219B and 555, were grown in two environments. Measurements were made on days to 50 per cent bloom. Estimates of standard errors were calculated from observations recorded on a number of individuals within each inbred line.

		Inbred lines	
		555	2219B
Environ-	1	93.0 ± 1.25	69.5 ± 2.25
ments	2	90.0 ± 0.85	60.0 ± 0.65

Estimates of parameters m, $[d]$, e_1 and gd_1 are obtained as:

$$m = \frac{1}{4}(93.0 + 69.5 + 90.0 + 60.0) = 78.125$$

$$[d] = \frac{1}{4}(93.0 - 69.5 + 90.0 - 60.0) = 13.375$$

$$e_1 = \frac{1}{4}(93.0 + 69.5 - 90.0 - 60.0) = 3.125$$

$$gd_1 = \frac{1}{4}(93.0 - 69.5 - 90.0 + 60.0) = -1.625$$

The standard error for these parameters is got as:

$$(1.25 + 2.25 + 0.85 + 0.65)^{1/2}$$
$$= 2.236$$

Values of e_1 and gd_1 are non-significant.

The formula used to calculate estimate of gd_1 is a scaling test which tells us whether the model which assumes absence of genotype × environment interaction is adequate or not. Estimates of these parameters could be obtained by means of procedure advocated for joint scaling test also.

If the F_1 of these two inbred lines is also grown along with the parents in two environments the mean measurements could be linearly expressed as:

Environment	Genotype *Aa*
X	$h + e_1 + gh_1$
Y	$h - e_1 - gh_1$

When several loci are considered h is replaced by $[h]$. The parameters $[h]$ and g_{h1} can be estimated only when F_1 is grown along with two parents.

The inbred lines and F_1 between them could be grown in several environments.

The mean expressions of two inbred lines say P_1 and P_2 and F_1 grown in *j*th environment could be expressed as:

$$\overline{P}_{1j} = m + [d] + e_j + gd_j$$

$$\overline{P}_{2j} = m - [d] + e_j - gd_j \text{ and}$$

$$\overline{F}_{1j} = m + [h] + e_j + gh_j ,$$

where m is the mid-parental value averaged over all the environments, $[d]$ is half the difference between the two inbrd lines averaged over all the environments, $[h]$ is the average deviation of F_1 from mid-point over all the environments. Sum of all the *e*s is zero and likewise sum of all *gd*s and the *gh*s over all the environments is zero.

Bucio Alanis and Hill (1966) observed that the regression of *gs* on corresponding *es* were significant and linear. Thus,

$$b_d = \frac{gd_j}{e_j}$$

$\therefore \qquad b_d e_j = gd_j$

Likewise

$$b_h = \frac{gh_j}{e_j}$$

$\therefore \qquad b_h e_j = gh_j$

Hence the mean expressions of P_1, P_2 and F_1 in jth environment could be linearly expressed as:

$$\begin{aligned}\overline{P}_{1j} &= m + [d] + e_j + gd_j \\ &= m + [d] + e_j + b_d e_j \\ &= m + [d] + (1 + b_d)e_j\end{aligned}$$

Similarly $\overline{P}_{2j} = m - [d] + (1 - bd)e_j$, and

$$\begin{aligned}\overline{F}_{1j} &= m + [h] + e_j + gh_j \\ &= m + [h] + e_j + b_h e_j \\ &= m + [h] + (1 + b_h)e_j\end{aligned}$$

Perkins and Jinks (1968) developed an analysis known as joint regression analysis, based on theory developed by Bucio Alanis (1966) and Bucio Alanis and Hill (1966), to measure genotype-environment interaction and identify stable genotypes involving several inbred lines and their crosses. The model upon which their analysis is based is:

$$Y_{ij} = \mu + d_i + E_j + g_{ij} + e_{ij}$$

where Y_{ij} is the performance of ith line in jth environment, μ is the grand mean overall the lines and all the environments, d_i is the additive genetic contribution to the ith line, E_j is the additive environmental contribution of jth environment, g_{ij} is the genotype-environmental interaction of ith line and e_{ij} is the experimental error of ith line in jth environment. They regarded d_i, E_j and g_{ij} as fixed effects, so that

$$\sum_i d_i = 0, \sum_j E_j = 0 \text{ and } \sum_{ij} g_{ij} = 0$$

Thus g_{ij} can be expressed as:

$$Y_{ij} - \mu - d_i - E_j$$

And since genotype-environment interaction shows linear regression on environmental effects:

$$g_{ij} = \beta_i E_j + \delta_{ij}$$

where β_i is the linear regression coefficient for *i*th line and δ_{ij} is deviation from the regression line for *i*th line in *j*th environment.

Perkins and Jinks (1966) showed that

$$1+\beta_i = \frac{\sum\limits_j Y_{ij} E_j}{\sum\limits_j (E_j)^2}.$$

This is similar to b_i given by Eberhart and Russell (1966). Therefore,

$$1+\beta_i = b$$

$$\therefore \quad \beta_i = b-1$$

Since variance due to genotype-environment interaction is more important, Perkins and Jinks (1968) proposed that regression of genotype × environment interaction on environmental index should be obtained rather than regression of mean performance (Y_{ij}) on environmental index as is done for Eberhart and Russell's (1966) analysis.

Weaknesses of Conventional Regression Models

Two major weaknesses of conventional regression analysis are:

(i) Use of non-independent environmental values, and
(ii) Linearity of genotypic response to environmental values.

9

PATH ANALYSIS

9.1 Genotypic Correlations

Very often it is observed that change in one variable is accompanied by change in another variable. For example, seed yield in linseed is influenced by the number of capsules per plant. Such characters are said to be correlated. When an increase in one variable is accompanied by increase in another correlated variable the correlation is positive. On the other hand, when increase in one variable is accompanied with decrease in another variable the correlation is negative.

The degree of correlation between two variables is measured by a correlation coefficient (p) and defined as:

$$\frac{\sigma_{xy}}{\sigma_x \cdot \sigma_y} \qquad (1)$$

where $\sigma_{xy} = \dfrac{\Sigma(x-\bar{x})(y-\bar{y})}{N}$

In this expression σ_{xy} is known as covariance between x and y variables. Sign of σ_{xy} may be positive or negative. Coefficient of correlation can, therefore, take a positve or negative sign. Estimate of p calculated from a sample is denoted by r. Whether positive or negative σ_{xy} does not exceed $\sigma_x \sigma_y$ and consequently the correlation coefficient necessarily varies between + 1 and – 1. The coefficient of correlation expresses association between two variables, but tells us nothing about the causal relations of variables, *i.e.*, which variable is dependent and which is independent.

Correlation coefficient is not associated with the units of measurements such as gram, kilogram, litres, *etc*.

Coefficient of correlation indicates the relationship between two variables, however, it provides no information regarding the extent of change in one variable resulting from change in another variable. It is the regression coefficient, which measures rate of change in one variable (the dependent variable) per unit rate of change in another variable (the independent variable). Detailed procedure of regression analysis is available in almost all the books of statistics. The regression coefficient, unlike the correlation coefficient, is not free from units of measurement.

In genetic studies it is not uncommon to find correlation between two or more characters. Genotypic correlation between two or more characters may result from pleiotropic effects of genes or linkage of genes governing inheritance of two or more characters. Correlation due to linkage is relatively ephemeral. On the other hand, correlation arising from pleiotropy is long lasting.

Correlation resulting from pleiotropy is the net effect of all the segregating genes that influence both the attributes. For example, some genes may increase expression of both the characters, however, among the remaining genes some may increase manifestation of one character but decrease the other.

Correlation between two or more characters can also arise from environmental agencies. Correlation resulting from environmental agencies is also a net effect, since some environmental effects may increase both the characters whereas some may tend to increase one but decrease the other character.

In many cases, the value of a variable is determined by many interacting variables, which calls for an extension of the concept of simple correlation and regression to more than two variables. This requires an introduction of the concept of partial correlation coefficient and partial regression coefficient. Partial correlation coefficient between any two variables measures the correlation coefficient between two variables after elimination of the effects of other variables in the system. Similarly, partial regression coefficient measures the rate of change in one variable per unit rate of change in the other variable, when rest of the variables in the system are held constant.

Association between two characters that we observe and measure is the phenotypic correlation. Phenotypic correlation is estimated from the phenotypic values observed on a number of individuals for a pair of characters. Since the phenotypic value is determined by genotypic value and environmental deviations, the phenotypic correlation is also determined by these agencies. Thus, we may find a correlation between the breeding values of two characters which will provide an estimate of genotypic correlation. Theoretically it is also possible to find correlation between the dominance deviations of two characters. Likewise, it may be theoretically possible to obtain an estimate of correlation between the non-allelic interaction deviations. Environmental correlation of two variables comprises of correlation due to environmental agencies and that due to non-additive genetic causes. The phenotypic correlation coefficient (r_{pxy}) may be obtained as:

$$\frac{Cov_{Pxy}}{\sigma_{Px} \cdot \sigma_{Py}}$$

where Cov_{pxy} is an estimate of phenotypic covariance between the two variables x and y, σ_{px} and σ_{py} denote the estimates of phenotypic standard deviations of x and y, respectively. Phenotypic covariance is made up of two components, *viz.* one attributable to the genetic causes (Cov_{Axy}) and the other to the environmental components (Cov_{Exy}). Provided that the genetic and environmental effects are not correlated, the phenotypic correlation (r_{Pxy}) is expressible as:

$$\frac{Cov_{Axy} + Cov_{Exy}}{\sigma_{Px} \cdot \sigma_{Py}} \tag{2}$$

We know that heritability (h^2) in the narrow sense, is a ratio of additive genetic variance to the phenotypic variance, *i.e.*, σ^2_A / σ^2_P. Therefore, the phenotypic variance can be expressed as:

$$\frac{\sigma^2_A}{h^2} \tag{3}$$

and hence $\sigma_P = \sigma_A / h$. Thus r_{Pxy} may be expressed alternatively as:

$$\frac{Cov_{A_{xy}}}{\sigma_{Px} \cdot \sigma_{Py}} + \frac{Cov_{E_{xy}}}{\sigma_{px} \cdot \sigma_{Py}} \tag{4}$$

$$= \frac{Cov_{A_{xy}}}{\frac{\sigma_{A_x}}{h_x} \cdot \frac{\sigma_{A_y}}{h_y}} + \frac{Cov_{E_{xy}}}{\sigma_{P_x} \cdot \sigma_{P_y}}$$

$$= h_x \cdot h_y \, r_{A_{xy}} + \frac{Cov_{E_{xy}}}{\sigma_{P_x} \cdot \sigma_{P_y}}$$

Like the heritability (h^2), e^2 is also a ratio. It is a ratio of environmental variance $\left(\sigma_E^2\right)$ to phenotypic variance $\left(\sigma_P^2\right)$. e^2 can be also expressed as $(1 - h^2)$. And since $e^2 = (1 - h^2) = \sigma_E^2 / \sigma_P^2, \sigma_P^2 = \sigma_E^2 / e^2$. And hence $\sigma_P = \sigma_E / e$.

Thus r_{Pxy} can be expressed as:

$$h_x \cdot h_y \cdot r_{Axy} + e_x \cdot e_y \cdot r_{Exy} \tag{5}$$

where r_{Axy} and r_{Exy} donote the coefficients of correlation due to breeding values and environmental causes, respectively. If the two characters have high heritabilities, the correlation due to environmental agencies will be relatively less important. The genotypic and the environmental correlation coefficients may bear different signs. Magnitudes of these correlation coefficients may also be different. Difference in the signs of the genotypic and environmental correlations suggests that both the agencies are probably influencing different physiological mechanisms.

How to arrive at the estimates of genotypic correlations? In practice it is the total genotypic correlation which is estimated, rather than the correlation between breeding values of two variables. A number of genotypes, which form the experimental material, are planted in an appropriate experimental design and observations are recorded on individuals for characters of interest. Analysis of covariance is then computed from the data recorded on individuals for two characters (*x* and *y*). Total covariation is then partitioned into components attributable to replications, genotypes and error. Estimate of genotypic covariance between two variables is then obtained as:

$$Cov_{g_{xy}} = \frac{\text{Mean sum of cross products for genotypes} - \text{Mean sum of cross products for error}}{\text{Number of replications}}$$

Estimates of the genotypic variances of two attributes (x and y) are obtained as described in Chapter 4. The genotypic correlation is then calculated as:

$$r_{g_{xy}} = \frac{Cov_{g_{xy}}}{\sigma_{g_x} \cdot \sigma_{g_y}}$$

Estimate of environmental correlation may be obtained by subtracting the genotypic correlation from the corresponding phenotypic correlation.

9.1.1 *Worked Example*

Twenty-eight genotypes of sorghum were grown in a randomised block design with two replications. Data were recorded on grain yield per plant (g) and 1000-grain weight (g) (Table 9.1).

Data for grain yield/plant and 1000-grain weight were analysed separately (Tables 9.2 and 9.3). The results of analysis suggested that there were significant differences among the 28 genotypes for grain yield/plant and 1000-grain weight. As described in Chapter 4, the estimate of genotypic variance for grain yield (σ_g^2) is obtained from mean squares in Table 9.2 as:

$$\sigma_g^2 = \frac{563.7174 - 84.1374}{2}$$

$$= 239.79$$

Estimate of genotypic variance for 1000-grain weight is also calculated similarly, using the values of mean squares in Table 9.3. The estimate of σ_g^2 for 1000-grain weight is found to be 8.075.

Steps involved in the calculation of various sums of cross products for analysis of covariance are shown below:

$$\text{Correction Factor} = \frac{(\text{Grand total of Yield}) \times (\text{Grand total of 1000-grain wt})}{\text{No. of replications} \times \text{No. of genotypes}}$$

$$= \frac{3018.698 \times 1238.79}{2 \times 28}$$

$$= 66777.3731$$

TABLE 9.1: Grain yield/plant (g) and 1000-grain weight (g) of 28 genotypes of sorghum

Sl No.	Grain yield/plant (g)			1000-grain weight (g)		
	Rep 1	Rep 2	Total	Rep 1	Rep 2	Total
1.	40.136	44.954	85.090	17.13	19.48	36.61
2.	50.002	43.280	93.282	18.64	20.71	39.35
3.	32.530	17.842	50.372	17.86	14.95	32.81
4.	21.728	13.398	35.126	14.07	12.39	26.46
5.	50.002	26.324	76.326	22.66	22.45	45.11
6.	38.776	35.098	73.874	25.03	22.01	47.04
7.	33.134	26.012	59.146	23.63	23.94	47.57
8.	112.420	69.152	181.572	25.74	22.40	48.14
9.	78.828	89.560	168.388	21.82	23.20	45.02
10.	51.956	60.276	112.232	21.87	19.96	41.83
11.	79.260	62.474	141.734	24.71	20.22	44.93
12.	63.214	66.046	129.260	25.73	24.13	49.86
13.	66.928	59.522	126.450	26.23	24.68	50.91
14.	64.772	68.090	132.862	19.96	20.78	40.74
15.	69.772	66.174	135.946	22.43	21.71	44.14
16.	59.392	78.075	137.467	23.24	25.90	49.14
17.	53.334	63.860	117.194	25.74	27.63	53.37
18.	62.884	61.885	124.769	27.58	27.16	54.74
19.	43.720	56.798	100.518	17.59	21.89	39.48
20.	55.874	58.016	113.890	20.09	19.32	39.41
21.	66.974	71.296	138.270	24.23	23.53	47.76
22.	58.042	67.376	125.418	23.70	23.58	47.28
23.	49.610	35.084	84.694	21.53	17.51	39.04
24.	56.226	40.908	97.134	23.08	18.63	41.71
25.	55.284	46.752	102.036	23.39	22.50	45.89
26.	52.364	47.014	99.378	22.97	22.42	45.39
27.	38.820	48.192	87.012	22.37	24.01	46.38
28.	48.146	41.112	89.258	24.18	24.50	48.68
Total	1554.128	1464.57	3018.698	627.20	611.59	1238.79

TABLE 9.2 : ANOVA for grain yield/plant (g)

Source	*df*	*SS*	*MS*
Replications	1	143.22	143.22
Genotypes	27	15220.37	563.7174
Error	27	2271.71	84.1374

TABLE 9.3: ANOVA for 1000-grain weight (g)

Source	*df*	*SS*	*MS*
Replications	1	4.352	4.352
Genotypes	27	503.015	18.630
Error	27	67.459	2.480

Total sum of cross products =

$$(40.136 \times 17.13) + (50.002 \times 18.64) \ldots + (41.112 \times 24.50)$$
$$- \text{Correction factor}$$
$$= 68555.7898 - 66777.3731$$
$$= 1778.4167$$

Replication sum of cross products =

$$\frac{1}{28}[1554.128 \times 627.20 + 1464.570 \times 611.59] - CF$$
$$= 66802.3374 - 66777.3731$$
$$= 24.9643$$

Genotype sum of cross products =

$$\frac{1}{2}[(85.090 \times 36.61) + (93.282 \times 39.35) + \ldots$$
$$+ (89.258 \times 48.68)] - CF$$
$$= 1493.5457$$

Error sum of cross product is got as a difference. Thus,

Error SCP = Total SCP – (Replication SCP + Genotype SCP)

$$= 1778.4167 - 24.9643 - 1493.5457$$
$$= 259.9067$$

The analysis of covariance table is set up as shown in Table 9.4.

TABLE 9.4 : Analysis of covariance for grain yield and 1000-grain weight of sorghum

Source	*df*	*SCP*	*MSCP*
Replications	1	24.9643	24.9643
Genotypes	27	1493.5457	55.3165**
Error	27	259.9067	9.6261

The genotypes *MSCP* is highly significant when tested against error *MSCP*. This significance implies significant covariance of grain yield/plant and 1000-grain weight in the present set of experimental material. Estimate of the genotypic covariance is obtained from the values of genotypes *MSCP* and error *MSCP* as:

$$\frac{55.3165 - 9.6261}{2}$$
$$= 22.8452$$

Estimate of the genotypic correlation between grain yield/plant and 1000-grain weight in the genetic material being investigated is, therefore,

$$\frac{+22.8452}{\sqrt{(239.79 \times 8.075)}}$$
$$= +0.5191$$

Positive genotypic correlation suggests that the genes which tend to enhance 1000-grain weight also increase grain yield/plant. However, from these results it may not be possible to say with certainty whether the correlation is a consequence of linkage between the two sets of genes or pleiotropic effect of a given set of genes.

9.2 Path Coefficients

Plant breeders have to deal with correlated characters during the improvement programmes. For example, yield of economically important characters, such as the grain yield in cereals, yield of the lint in cotton, *etc*., are influenced by the component characters. In wheat, for example, it is known that the kernel yield is determined by the number of tillers/plant, number of kernels/spike, 1000-kernel weight, *etc*. Grafius (1959) expressed his opinion that there may not be genes for yield *per se*, rather there could be genes which govern the inheritance of component characters. Therefore, rapid improvement in yield is expected to result if selection is practised for component characters. Rate of improvement is expected to be rapid if differential emphasis is laid on the component characters during selection. The basis of differential emphasis could be the degree of influence of component characters on the economic character of interest.

The degree of influence of one variable on the other can be expressed in quantitative terms. "Path coefficient" analysis, a method developed by Sewall Wright (1921) is very efficient in this respect. Dewey and Lu (1959) employed this method for the first time in plants to disentangle the direct and indirect influences of components of seed yield.

Path analysis is a special type of multi-variate analysis, which deals with a "closed" system of variables, which are linearly related. What do we mean by a "closed" system of variables? By a closed system of variables is meant that each variable in the system is either a linear combination of some other variables in the system or is one of the basic factors in the system. In other words, the system is formally complete, including all the basic factors (the "causes") and their resultant variables (the "effects"). Suppose X_0 is a character, which is linearly determined by correlated variables X_1, X_2 and X_3. Because of the closed system, a path diagram can be formulated as (Fig. 9.1):

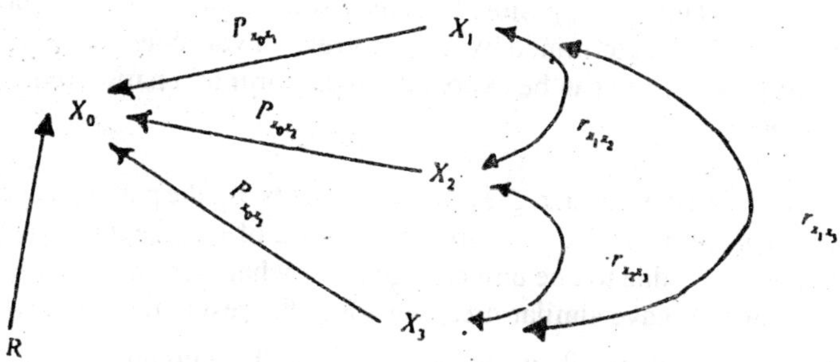

FIG. 9.1: *Path diagram showing the direct and indirect influences of causal factors (X_1, X_2, X_3) on a dependent character (X_0).*

In Fig. 9.1 symbols $P_{x_0:x_1}$, $P_{x_0:x_2}$, and $P_{x_0:x_3}$, represent path coefficients from causes X_1, X_2 and X_3, respectively, $r_{x_1x_2}$, $r_{x_1x_3}$ and $r_{x_2x_3}$ are the correlation coefficients and R is variation in X_0 that is due to those agencies which are not known. It is a convention to use a double headed arrow for correlation coefficient and unidirectional arrow for the direct path of influence from one variable in the system to the dependent variable. If we denote the standard deviation of X_0 by a symbol σ_{x_0} and the standard deviation of X_0 due to the influence of X_1 by $\sigma_{x_0:x_1}$, such that all the other causes (except the X_1) are kept constant but the variation of X_1 is as great as before, the path-coefficient for path from cause X_1 to X_0 is defined as:

$$p(X_0 \leftarrow X_1) = P_{x_0:x_1} = \frac{\sigma_{x_0:x_1}}{\sigma_{x_0}}$$

When this definition is given, it is assumed that the direct effect along a given path can be measured by standard deviation remaining in X_0 after all the other paths of influence are eliminated, while variation of the cause back of the given path (*i.e.*, variation of X_1) is kept as great as ever, regardless of its relationships to the other causes which have been made constant.

At times, breeders have to predict the value of a dependent variable, say X_0, given the values of other variables, *viz.* $X_1, X_2, X_3, \ldots, X_n$. Sometimes they are interested in the variation of X_0 that is attributable to variation in $X_1, X_2, X_3, ..., X_n$. How is it possible? Let us assume a simple model such that a character X_0 is determined by three correlated variables, *viz.* X_1, X_2 and X_3. This relationship can be expressed in the form of a partial regression equation as:

$$X_0 = \mu + \beta_1 X_1 + \beta_2 X_2 + \beta_3 X_3 + R \tag{6}$$

where $\beta_1, \beta_2, \beta_3$ are the partial regression coefficients. β_1, the partial regression coefficient of X_0 on X_1, measures the amount of change that can be brought about in X_0 due to one unit change in X_1, when X_2 and X_3 are held constant. β_2 and β_3 have similar meanings. R is the residual component. The constants μ, β_1, β_2 and β_3 are so calculated that the amount $(X_0 - \hat{X}_0)^2$ is a minimum. $\hat{X}_0$ is the expected value of X_0 that is calculated on the basis of equation (6). The regression coefficients are associated with physical units, such as y kilogram increase in yield resulting from x cm increase in plant height. The values of $\beta_1, \beta_2, \beta_3$, therefore, depend not only upon the influence of X_1, X_2, X_3 on X_0 but also upon the actual physical units employed to measure these variables, although the influences of X_1, X_2 and X_3 remain same. If the values of variables are expressed in terms of "standardised" units, the physical units associated with regression coefficients will vanish, which will enable us to compare the influences of two or more independent variables on the dependent variable. The dependent variable X_0 was expressed in equation (6) as:

$$X_0 = \mu + \beta_1 X_1 + \beta_2 X_2 + \beta_3 X_3 + R$$

The value of μ can, therefore, be estimated as:

$$\mu = \overline{X}_0 - \hat{\beta}_1 \overline{X}_1 - \hat{\beta}_2 \overline{X}_2 - \hat{\beta}_3 \overline{X}_3 \tag{7}$$

where $\hat{\beta}_1, \hat{\beta}_2$ and $\hat{\beta}_3$ donote the estimates of β_1, β_2 and β_3, respectively. If we substitute this value of μ in equation (6) we get:

$$X_0 = \overline{X}_0 - \beta_1 \overline{X}_1 - \beta_2 \overline{X}_2 - \beta_3 \overline{X}_3 + \beta_1 X_1 + \beta_2 X_2 + \beta_3 X_3 + R$$

or $(X_0 - \overline{X}_0) = \beta_1 (X_1 - \overline{X}_1) + \beta_2 (X_2 - \overline{X}_2) + \beta_3 (X_3 - \overline{X}_3) + R$

Standardising the variables in expression given above will result in

$$\frac{X_0 - \overline{X}_0}{\sigma_{x_0}} = \frac{\beta_1 \sigma_{x_1}}{\sigma_{x_0}} \left(\frac{X_1 - \overline{X}_1}{\sigma_{x_1}} \right) + \frac{\beta_2 \sigma_{x_2}}{\sigma_{x_0}} \left(\frac{X_2 - \overline{X}_2}{\sigma_{x_2}} \right) +$$

$$\frac{\beta_3 \sigma_{x_3}}{\sigma_{x_0}} \left(\frac{X_3 - \overline{X}_3}{\sigma_{x_3}} \right) + \frac{R}{\sigma_{x_0}} \tag{8}$$

When the variables are expressed as deviation from their respective means and also in terms of standardised units, their means will be zero and the variance will be equal to unity. Thus, if we donote $X_1 - \overline{X}_1 / \sigma_{x_0}$ by a lower case letter x_1, the mean of x_1s will be zero and the variance unity. Let us replace the expression $\beta_1 \sigma_{x_1} / \sigma_{x_0}$ in this equation by a term $P_{x_0 : x_1}$ which is a standardised partial regression coefficient. It is called as the "path coefficient". In the like manner, terms $\beta_2 \sigma_{x_2} / \sigma_{x_0}, \beta_3 \sigma_{x_3} / \sigma_{x_0}$, could be replaced by $P_{x_0 : x_2}$ and $P_{x_0 : x_3}$, respectively. It should be pointed out that the path coefficients have a direction similar to the regression coefficients, *i.e.*, they may bear a positive or a negative sign. Unlike the correlation coefficients, the path coefficients could be greater or lesser than unity.

For prediction of X_0 from the values of X_1, X_2 and X_3, we need estimates of regression coefficients, *viz.* β_1, β_2 and β_3. Three simultaneous equations are required to estimate three unknowns, *viz.* β_1, β_2 and β_3. These unknowns are estimated according to the principles of least square analysis. The three normal equations are:

$$\beta_1 \sigma_1^2 + \beta_2 \sigma_{12} + \beta_3 \sigma_{13} = \sigma_{10}$$

$$\beta_1 \sigma_{21} + \beta_2 \sigma_2^2 + \beta_3 \sigma_{23} = \sigma_{20}$$

$$\beta_1 \sigma_{31} + \beta_2 \sigma_{32} + \beta_3 \sigma_3^2 = \sigma_{30} \tag{9}$$

where σ_{10}, σ_{20}, σ_{30} are the estimates of covariances between X_0 and X_1, X_2 and X_3, respectively. $\sigma_{12} = \sigma_{21}$, $\sigma_{13} = \sigma_{31}$ and $\sigma_{23} = \sigma_{32}$ are the estimates of covariances. σ_1^2, σ_2^2 and σ_3^2 are estimates of variances of the variables X_1, X_2 and X_3, respectively. We know that the estimate of correlation coefficient is calculated by dividing the covariance by the product of corresponding estimates of standard deviations. Thus $r_{x_0 x_1}$ is obtained as:

$$\frac{Cov_{(x_0 . x_1)}}{\sigma_{x_0} \cdot \sigma_{x_1}}$$

$\therefore \quad Cov_{(x_0 . x_1)} = r_{x_0 x_1} \sigma_{x_0} \cdot \sigma_{x_1}$. Substitution of similar values for covariances in equation (9) gives:

$$\beta_1\sigma_1^2 + \beta_2\sigma_{12} + \beta_3\sigma_{13} = r_{10}\cdot\sigma_0\cdot\sigma_1$$
$$\beta_1\sigma_{21} + \beta_2\sigma_2^2 + \beta_3\sigma_{23} = r_{20}\cdot\sigma_0\cdot\sigma_2$$
$$\beta_1\sigma_{31} + \beta_2\sigma_{32} + \beta_3\sigma_3^2 = r_{30}\cdot\sigma_0\cdot\sigma_3 \tag{10}$$

We shall deal with first of these equations and simplify it further. Other equations are also simplified in similar manner. The expression σ_1^2 in first equation can be replaced by $\sigma_1 \cdot \sigma_1$ and, therefore, the equation can be expressed as:

$$\frac{\beta_1\sigma_1 . \sigma_1}{\sigma_0\sigma_1} + \frac{\beta_2\sigma_{12}}{\sigma_0\sigma_1} + \frac{\beta_3\sigma_{13}}{\sigma_0\sigma_1} = r_{10}$$

or
$$\frac{\beta_1\sigma_1}{\sigma_0} + \frac{\beta_2\sigma_{12}}{\sigma_0\sigma_1} + \frac{\beta_3\sigma_{13}}{\sigma_0\sigma_1} = r_{10}$$

Now, if we multiply the second and the third elements of this equation by σ_2/σ_2 and σ_3/σ_3, respectively, we get:

$$\frac{\beta_1\sigma_1}{\sigma_0} + \frac{\beta_2\sigma_{12}\sigma_2}{\sigma_0\sigma_1\sigma_2} + \frac{\beta_3\sigma_{13}\sigma_3}{\sigma_0\sigma_1\sigma_3} = r_{10}$$

or
$$P_{x_0x_1} + \frac{\beta_2\sigma_2}{\sigma_0} r_{12} + \frac{\beta_3\sigma_3}{\sigma_0} r_{13} = r_{10}$$

or
$$P_{x_0x_1} + P_{x_0x_2} r_{12} + P_{x_0x_3} r_{13} = r_{10}$$

In similar manner, we simplify equations two and three of (10) and find that r_{20} and r_{30} also have three components. If we denote $P_{x_0x_1}$, $P_{x_0x_2}$ and $P_{x_0x_3}$ by symbols P_{10}, P_{20} and P_{30}, respectively, for the sake of brevity, the equations of (10) could be expressed as:

$$\hat{P}_{10} + \hat{P}_{20}r_{12} + \hat{P}_{30}r_{13} = r_{10}$$
$$\hat{P}_{10}r_{21} + \hat{P}_{20} + \hat{P}_{30}r_{23} = r_{20}$$
$$\hat{P}_{10}r_{31} + \hat{P}_{20}r_{32} + \hat{P}_{30} = r_{30} \tag{11}$$

These equations point to the fact that similar to the analysis of variance, which partitions total variation observed for an attribute into its component causes, the correlation coefficient can also be partitioned into its component causes. Thus r_{10}, which is the correlation between variables X_0 and X_1, comprises of P_{10}, which is the direct path of X_1 to X_0, $P_{20}\, r_{12}$ and $P_{30}\, r_{13}$. The latter two expressions specify the indirect paths from variables through X_1 and X_2 and X_1 and X_3, respectively. Thus path analysis is analogous to the analysis of variance and may be called as "analysis of correlation" (Li, 1956).

Since X_0 depends upon three correlated variables X_1, X_2 and X_3, as mentioned in the beginning of this section, variation in X_0 can be linearly expressed as:

$$\sigma^2_{x_0} = \beta_1^2\sigma^2_{x_1} + \beta_2^2\sigma^2_{x_2} + \beta_3^2\sigma^2_{x_3} + 2\beta_1\beta_2\sigma_{x_1x_2}$$

$$+2\beta_1\beta_3\sigma_{x_1x_3} + 2\beta_2\beta_3\sigma_{x_2x_3} + \sigma^2_R$$

and since $\sigma_{x_1x_2}$, $\sigma_{x_1x_3}$ and $\sigma_{x_2x_3}$ are covariances, they could be alternatively expressed as $r_{12}\sigma_1\sigma_2$, $r_{13}\sigma_1\sigma_3$ and $r_{23}\sigma_2\sigma_3$, respectively. Hence $\sigma^2_{x_0}$ can be linearly expressed as

$$\sigma^2_{x_0} = \beta_1\sigma^2_{x_1} + \beta_2\sigma^2_{x2} + \beta_3\sigma^2_{x3} + 2\beta_1\beta_2 r_{12}\sigma_{x1}\sigma_{x2}$$

$$+2\beta_1\beta_3 r_{13}\sigma_{x1}\sigma_{x3} + 2\beta_2\beta_3 r_{23}\sigma_{x2}\sigma_{x3} + \sigma^2_R$$

If both the sides are divided by $\sigma^2_{x_0}$, we get:

$$1 = \frac{\beta_1\sigma^2_{x_1}}{\sigma^2_{x_0}} + \frac{\beta_2\sigma^2_{x2}}{\sigma^2_{x_0}} + \frac{\beta_3\sigma^2_{x3}}{\sigma^2_{x_0}} + \frac{2\beta_1\beta_2 r_{12}\sigma_{x1}\sigma_{x2}}{\sigma^2_{x_0}}$$

$$+\frac{2\beta_1\beta_3 r_{13}\sigma_{x1}\sigma_{x3}}{\sigma^2_{x_0}} + \frac{2\beta_2\beta_3 r_{23}\sigma_{x2}\sigma_{x3}}{\sigma^2_{x_0}} + \sigma^2_R \tag{12}$$

The terms $\frac{\beta_1\sigma^2_{x1}}{\sigma^2_{x_0}}$, $\frac{\beta_2\sigma^2_{x_2}}{\sigma^2_{x_0}}$ and $\frac{\beta_3\sigma^2_{x3}}{\sigma^2_{x_0}}$ in equation (12) could be replaced by P^2_{10}, P^2_{20} and P^2_{30}, respectively, because the terms $\frac{\beta_1\sigma_{x_1}}{\sigma_{x_0}}$, $\frac{\beta_2\sigma_{x_2}}{\sigma_{x_0}}$ and $\frac{\beta_3\sigma_{x_3}}{\sigma_{x_0}}$ were defined as path coefficients and symbolised as P_{10}, P_{20} and P_{30}, respectively. The expression $\frac{2\beta_1\beta_2\sigma_{x1}\sigma_{x2}r_{12}}{\sigma^2_{x_0}}$ can be alternately written as:

$$\frac{2\beta_1\sigma_{x1}\beta_2\sigma_{x2}r_{12}}{\sigma_{x_0}\sigma_{x_0}}$$

In this expression $\frac{\beta_1\sigma_{x1}}{\sigma_{x_0}}$ and $\frac{\beta_2\sigma_{x2}}{\sigma_{x_0}}$ are the paths and may, therefore, be replaced by symbols P_{10} and P_{20}, respectively. We can, therefore, write $\frac{2\beta_1\beta_2\sigma_{x1}\sigma_{x2}r_{12}}{\sigma^2_{x0}}$ alternatively as $2P_{10}P_{20}r_{12}$. Likewise $\frac{2\beta_1\beta_3\sigma_{x1}\sigma_{x3}r_{13}}{\sigma^2_{x0}}$ and $\frac{2\beta_2\beta_3\sigma_{x2}\sigma_{x3}r_{23}}{\sigma^2_{x0}}$ could be expressed as $2P_{10}P_{30}r_{13}$ and $2P_{20}P_{30}r_{23}$, respectively. In the light of these new expressions, equation (12) can also be written as:

$$1 = P^2_{10} + P^2_{20} + P^2_{30} + 2P_{10}P_{20}r_{12} + 2P_{10}P_{30}r_{13} + 2P_{20}P_{30}r_{23} + R^2 \quad (13)$$

Apart from the residual variation, which could arise from unknown and uncontrolled reasons, total variation of a dependent variable may be expressed as shown in equation (13). This theory can be extended to any number of variables of a closed system. The expression of equation (13) is a form of equation known as "coefficient of determination". The magnitude of residual variation could, therefore, be estimated as:

$$1 - P^2_{10} - P^2_{20} - P^2_{30} - 2P_{10}P_{20}r_{12} - 2P_{10}P_{30}r_{13} - 2P_{20}P_{30}r_{23} \quad (14)$$

According to this analysis, (P^2_{10}) per cent of the total variation of X_0 can be attributed to the direct effect of X_1, when other variables are held constant. Likewise (P^2_{20}) per cent and (P^2_{30}) per cent variation in X_0 can be accounted for by variations in X_2 and X_3, respectively. The indirect effects of X_1 on X_0 *via* X_2 and X_3 will be $2(P_{10}P_{20}r_{12})$ per cent and $2(P_{10}P_{30}r_{13})$ per cent, respectively. Similar interpretation can be made for variation in X_0

due to other variables.

This method permits breeders to identify relatively important components of a dependent variable, on the basis of their direct and indirect influences. This technique, therefore, enables differential emphasis to be laid on various component characters during selection.

9.3 Path Analysis

Based on the theory presented in section 9.2 correlation between a number of independent variables, which are the component characters, and the dependent variable can be partitioned into the components, attributable to the direct effects and the indirect influences. Dewey and Lu (1959) employed this procedure to disentangle the direct and the indirect influences of components of seed yield in case of crested wheat-grass. For this purpose genotypic correlations between all the characters being studied are obtained as described in section 9.1.1. If a character X_0 is determined by correlated characters X_1, X_2 and X_3, a path diagram may be formulated as described in section 9.2. A set of three simultaneous equations is then formulated from the path diagram (three equations, because values of three unknowns, *viz.* P_{10}, P_{20} and P_{30}, are to be calculated). Thus:

$$r_{x_0x_1} = P_{10} + P_{20}r_{x_1x_2} + P_{30}r_{x_1x_3}$$

$$r_{x_0x_2} = P_{10}r_{x_2x_1} + P_{20} + P_{30}r_{x_2x_3}$$

$$r_{x_0x_3} = P_{10}r_{x3}x_1 + P_{20}r_{x_3x_2} + P_{30} \qquad (15)$$

Information provided in equation (15) can be arranged in the matrix form as:

$$\underset{A}{\begin{bmatrix} 1 & r_{x_1x_2} & r_{x_1x_3} \\ r_{x_1x_2} & 1 & r_{x_2x_3} \\ r_{x_1x_3} & r_{x_3x_2} & 1 \end{bmatrix}} \underset{B}{\begin{bmatrix} \hat{P}_{10} \\ \hat{P}_{20} \\ \hat{P}_{30} \end{bmatrix}} = \underset{C}{\begin{bmatrix} r_{x_0x_1} \\ r_{x_0x_2} \\ r_{x_0x_3} \end{bmatrix}} \qquad (16)$$

Matrix A is symmetrical about the diagonal elements. The diagonal elements in this matrix represent the direct effects of X_1, X_2 and X_3, respectively on X_0. All the direct effects have been replaced by unity in this matrix. Elements of the column matrix B specify the path coefficients to be estimated. The column matrix C represents the estimated values of genotypic correlation coefficients between the dependent variable X_0, and the component variables, *i.e.*, X_1, X_2 and X_3. Estimates of unknowns are, therefore, calculated as:

$$B = A^{-1} C,$$

where A^{-1} is the inverse of matrix A. This may be obtained as described in the Appendix of Chapter 3. The indirect effects are calculated from the three simultaneous equations, after substituting the values of P_{10}, P_{20} and P_{30} in these equations. Residual variation can be estimated as described in section 9.2 [equation (14)]

9.3.1 *Worked Example*

Twenty-eight genotypes of sorghum were planted in randomised block design with two replications. Observations were recorded on (i) grain yield/plant (g), (ii) number of grains/panicle, (iii) 1000-grain weight (g), (iv) plant height (cm), and (v) days to 50 per cent flowering. Simple genotypic correlations among these characters were estimated as described in section 9.1 (Table 9.5).

TABLE 9.5: Genotypic correlations in sorghum

	0	1	2	3	4
	Grain Yield	No. of grains	1000-grain weight	Plant height	Days to 50% flower
Grain yield	–	+ 0.9437	+ 0.5199	+ 0.7923	– 0.1867
No. of grains	–	–	+ 0.2288	+ 0.5936	– 0.0520
1000-grain wt	–	–	–	+ 0.7451	+ 0.1194
Plant height	–	–	–	–	−0.6246
Days to 50 % flower	–	–	–	–	–

From the information provided in Table 9.5 (Fig. 9.2) is constructed as shown below:

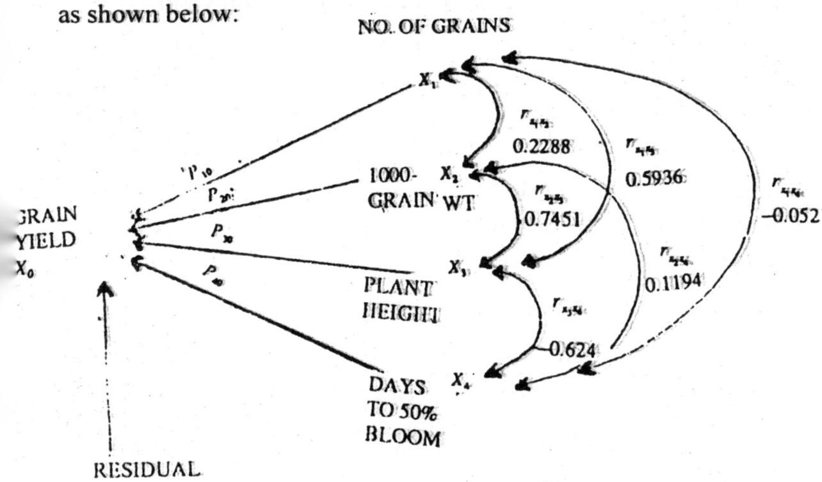

FIG. 9.2 : Path diagram for grain yield of sorghum

A set of simultaneous equations is set up for the estimation of four unknowns, *viz.* P_{10}, P_{20}, P_{30} and P_{40} on the basis of information provided in Table 9.5 and Fig. 9.2 Thus,

$$\begin{aligned}
r_{10} &= P_{10} + P_{20}r_{12} + P_{30}r_{13} + P_{40}r_{14}\\
r_{20} &= P_{10}r_{21} + P_{20} + P_{30}r_{23} + P_{40}r_{24}\\
r_{30} &= P_{10}r_{31} + P_{20}r_{32} + P_{30} + P_{40}r_{34}\\
r_{40} &= P_{10}r_{41} + P_{20}r_{42} + P_{30}r_{43} + P_{40}
\end{aligned}$$

Values of various correlation coefficients are substituted in these simultaneous equations. Thus,

$$\begin{aligned}
0.9437 &= P_{10} + 0.2288\,P_{20} + 0.5936\,P_{30} + (-0.052)\,P_{40}\\
0.5199 &= 0.2288\,P_{10} + P_{20} + 0.7451\,P_{30} + 0.1194\,P_{40}\\
0.7923 &= 0.5936\,P_{10} + 0.7451\,P_{20} + P_{30} + (-0.6246)\,P_{40}\\
-0.1867 &= -0.0520\,P_{10} + 0.1194\,P_{20} + (-0.6246)\,P_{30} + P_{40}
\end{aligned} \quad (17)$$

Although the set of simultaneous equations can be solved in several different ways, we shall employ matrix method. Arrange the information of equation (17) in the matrix form as:

$$\underset{A}{\begin{bmatrix} 1 & 0.2288 & 0.5936 & -0.052 \\ 0.2288 & 1 & 0.7451 & 0.1194 \\ 0.5936 & 0.7451 & 1 & -0.6246 \\ -0.052 & 0.1194 & -0.6246 & 1 \end{bmatrix}} \underset{B}{\begin{bmatrix} P_{10} \\ P_{20} \\ P_{30} \\ P_{40} \end{bmatrix}} = \underset{C}{\begin{bmatrix} 0.9437 \\ 0.5199 \\ 0.7923 \\ -0.1867 \end{bmatrix}}$$

The next step is to get the inverse of matrix A, *i.e.*, A^{-1}. Method described in Chapter 3 is used for this purpose. Matrices A^{-1}, C and B are now arranged as:

$$\underset{A^{-1}}{\begin{bmatrix} 0.3550 & -1.5977 & 1.8199 & 1.3456 \\ -1.5977 & -1.4806 & 3.4592 & 2.2539 \\ 1.8199 & 3.4592 & -4.6825 & -3.2423 \\ 1.3456 & 2.2539 & -3.2423 & -1.2241 \end{bmatrix}} \underset{C}{\begin{bmatrix} 0.9437 \\ 0.5199 \\ 0.7923 \\ -0.1867 \end{bmatrix}} = \underset{B}{\begin{bmatrix} P_{10} \\ P_{20} \\ P_{30} \\ P_{40} \end{bmatrix}}$$

Estimates of the four path coefficients are obtained as:

$$P_{10} = (0.3550 \times 0.9437) + (-1.5977 \times 0.5199) + (1.8199 \times 0.7923) + (1.3456 \times -0.1867) = 0.6951$$

$$P_{20} = (-1.5977 \times 0.9437) + (-1.4806 \times 0.5199) + (3.4592 \times 0.7923) + (2.2539 \times -0.1867) = 0.0425$$

$$P_{30} = (1.8199 \times 0.9437) + (3.4592 \times 0.5199) + (-4.6825 \times 0.7923) + (-3.2423 \times -0.1867) = 0.4112, \text{ and lastly}$$

$$P_{40} = (1.3456 \times 0.9437) + (2.2539 \times 0.5199) + (-3.2423 \times 0.7923) + (-1.2241 \times -0.1867) = 0.1013$$

Estimates of path coefficients are then substituted at appropriate places in the equations of (17). It is now an easy matter to estimate the indirect effects. Let us, for the purpose of illustration, take first of the four equations in (17). Thus,

$$r_{10} = P_{10} + P_{20}r_{12} + P_{30}r_{13} + P_{40}r_{14}$$

$$0.9437 = 0.6951 + (0.0425 \times 0.2288)$$

$+(0.4112\times 0.5936)+(0.1013\times -0.0520)$
$0.9437=0.6951+0.0097+0.2441-0.0052$

Thus, the genotypic correlation between grain yield and number of grains has four components, *viz.*

(i)	Direct effect of number of grains, P_{10}	0.6951
(ii)	Indirect effect of number of grains *via* 1000-grain weight, $P_{20}r_{12}$	0.0097
(iii)	Indirect effect of number of grains *via* plant height, $P_{30}r_{13}$	0.2441
(iv)	Indirect effect of number of grains *via* days to 50 per cent flowering, $P_{40}r_{13}$	–0.0052
	Total	0.9437

Since the genotypic correlation between a dependent variable and a given component comprises of the direct effect of the given component and its indirect effects, sum of all the effects should be equal to the genotypic correlation.

The indirect effects of other components are also estimated as described for the number of grains. A table of path analysis is then prepared (Table 9.6).

TABLE 9.6: Path analysis of grain yield in sorghum

S. No.	Cause of the effect		
1.	Correlation between yield and No. of grains	r_{10}	0.9437
	(a) Direct effect	P_{10}	0.6951
	(b) Indirect effect via 1000-grain weight	$P_{20}r_{12}$	0.0097
	(c) Indirect effect via plant height	$P_{30}r_{13}$	0.2440
	(d) Indirect effect via days to 50 per cent flowering	$P_{40}r_{14}$	– 0.0052
			0.9436
2.	Correlation between yield and 1000-grain wt	r_{20}	0.5199
	(a) Direct effect	P_{20}	0.0425
	(b) Indirect effect via No. of grains	$P_{10}r_{12}$	0.1590
	(c) Indirect effect via plant height	$P_{30}r_{23}$	0.3063
	(d) Indirect effect via days to 50 per cent flowering	$P_{40}r_{24}$	0.0120
			0.5198

S. No.	Cause of the effect		
3.	Correlation between yield and plant height	r_{30}	0.7923
	(a) Direct effect	P_{30}	0.4112
	(b) Indirect effect via No. of grains	$P_{10}r_{13}$	0.4126
	(c) Indirect effect via 1000 grain weight	$P_{20}r_{23}$	0.0316
	(d) Indirect effect via days to 50 per cent flowering	$P_{40}r_{34}$	−0.0632
			0.7922
4.	Correlation between yield and days to 50 per cent flowering	r_{40}	−0.1867
	(a) Direct effect	P_{40}	0.1013
	(b) Indirect effect via No. of grains	$P_{10}r_{14}$	−0.0361
	(c) Indirect effect via 1000-grain wt.	$P_{20}r_{24}$	0.0050
	(d) Indirect effect via plant height	$P_{30}r_{34}$	−0.2568
			−0.1866
5.	Residual causes of variation	P_x^2	0.0151

Residual variation is calculated as:

$$1 - P_{10}^2 - P_{20}^2 - P_{30}^2 - P_{40}^2 - 2P_{10}P_{20}r_{12} - 2P_{10}P_{30}r_{13}$$
$$-2P_{10}P_{40}r_{14} - 2P_{20}P_{30}r_{23} - 2P_{20}P_{40}r_{24} - 2P_{30}P_{40}r_{34}.$$

Substitute the values of P_{10}, P_{20}, P_{30}, P_{40} and various indirect effects in this equation. Thus

$$1-(0.6951)^2-(0.0425)^2-(0.4112)^2-(0.1013)^2$$
$$-2(0.6951\times 0.0425\times 0.2288)-2(0.6951\times 0.4112\times 0.5936)$$
$$-2(0.6951\times 0.1013\times -0.052)-2(0.0425\times 0.4112\times 0.7451)$$
$$-2(0.0425\times 0.1013\times 0.1194)-2(0.4112\times 0.1013\times -0.6246)$$
$$=0.0151$$

Results of path analysis reveal that number of grains is an important component of grain yield, because it has relatively large positive and direct effect. This direct influence is also reinforced by its indirect effect through plant height. The magnitude of direct effect of plant height is next to number of grains and hence may be regarded as another important character influencing grain yield. Although the correlation between yield and 1000- grain weight is positive and considerably large, the direct effect of this attribute on yield is negligible. Large positive correlation resulted from the indirect influence *via* plant height and also number of grains. The negative correlation between grain yield and days to 50 per cent flowering seems to be a consequence of negative indirect influence *via* plant height. This point needs consideration, because direct effect of days to 50 per cent flowering is positive in direction. Path analysis thus enables us to disentangle the direct and indirect influences of component characters. On the basis of these influences, differential emphasis can be laid on different characters during selection.

10

SELECTION

10.1 Change of Gene Frequency

Basically there are only two things that breeders can do to improve the genetically variable population. Firstly, they can decide which individuals will be allowed to produce next generation and within limits which of these individuals will be allowed to produce many and which few offspring. This is selection. Non-random differential reproduction is called as selection. Secondly, breeders can decide how the selected individuals will be mated to each other to generate further genetic variability.

In the course of evolution as well as in the crop improvement programmes, populations are constantly being sifted towards superior types. Primary force in this processes of continuous sifting is selection. Before considering the effects of selection two basic properties of selection should be kept in mind. These are:

(i) Selection can act effectively only on heritable differences, and
(ii) Selection cannot create variability but can act on heritable variability already existing in the population.

Fundamental effect of selection is to change the frequencies with which various genes or combinations of genes occur in the population. Three phenotypically observable responses to selection are:

(i) Change in the proportion of previously existing genotypes accompanied with shift in the population mean.
(ii) Appearance of new genotypes, and
(iii) Change in the variability of the character in the population.

Although the basic effect of selection is to change the gene frequencies, changes of gene frequencies themselves are almost completely hidden from us for genes concerned with quantitative characters because we cannot measure the effect of individual genes concerned with these characters. Hence, effects of selection are described in a different manner. The effects of selection on quantitative characters can be measured in terms of change in the genetic properties of population, such as means, variances and covariances, without forgetting the fact the underlying cause of change in these properties is the change of gene frequencies.

Change of gene frequencies is brought about by artificial and natural forces of selection. Artificial selection, that is selection resulting from action of breeder in the choice of parents, produces its change of gene frequencies by separating the adult individuals of parental generation into two groups, *viz.*, the selected and discarded, that differ in gene frequencies. Natural selection operates through differences of fertility among the individuals of parental generation and/or differences of viability among the individuals of their progeny. In this way there are three stages at which selection can operate and bring about change of gene frequencies:

(i) Through artificial selection among the adult individuals of parental generation,
(ii) Through natural differences of fertility also among the adult individuals of parental generation, and
(iii) Through natural differences of viability among the individuals of progeny generation.

In nature, selective pressures are exclusively those which are associated with survival. Characteristics that make a domesticated species useful to man may not be necessarily associated with survival. In fact, quite the reverse may be true for some characters. But in some cases characters that contribute to survival in wild species may also be associated with basic adaptation and productiveness of these species under cultivation. In nature, among the other things, survival of plants depends upon two factors:

(i) Number of (and not the weight) seeds each type produces, and
(ii) Proportion of seeds of each type that reach matutiy and produce offspring.

Both these factors are in themselves summaries of a large number of genetic and environmental factors (and their interactions), some of which may be known but most of which escape our powers of measurement and detection.

Usually it is assumed that all the individuals in a population contribute equal number of offspring to the next generation. However, individuals differ in their fertility and/or viability and they, therefore, contribute unequally to the next generation. Proportionate contribution of offspring to the next generation is called as "fitness" of an individual, or sometimes the "adpative value" or "selective value". One of the most important causes for change in the frequency of a gene lies in differences in the ability of its carriers to produce surviving offspring. If the individuals carrying gene A are more successful in reproduction than individuals carrying its allele a, the frequency of the former will tend to be larger than the latter. A wide variety of mechanisms responsible for modifying the reproductive success of genotypes are known collectively as selection. If the differences of fitness are in any way associated with presence or absence of a particular gene in individual's genotype, selection operates on that gene. When a gene is subject to selection its frequency in offspring generation differs from that in the parental generation because parents of different genotypes pass on their genes unequally to the next generation. In this way selection causes change of gene frequency and consequently the genotype frequency.

The fitness of an individual, which is the relative reproductive success, can be simply measured by comparing the number of offspring produced by one genotype with those produced by another. For example, let us suppose that the individuals of genotype A produce 100 offspring that reach maturity while individuals of genotype a produce only 90 in the same environment. The reproductive success of a is reduced by 10 offspring or by a fraction $10/100 = 0.1$. Thus genotype A possesses superior adpative value relative to a. The force acting to reduce adaptive value of a genotype is called as coefficient of selection, s. The strength of selection, which is measured in terms of coefficient of selection (s),, is the proportionate reduction in the gametic contribution of a particular genotype as compared to the standard, which is usually the most favoured. The contribution of favoured genotype, measured in terms of fitness, is taken to be 1. The fitness of unfavoured genotype, which is reduced by s, is measured as $1—s$.

The fitness of a genotype with respect to a particular locus is not necessarily same in all individuals because it depends upon the environmental circumstances in which the individual lives, and also upon the genotypes with respect to other loci. When we assign certain fitness to a genotype, it refers to the average fitness of that genotype in the population as a whole.

Now let us consider the effects of selection. We shall assume a simple genetic situation, *i.e.*, a single locus with two alleles (A_1 and A_2) to explain how change of gene frequency is brought about by selection. As pointed out previously selection may operate at two stages, *viz.*, gametic and zygotic.

10.1.1 *Selection at Gametic Stage*

When selection operates at gametic stage, there is no discrimination between the dominant and recessive genes because phenotypes of both the genes are expressed in haploid gametes. Selection can, therefore, be successfully exercised for either of the genes without error. How much is the change produced by selection at gametic stage? To describe the effects of selection at gametic stage let us assume that there are two alleles at a locus, *i.e.* A_1 and A_2. If the fitness of gene A_1 is 1.0 and that of A_2 is $1-s$, frequencies of these genes in next generation could be obtained as:

	Genotypes of gametes		Total
	A_1	A_2	–
Initial frequency	p_o	q_o	1
Fitness	1	$1-s$	–
Frequency after selection	p_o	$q_o(1-s)$	$p_o + q_o - sq_o$ $= (1-sq_o)$

If gene A_2 is lethal *i.e.*, $s = 1$, this gene will be eliminated in the next generation. However, if s is less than 1, gene A_2 will persist for some time in the population. What will be the frequency of gene A_2 after one generation of selection, if s is less than 1? How much will be the change in frequency of gene A_2 after one generation of selection? Let us find out. From the table presented above it appears that the frequency of gene A_2 after one generation of selection will be:

$$q_1 = \frac{(1-s)q_0}{1-sq_0}$$

The change of gene frequency (Δq) will be the difference between new frequency of this gene (q_1) and frequency before selection (q_0). Thus,

$$\Delta q = q_1 - q_0$$

$$= \frac{q(1-s)}{(1-sq)} - q_0$$

$$= \frac{q - sq - [q(1-sq)]}{1-sq}$$

$$= \frac{q - sq - q + sq^2}{1-sq}$$

$$= \frac{-sq(1-q)}{1-sq} \quad \text{... (1)}$$

What does the expression (1) suggest? The negative sign implies that the change will be in negative direction, which will tend to diminish the frequency of gene A_2. For example, if the frequencies of genes A_1 and A_2 are 0.40 and 0.60, respectively, and the coefficient of selection against A_2 is 0.20, Δq after one generation of selection will be:

$$\frac{-sq(1-q)}{1-sq}$$

$$= \frac{-(0.20 \times 0.60)(1-0.60)}{1-(0.20 \times 0.60)}$$

$$= \frac{-0.048}{0.88}$$

$$= -0.0545$$

Thus, in the next generation, frequency of gene A_2 will, be reduced by 0.0545. The new frequency of A_2 will, therefore, be 0.60–0.0545 = 0.5455 or roughly 0.55.

Expression (1) also suggests that the change of gene frequency resulting from selection depends not only upon the coefficient of selection s, but also the initial gene frequency.

10.1.2 *Zygotic Selection*

In most of the higher plants and animals selection operates at zygotic stage. To describe the effects of selection at zygotic level let us consider a single locus with two alleles, *i.e.*, A_1 and A_2. With respect tc this locus there will be three genotypes. Among other things, effectiveness of selection at zygotic level depends upon the degree of dominance. The reason is obvious. If gene A_1 is completely dominant, A_2 will be shielded from selection in heterozygote, *i.e.*, A_1A_2.

Let us derive change in the frequency of gene A_2 (*i.e.* Δq), when selection operates against A_2A_2. The discussion refers to the population in Hardy-Weinberg equilibrium. To begin with let us assume that gene A_2 is lethal, *i.e.*, $s = 1$. Frequency of gene A_2 after one generation of selection can be got from following table.

	Genotypes			Total
	A_1A_1	A_1A_2	A_2A_2	
Initial frequency	p_0^2	$2p_0q_0$	q_0^2	
Fitness	1	1	$1-s=0$	
Frequency after selection	p_0^2	$2p_0q_0$	0	$p_0^2 + 2p_0q_0$ $= p_0(p_0 + 2q_0)$. and since $p_0 + q_0 = 1$ $= p_0(1+q_0)$

Frequency of gene A_2 in the next generation (q_1) will be:

$$q_1 = \frac{p_0 q_0}{p_0(1+q_0)}$$

$$= \frac{q_0}{(1+q_0)}$$

Change of gene frequency (Δq) resulting from one generation of selection is, therefore,

$$\Delta q = q_1 - q_0$$

$$= \frac{q}{1+q} - q$$

$$= \frac{q-[q(1+q)]}{1+q}$$

$$= \frac{q-q-q^2}{1+q}$$

$$= \frac{-q^2}{1+q} \quad \text{... (2)}$$

Expression (2) suggests that the frequency of gene A_2 will diminish as a result of selection. If the initial frequency of A_2 is large, change of gene frequency will be relatively larger in magnitude. On the other hand, if q_0 is small, some of the A_2 genes will be sheltered in heterozygotes and will be shielded from selection. Hence, total elimination of recessive lethal gene is very difficult when it is rare because when it is rare it is in heterozygotes. Also note that when q decreases to small fractions, the change in each generation is approximately equal to q^2 because the denominator $(1+q)$ is not much different from unity.

Let us consider another situation where the coefficient of selection for A_2A_2 is not unity. When $s \neq 1$, the change of gene frequency, *i.e.*, Δq, resulting from one generation of selection can be derived from the following table:

	Genotypes			Total
	A_1A_1	A_1A_2	A_2A_2	
Initial frequency	p_0^2	$2p_0q_0$	q_0^2	1
Fitness	1	1	1–s	
Frequency after selection	p_0^2	$2p_0q_0$	q_0^2 (1–s)	$1-sq_0^2$

Frequency of gene A_2 after one generation of selection (q_1) will, therefore, be:

$$q_1 = \frac{pq+q^2(1-s)}{1-sq^2}$$

The change of gene frequency (Δq) after one generation of selection can be got as:

$$\Delta q = q_1 - q_0$$

$$= \frac{pq+q^2-sq^2}{1-sq^2} - q$$

$$= \frac{pq+q^2-sq^2-[q(1-sq^2)]}{1-sq^2}$$

$$= \frac{pq+q^2-sq^2-q+sq^3}{1-sq^2}$$

$$= \frac{-sq^2(1-q)+q(p+q-1)}{1-sq^2}, \text{ and since } p+q=1$$

$$= \frac{-sq^2(1-q)}{1-sq^2} \qquad \text{... (3)}$$

Expression (3) suggests that change of gene frequency depends not only on the degree of dominance and coefficient of selection but also on the initial gene frequency. Here it was assumed that gene A_1 was completely dominant.

Falconer (1960) has shown that (i) selection is most effective at intermediate gene frequencies, and (ii) selection for or against recessive gene is extremely ineffective when recessive gene is rare, because when it is rare it is present in heterozygotes.

From the expressions derived in (2), (3) it is clear that selection causes change in the frequency of favoured allele. The frequency of favoured allele increases in the selected population. In several cases of selection experiments, progress in improvement is slow at first because the frequency of genes for which selection is practiced is low in the initial population. But as the frequency of desired allele increases, the rate of progress improves, reaching a maximum, after which it declines. This does not depend upon the degree of dominance. Dominance alters the frequency of gene being favoured. As the frequency of gene changes (say q) the change of gene frequency, expressed as Δq also exhibits change, because it depends upon the amount of free variability that is available for selection. For example, in a population which has attained Hardy-Weinberg equilibrium, allele a will be found in aa and Aa genotypes with the frequencies q^2 and pq respectively. Gene a will be shielded by the dominant gene A in heterozygote and hence will not be freely available for selection. As the genes become homozygous, their availability for selection increases.

There may be situations where dominant allele is not favoured and the recessive allele is favoured. In this case selection will be more effective because dominant gene is subject to selection in all the genotypes. For example, if dominant gene is completely lethal, its frequency will be reduced to zero after one generation of selection. It can be easily confirmed that when selection operates against A_1 - genotypes, Δp (*i.e.* change in the frequency of allele A_1) will be:

$$\frac{-sp(1-p)^2}{1-sp(2-p)}$$

However, if our interest is in the frequency of allele A_2, it can be verified that Δq will be:

$$\frac{sq^2(1-q)}{1-s(1-q^2)}$$

after one generation of selection against A_1.

Finally, if selection operates against gene A_2 and there is no dominance, the fitness of A_1A_1, A_1A_2 and A_2A_2 will be 1, $1-\frac{1}{2}s$ and $1-s$, respectively. Change in the frequency of gene A_2, *i.e.*, Δq, resulting from one generation of selection against A_2A_2 will be:

$$-\frac{\frac{1}{2}sq(1-q)}{1-sq}$$

We have been considering the effects of selection operating on a gene which is partially or completely dominant with respect to fitness. Consequences of selection against partially or completely dominant genes are same, *i.e.* elimination of the gene against which selection is operating and establishment or fixation of favoured allele. There are various conditions, however, which permit both the alleles at a locus to remain indefinitely in population, provided selection coefficients remain constant. One such condition is known as overdominance and exists when the heterozygote has superior reproductive fitness than either of the homozygotes.

Let us examine the consequences of this form of selection. Assume that the hetrozygote A_1A_2 has an adaptive value of 1 while the fitnesses of A_1A_1 and A_2A_2 are reduced by coefficients of selection s_1 and s_2, respectively. Frequency of gene A_2 after one generation of selection can be obtained from the table presented below.

	Genotypes			Total
	A_1A_1	A_1A_2	A_2A_2	
Initial frequency	p^2	$2pq$	q^2	1
Fitness	$1-s_1$	1	$1-s_2$	
Frequency after selection	$p^2(1-s_1)$	$2pq$	$q^2(1-s_2)$	$1-s_1p^2-s_2q^2$

Frequency of gene A_2 in the new population (q_1) is, therefore,

$$\frac{pq+q^2(1-s_2)}{1-s_1p^2-s_2q^2}$$

Change in the frequency of gene A_2 (Δq) after one generation of selection is, therefore,

$$\frac{pq(s_1p-s_2q)}{1-s_1p^2-s_2q^2} \quad \text{... (4)}$$

When selection favours heterozygote, gene frequency attains an equilibrium at an intermediate value, both alleles remaining in the population, even without mutation. When Δq is zero, equilibrium is reached and there is no change in the frequencies of genes. There are three possible conditions which are likely to cause the numerator to be equal to zero and, therefore, $\Delta q = 0$. These are:

(i) Frequency of allele $A_1 = 0$
(ii) Frequency of allele $A_2 = 0$ and
(iii) $s_1p = s_2q$.

Under first two conditions, both the alleles will not be present in the population at the same time, and the equilibrium will be absent. The third condition is $s_1p = s_2q$, so that $\Delta q = pq(0) = 0$. Frequency of gene A_2 at equilibrium can be derived as:

$$s_1p = s_2q$$
$$s_1(1-q) = s_2q$$
$$s_1 - s_1q = s_2q$$
$$\therefore\ s_1 = s_2q + s_1q \text{ and}$$
$$s_1 = q(s_2 + s_1)$$

$$\therefore q = \frac{s_1}{s_1+s_2} \quad \text{... (5)}$$

Frequency of gene A_1 at equilibrium is $s_2/s_1 + s_2$.

If s_1 and s_2 are constant values, both p and q will reach stable equilibrium. However, if q departs from this equilibrium value, selection pressure will force it back. If q is less than its equilibrium value, Δq will be positive. When q is larger than its equilibrium value, Δq will be negative.

This point will be clear to the reader with an example. Suppose the frequencies of genotypes A_1A_1, A_1A_2, and A_2A_2 are 0.40, 0.40 and 0.20, respectively and that $s_1 = 0.10$ and $s_2 = 0.20$. Expected frequency of gene A_2 at equilibrium is

$$q = \frac{s_1}{s_1 + s_2}$$

$$= \frac{0.1}{0.1 + 0.2}$$

$$= 0.33$$

However, in the base population frequency of this gene is:

$$0.2 + 0.2 = 0.4$$

Frequency of gene A_2 in the population being considered is more than the expected value at equilibrium. Change of gene frequency will, therefore, be negative as shown below

$$\Delta q = \frac{pq(s_1 p - s_2 q)}{1 - s_1 p^2 - s_2 q^2}$$

$$= \frac{0.6 \times 0.4[(0.1 \times 0.6) - (0.2 \times 0.4)]}{1 - (0.1 \times 0.6^2) - (0.2 \times 0.4^2)}$$

$$= -0.0051$$

The change of gene frequency will be negative so long q does not reach its equilibrium frequency, *i.e.*, 0.33.

Three or more alleles at a locus are maintained in the same way, provided the heterozygote of any pair is superior in fitness to both the homozygotes of that pair. A feature of the equilibrium worthy of note is that the gene frequency depends not on the degree of superiority of the heterozygote but on the relative disadvantage of one homozygote compared with that of the other. Maintenance of different genotypes, with respect to a single locus, is an example of "balanced polymorphism" a term coined by Ford (1940) to describe the preservation of genetic variability (polymorphism) through selection. Existence in the population of individuals with readily observable differences caused by genes at intermediate frequencies is called as polymorphism. There are many causes for polymorphism. Some of them are listed below:

(i) Relatively small heterozygous advantage may enable genes that are otherwise lethal to remain in the population.

(ii) Selection coefficient may change so that genes detrimental at one time are advantageous at another time. Thus the force of selection operating against a gene may be reversed before the gene is eliminated.

Selection coefficients may vary from one environment to other. A population which is growing over wide agro-ecological situations, therefore, maintains a variety of genotypes, each of which is superior in a particular habitat.

(iii) Interaction between gene loci may also result in polymorphism. For example, if the heterozygous combination at two loci, *viz.* A, a and B, b, is superior in replusion phase, all the four alleles will be maintained in the population.

10.1.3. *Number of Generations*

How many generations of selection would be required to attain a desired change in the frequency of a gene? Selection against a dominant gene leads to its elimination from the population at a faster pace than selection against a recessive gene. The reason being that the recessive gene is sheltered by it's dominant allele in heterozygote and hence protected from selection. Frequency of recessive gene will, therefore, change gradually.

Let us derive the expression for number of rounds of selection required to produce change in the frequency of recessive lethal gene. Imagine that gene A_2 is lethal. Then the contribution of homozygote A_2A_2 to the next generation will be reduced by an amount s. Fitness of this genotype will, therefore, be $1-s$. Frequency of gene A_2 in the new population will be:

$$\frac{pq + q^2(1-s)}{1-sq^2}$$

When a gene is lethal, s is equal to 1. Substitute this value in the expression given above. q_1 will, therefore, be:

$$\frac{q_0}{1+q_0}$$

where q_o is the frequency of gene A_2 in the base population. It can be verified that after two generations of selection against gene A_2 the frequency of this gene (q_2) will be:

$$q_2 = \frac{q_1}{1+q_1}$$

Substituting the value of q_1 in this expression we get

$$\frac{\dfrac{q_0}{1+q_0}}{1+\dfrac{q_0}{1+q_0}}$$

Upon simplification q_2 is found to be: $q_o/1 + 2q_o$.

So in general, frequency of gene A_2 after n generations of selection (q_n) will be:

$$q_n = \frac{q_0}{1+nq_0} \qquad \text{... (6)}$$

Expression in (6) could be used to calculate number of generations (n) required to produce a given change of gene frequency. Thus,

$$q_n(1 + nq_o) = q_o$$

$$q_n + nq_nq_o = q_o$$

$$nq_nq_o = q_o - q_n$$

$$\therefore \quad n = \frac{q_0 - q_n}{q_0q_n}$$

or

$$\frac{1}{q_n} - \frac{1}{q_0} \qquad \text{... (7)}$$

10.2 Response to Selection

The most important consequence of change in the frequency of gene is the change in the frequencies of genotypes. And since the effects of selection are exerted by changing the frequencies with which various genes or combinations of genes occur, selection leads to change in the genotype frequencies and consequently the observable genetic properties of a population. Change produced by selection, in which a breeder is chiefly interested, is the change of population mean, which is known as 'response' to selection. Response may be defined as the difference between mean phenotypic value of offspring of selected parents and whole of the parental generation before selection. It is assumed here that the individuals to be employed as parents are selected from the parental generation on the basis of their own phenotypic values. Mean phenotypic value of individuals selected to be the parents expressed as deviation from population mean *i.e.*, mean of all the individuals in the parental generation before selection, is known as selection differential (Fig 10.1)

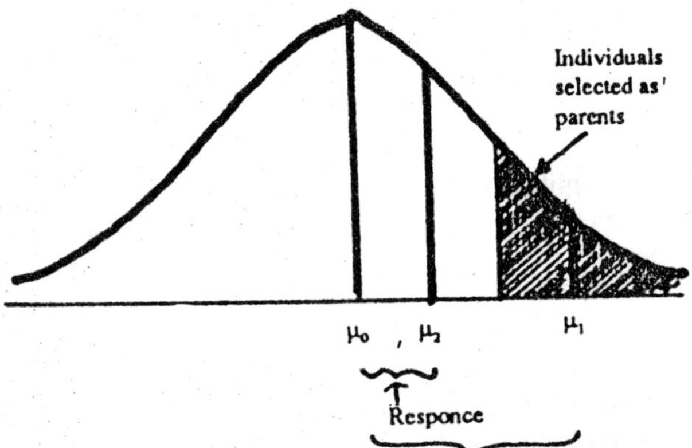

μ_o = Mean of initial parental population
μ_1 = Mean of individuals selected to be the parents
μ_2 = Mean of offspring of selected parents

FIG 10.1: *Response to selection and selection differential*

It was shown in section 4.8.1. that heritability can be estimated as regression of mean phenotypic value of offspring on their corresponding mid-parental values, *i.e.*, $b_{o\bar{p}}$. Therefore; the regression of response; which is the mean phenotypic value of offspring expressed as deviation from population mean, on the selection differential, which is measured as the difference between individuals selected as parents and the population mean, is equal to $b_{o\bar{p}}$ and consequently heritability (h^2). Thus heritability can also be expressed as:

$$h^2 = \frac{R}{S}, \qquad \text{... (8)}$$

where *R* and *S* denote the response and selection differential, respectively.

Thus we have the relationship.

$$h^2 = \frac{R}{S} = b_{0\bar{p}}$$

Expected response could, therefore, be obtained as:

$$R = h^2 S \qquad \text{... (9)}$$

or

$$R = b_{o\bar{p}} S$$

Relationship $R = b_{o\bar{p}}S$ is not a prediction equation but simply a description because the regression of offspring on their mid-parental values cannot be obtained unless selection is exercised in a given population and progeny of the selected parents raised. On the other hand, expression R = h^2S may be regarded as a prediction equation, where h^2 is the estimate of heritability in parental generation. Gene frequencies are known to influence the magnitude of components of genotypic variance (section 4.3). And since heritability depends upon the relative magnitudes of these components, heritability will change as a consequence of change of gene frequencies brought about by selection. For this reason, the estimates of heritabilities of parental and progeny generations are expected to be different. Experiments have, nevertheless, indicated that response is usually maintained with little change over several generations. In practice, therefore, prediction of response may be expected to hold good for several generations.

Breeders make all the endeavours to improve the magnitude of response to selection. Expression (9) suggests that the response depends upon two factors, *viz.* the heritability and the selection differential. Response to selection could be augmented if heritability and/or selection differential are improved. Magnitude of selection differential is usually known after individuals to be employed as parents have been selected from the population. Since selection differential is defined as difference between the mean phenotypic value of the individuals selected to be the parents and whole of the parental generation before selection, the magnitude of selection differential is governed by the variability in the initial population and the proportion of individuals selected as parents. For a given intensity of selection that is applied to two populations, one should not be surprised to find that the magnitude of response is relatively larger for a population that has more variability (measured as standard deviation). On the other hand, if two populations have same standard deviation for a given character, the magnitude of response will be larger for the population which has been subjected to more stringent selection, *i.e.*, less proportion of individuals have been selected from the population to be used as parents.

Standard deviation, which is a measure of variability, is property of a character as well as the population. It is associated with physical units of measurement, such as grammes, centimetres, litres, *etc.* Response to selection is also associated with physical units of measurements. Hence, it may not be possible to compare the response observed for two or more characters measured in different units. However, response to selection could be generalised if the response and the selection differential are expressed in "standardised" units, *i.e.*, in terms of standard deviation. Thus R/σ_p is a generalized measure of response, which enables comparisons among the responses observed for different characters and different populations. Likewise, S/σ_p, is the generalised measure of selection differential, which permits us to compare different methods of selection. The standardised selection differential, S/σ_p, is called as the intensity of selection and symbolised as i. Thus, the response in terms of standardised units is expressed as:

$$\frac{R}{\sigma_P} = \frac{S}{\sigma_P}.h^2, \quad \text{and since} \frac{S}{\sigma_P} = i,$$

$$R = i\,\sigma_p h^2 \qquad \dots (10)$$

Heritability is a ratio of additive genetic variance to phenotypic variance, *i.e.* σ_A^2 / σ_P^2. Therefore, expression (10) can also be written as:

$$R = i\sigma_A h \qquad \dots (11)$$

Now let us assume that the phenotypic values of individuals in the populations are normally distributed with mean μ and standard deviation σ_p. Let x denote the point of truncation (Fig 10.2), such that all the individuals with phenotypic values greater than x are selected. If the mean values of initial population and selected individuals are represented by μ_0 and μ_1, respectively, the selection differential S is given by $\mu_1 - \mu_0$. It follows from one of the important properties of normal distribution that

$$\frac{S}{\sigma_p} = i = \frac{Z}{p}, \qquad \dots (12)$$

where Z is the height of the ordinate at the point of tuncation and p is the proportion of individuals selected (having a value greater than say

x). Thus, if the proportion of individuals to be selected is known, it is possible to determine by how many standard deviations the mean of selected individuals will deviate from the mean of entire population before selection. Breeders can increase the selection differential by increasing the heritable variation (or heritability) in the population and/or increasing the intensity of selection. There are several ways by which a breeder can generate more variability. However, it may not be possible to increase the intensity of selection beyond a certain limit. Why? There are two reasons. Firstly, a certain proportion of individuals in the population must be retained if the population size is to be maintained. For example, if all the plants in the population are to be saved to maintain the size of population, selection intensity will be zero. However, if the species is prolific, selection differentials up to several hundreds is possible. Let us assume that it is not possible to grow more than 500 plants in anyone generation. If it is desired to save extreme five per cent plants (*i.e.*, 25 plants), which are most desirable for the character to be improved, selected plants should produce on an average 20 offspring so that the population size is maintained. If the selection limit is set to the extreme one per cent individuals, *i.e.*, 5 p , selected plants must produce 100 offspring on an average. For most plant species selection differentials of this magnitude pose no real problem, but in breeding of some plant species and in breeding of the large domestic animals, this is not possible. Population size is also important in connection with inbreeding. And hence there is a limit beyond which *i* cannot be increased.

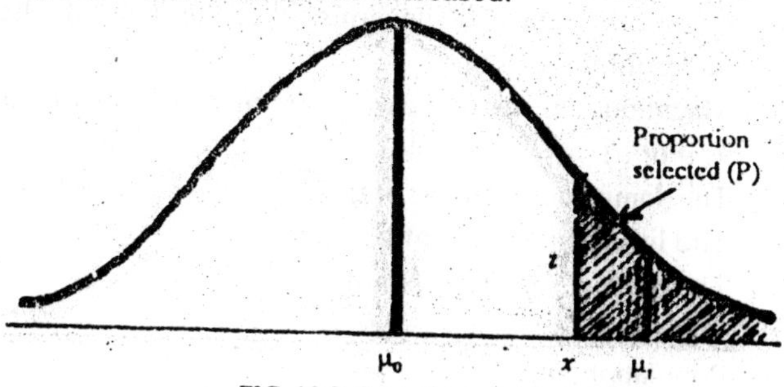

FIG. 10.2: *Selection intensity*

Secondly, breeders are concerned with improvement of two or more characters simultaneously. This influences the intensity of selection that is actually effective. Suppose we wish to improve two characters x and y

simultaneously. If it is desired to select extremely superior five per cent plants for both characters we may have to reject some plants which are superior for x but not for y and *vice versa*. Then breeder has to relax intensity of selection for individual character. In general, when attention is to be paid during selection to n characters simultaneously and x per cent population is to be saved to maintain the population size, the intensity of selection for anyone character is given by $n\sqrt{x}$, (Allard, 1960). Thus simultaneous selection for two or more characters imposes restriction on the intensity of selection.

Response to selection cannot be expected to continue indefinitely. It is expected that sooner or later all the favourable genes, originally segregating, will be brought to fixation. As they approach fixation, genetic variance will decline and the response will diminish. When the fixation is complete response will cease and the population may then fail to respond to selection in the opposite direction also.

10.2.1 *The speed of advance under selection*

Any breeding programme aims to accomplish the desired level of improvement in plants as early as possible. The speed with which this could be achieved depends upon several factors among which following are important:

(i) Number of gene pairs governing the inheritance of character under improvement.
(ii) Magnitude of effect of genes on the character (measured either as *a* or *d*)
(iii) The dominance relations of genes, *i.e.* the magnitude of *d* or *h*.
(iv) The linkage relations of genes
(v) The narrow sense heritability
(vi) Intensity of selection
(vii) Population size

Not only the limit of improvement of a character is determined by the number of gene pairs governing the inheritance of a character but also the speed of progress. If a single gene pair governs the inheritance of a character, about 25 per cent plants in the F_2 generation will be homozygous for desirable gene. If there is no dominance, *AA* and *Aa* could be distinguished and selection of *AA* (if desirable, or *aa* if it is desirable) would lead to immediate fixation of a character and attainment of improvement. On the other hand, when *n* gene pairs govern the inheritance, one plant out of 4^n will be homozygous for desirable genes in the F_2 generation. Since very large poulations of F_2s are seldom grown by the breeders, there is little chance of selecting such a plant and immediate achievement of goal. Moreover due to considerable influence of nonheritable agencies on quantitative characters, it is sometimes difficult to differentiate plants possessing superior combinations of genes from those plants which are growing in favourable environments. Consequently, number of genes limit the speed of progress.

Linkage among the genes with desirable and undesirable effects on characters also determine the speed with which a breeder can achieve his goal. Quantitative characters are governed by several genes with small, similar and cumulative effects. Many of these genes are located on the same chromosome. These are consequently linked. Strength of linkage between the genes with desirable and undesirable influences on the trait will decide how quickly desirable recombinants will be isolated. More closely the genes are placed, stronger is the linkage and lesser are the chances that in early segregating generations recombinant plants with desirable gene combinations are obtained. Of course, this will also depend upon the breeding procedure.

Plants are selected from segregating material on the basis of their phenotypic values. However, it is the genotype of plant which determines the progress attained. Correspondence between genotypic value and phenotypic value is measured as broad sense heritability. In other words, the proportion of heritable variance that makes up the phenotypic variance. A breeder may not realize progress in improvement of a trait if inheritance is largely governed by nonheritable agencies. For example, two plants of wheat may have superior phenotypes because of different reasons. One may possess superior genetic architecture whereas another in it's vicinity may have superior environment around it. Only progeny test can distinguish between the two causes of superiority. Moreover it is the additive component of genotypic variation that is fixable. Selection can take advantage of this component of variation for development of superior true breeding variety. Consequently, narrow sense heritability determines the speed of advance during selection.

It was shown in section 10.2 that response to selection is dependent on selection intensity and narrow sense heritability. Thus intensity of selection also determines the speed of genetic advance. Since the compoenents of genotypic variation, such as additive and dominance, are influenced by gene frequency and degree of dominance (section 4.3), these could also be regarded as factors restricting the speed of progress during selection.

Population size is also an important factor. As the number of gene pairs influencing the inheritance of a character increases, the proportion of plants homozygous for all the desirable genes will be relatively rare. Very large segregating populations are seldom grown and hence plants homozygous for all the desirable genes may be rarely expected in segregating population. Breeder has to be content with plants closer to superiority, although they may be heterozygous.

10.2.2 *Correlated Response to Selection*

Two or more characters are correlated because genes influencing these characters are located on the same chromosome. Therefore, change in the mean expression of one character, resulting from selection for that character, also causes change in the mean measurements of correlated character or characters. This is known as correlated response to selection. How much is the correlated response for character Y, when character X is actually selected? Let us derive the correlated response of Y. The expected response of X is;

$$R_x = i_x \sigma_{Ax} h_x$$

Correlated response of Y will be given by the regression of breeding value of Y on the breeding value of X, (b_{AXY}). Thus,

$$b_{AXY} = \frac{\sigma_{AXY}}{\sigma^2_{AX}} \qquad \text{... (13)}$$

Where σ_{AXY} is the covariance of breeding values of Y with X and σ^2_{AX} is the variance of breeding values of character X. If the numerator as well as the denominator of (13) are multiplied with σ_{AY} we get:

$$\frac{\sigma_{A_{XY}}}{\sigma_{A_X}\sigma_{A_X}}\frac{\sigma_{A_Y}}{\sigma_{A_Y}}=r_{A_{XY}}\frac{\sigma_{A_Y}}{\sigma_{A_X}} \quad \text{... (14)}$$

The correlated response of Y is, therefore, given by

$$CR_Y = b_{A_{XY}} R_X$$

$$= r_{A_{XY}} \frac{\sigma_{A_Y}}{\sigma_{A_X}} i_X \sigma_{A_X} h_X$$

$$= i_X \sigma_{A_Y} h_X r_{A_{XY}} \quad \text{... (15)}$$

In section 10.2 it was shown that $\sigma_A = \sigma_p h$. If this value is substituted in (15) we get:

$$CR_Y = i_X h_X h_Y \sigma_{PY} r_{A_{XY}} \quad \text{... (16)}$$

This expression shows that correlated response can be predicted if genetic correlation and the heritabilities of two characters – in the present case X and Y – are known. Magnitude of correlated response will be relatively smaller if genetic correlation is low. If correlation between two characters is due to linkage the magnitude of correlated response will change from one generation to the next because of recombinations among the genes influencing the two characters.

At times breeders find it more convenient or economical to select a character Y, instead of the character X in which improvement is desired. This method of selection is known as indirect selection. The character, which is selected, is known as secondary character. In what circumstances indirect selection would be more efficient? Let us find out. Based on (15) the correlated response of X would be:

$$CR_X = i_Y \sigma_{A_X} h_Y r_{A_{XY}}$$

The expected response of character X resulting from direct selection is:

$$R_X = i_X \sigma_A h_X$$

The merit of indirect selection is, therefore, given by:

$$\frac{CR_X}{R_X} = \frac{i_Y \sigma_{A_X} h_Y r_{A_{XY}}}{i_x \sigma_{A_X} h_X}$$

$$= \frac{i_Y h_Y}{i_X h_X} r_{A_{XY}} \qquad \ldots (17)$$

If we assume that same intensity of selection is possible for both the characters (*i.e.*, X and Y), expression (17) suggests that indirect selection will be more efficient when the heritability of secondary character is larger in magnitude than the primary character and the genetic correlation between X and Y is high. Indirect selection will also be efficient when more stringent selection is possible for secondary character.

10.3 Selection for Multiple Characters

Economic value of a plant depends almost always upon several characters. For example, in cereals, grain yield, size of kernel, quality of kernel, plant height, resistance to insects and diseases, *etc.* determine the economic value of a plant. While selecting a desirable plant from segregating material a breeder has to give due consideration simultaneously to several attributes. An efficient selection procedure is, therefore, required which will enable a breeder to attain maximum improvement in the economic value of a plant, which is determined by several characters. Basically there are three selection methods which could be employed for improving several characters simultaneously. These are, tandem selection, independent culling levels and selection index (Hazel and Lush, 1943). Among these, selection index is more efficient and widely accepted by the plant breeders. This method will, therefore, be described in some detail.

10.3.1. *Tandem Selection*

In this method individual characters are improved successively. Character A is improved first, followed by character B and so on. As a first step, selection is practiced only for character A and, therefore, progress is equal to the response for this character alone. No progress should be expected for other characters (assuming no genetic correlation) during this period. Let us assume that economic value is determined by n characters. If only one character is improved for one generation, the expected genetic improvement in the economic value after n generations will be:

$$h_1^2 (P_1 - \bar{P}_1) + h_2^2 (P_2 - \bar{P}_2) + ... + h_n^2 (P_n - \bar{P}_n)$$

$$= \sum_j^n h_j^2 (P_j - \bar{P}_j)$$

If we assume that the heritability, variances and selection intensities for n characters being improved are same, the average change in the economic value per generation will be $i\sigma_p h^2$.

10.3.2 *Independent Culling Levels*

It is a method of selection in which the selected individuals have to surpass a certain minimum value for each of the characters to be improved. This minimum performance is independent between the characters. For example, a sorghum breeder may set a limit for selecting plants from segregating populations, such that only those plants will be selected which yield 50 grammes of grain per plant, mature in 95 to 100 days and the plants are 150 to 180 cm tall. He will then reject those plants which do not meet these standards. According to this selection scheme a plant which yields 80 grammes of grain, but is 190 cm tall and matures in about 140 days, is liable to be rejected. This selection method immediately reduces the selection intensity of individual characters. The more the number of characters to be considered larger will be the reduction in intensity of selection.

10.3.3 *Selection Index*

The aim of most breeding programmes is simultaneous improvement of several characters. An objective method involving simultaneous selection for several attributes then becomes necessary. It has been recognised that most rapid improvement in the economic value is expected from selection applied simultaneously to all the characters which determine the economic value of a plant, provided appropriate weights are assigned to each character according to their relative economic importance, heritability and correlations (both phenotypic and genotypic) between characters. Selection for economic value is thus a complex matter. If the component characters are combined together into a score or an index in such a way that when selection is applied to the index, as if index is the character to be improved, most rapid improvement of economic value is expected. Such an index was first proposed by Smith (1937) based on the "discriminant function" of Fisher (1936). Hazel (1943) also developed a method of index selection based on the path coefficients. In this chapter the method of selection developed by Smith (1937) will be described.

The characters of economic importance are mostly quantitative in nature. Phenotypic expression of such characters is influenced by heritable as well as non-heritable agencies, and hence it is difficult to determine the genetic worth of an individual plant unless we have adequate seed for planting a replicated trial. Breeders select plants on the basis of phenotypic values of the characters which in their opinion determine the economic value. There is no sound basis to assign more or less weights to the characters because the actual worth of characters is usually not known. Smith (1937) advocated use of "discriminant function" of the observable characters which will best indicate the genetic worth of a plant. How to develop discriminant functions?

Let us assume that the economic value of a plant is determined by three characters, *viz.* x_1, x_2 and x_3. Suppose that it is desired to select plants, the merit (H) of which is linearly expressed as:

$$H = a_1G_1 + a_2G_2 + a_3G_3 \qquad \text{... (18)}$$

If n characters determine the merit, linear function could be expressed as:

$$H = a_1G_1 + a_2G_2 + \ldots\ldots + a_nG_n \qquad \text{... (19)}$$

where $G_1, G_2, \ldots\ldots G_n$ represent the genotypic values of characters and $a_1, a_2 \ldots\ldots a_n$ denote the weights to be assigned to each of the character. Weights reflect the relative importance of each character and determine the total genetic advance to be expected through index selection as well as the gains in individual character. There is no way in practice to avoid use of weights because weights are also assigned while deciding the relative importance of different characters. In most of the cases weights are assigned on the basis of economic gain that is expected to result from one unit change in a given character relative to others. The relative market prices can also be taken into consideration for assigning weights. Since weights are assigned empirically, selection index changes according to the situations. Several efforts have been made to develop durable selection indices (Pesek and Baker, 1969 and 1970).

It may be pointed out that the requirement of linearity of a model is made to enable a mathematical solution (Kempthorne, 1957). However, depending upon how the characters combine indices could be developed which are linear or non-linear. Non-linear indices are employed in those situations where component characters combine in a multiplicative fashion. Kempthorne and Nordskog (1959) introduced the concept of "restricted selection indices", which enables us to restrict changes in some of the characters without affecting the development in others. This will facilitate differential improvements in various characters.

The merit, linearly described in equation (19), cannot be directly evaluated because only the phenotypic values are measured which may not truly represent the genotypic values. The phenotype (I) is linearly expressed as:

$$I = b_1x_1 + b_2x_2 + b_3x_3 \qquad \text{... (20)}$$

if the economic value is governed by three characters, and as:

$$I = b_1x_1 + b_2x_2 + \ldots\ldots + b_nx_n \qquad \text{... (21)}$$

when n characters are involved. Now the problem is to calculate values of b in such a manner that the regression of I on H will be maximum, so that selection of phenotypes using I as a discriminant function will ensure maximum gain. Maximising the regression of I on H yields three simultaneous equations (n equations for n characters):

$$b_1\sigma_1^2 + b_2\sigma_{12} + b_3\sigma_{13} = A_1$$

$$b_1\sigma_{21} + b_2\sigma_2^2 + b_3\sigma_{23} = A_2$$

$$b_1\sigma_{31} + b_2\sigma_{32} + b_3\sigma_3^2 = A_3 \qquad \text{... (22)}$$

where σ_1^2, σ_2^2 and σ_3^2 are the phenotypic variances of characters x_1, x_2 and x_3, respectively, and $\sigma_{12} = \sigma_{21}$, $\sigma_{13} = \sigma_{31}$ and $\sigma_{23} = \sigma_{32}$ symbolise the phenotypic covariances. A_1, A_2 and A_3 are estimated as:

$$A_1 = a_1G_1^2 + a_2G_{12} + a_3G_{13}$$

$$A_2 = a_1G_{21} + a_2G_2^2 + a_3G_{23}$$

$$A_3 = a_1G_{31} + a_2G_{32} + a_3G_3^2 \qquad \text{... (23)}$$

where a_1, a_2 and a_3 are the weights applied and G_1^2, G_2^2 and G_3^2 are the estimates of genotypic variances of characters x_1, x_2 and x_3, respectively. In expression (23), $G_{12} = G_{21}$, $G_{23} = G_{32}$ and $G_{13} = G_{31}$, and represent the estimates of genotypic covariances. Equations (22) and (23) are rearranged as:

$$b_1\sigma_1^2 + b_2\sigma_{12} + b_3\sigma_{13} = a_1G_1^2 + a_2G_{12} + a_3G_{13}$$

$$b_1\sigma_{21} + b_2\sigma_2^2 + b_3\sigma_{23} = a_1G_{21} + a_2G_2^2 + a_3G_{23}$$

$$b_1\sigma_{31} + b_2\sigma_{32} + b_3\sigma_3^2 = a_1G_{31} + a_2G_{32} + a_3G_3^2 \qquad \text{... (24)}$$

The set of equations in (24) can also be arranged in matrix form as:

$$\underset{X}{\begin{bmatrix} \sigma_1^2 & \sigma_{12} & \sigma_{13} \\ \sigma_{21} & \sigma_2^2 & \sigma_{23} \\ \sigma_{31} & \sigma_{32} & \sigma_3^2 \end{bmatrix}} \underset{b}{\begin{bmatrix} b_1 \\ b_2 \\ b_3 \end{bmatrix}} = \underset{G}{\begin{bmatrix} G_1^2 & G_{12} & G_{13} \\ G_{21} & G_2^2 & G_{23} \\ G_{31} & G_{32} & G_3^2 \end{bmatrix}} \underset{a}{\begin{bmatrix} a_1 \\ a_2 \\ a_3 \end{bmatrix}} \qquad \text{... (25)}$$

where the matrix X is a phenotypic variance-covariance matrix. Elements of matrix G are the estimates of genotypic variances and covariances and the elements of column vectors b and a represent the discriminant function coefficients and assigned weights, respectively. From the set of matrices in (25) estimates of bs are obtained as:

$$b = G.\, a\, .\, X^{-1} \qquad \text{... (26)}$$

where X^{-1} is the inverse of matrix X.

It should be pointed out that there are two ways in which weights could be assigned. Equal weights could be assigned to all the component characters without distinguishing their relative importance to the economic value. Since the means of component characters may differ, equal weighting may be obtained as:

$$a_1 = \frac{1}{\bar{x}_1}, a_2 = \frac{1}{\bar{x}_2}, a_3 = \frac{1}{\bar{x}_3}, \ldots. a_n = \frac{1}{\bar{x}_n}$$

Breeders should use reasoning and experience while assigning relative weights. Suppose three characters determine the economic value, *viz.*, grain yield/plant(x_1), chapati making quality (x_2) and resistance to rust (x_3). If ten units of improvement in chapati making quality results in economic gain equal to one kilogram of grain yield and 5 per cent reduction in rust incidence causes gains equal to one kilogram of grain, then the weights will be:

$$a_1 = \frac{1}{1}, a_2 = \frac{1}{10} \text{ and } a_3 = \frac{1}{-5}$$

$$= 1, \quad = 0.10, \quad = -0.20$$

The weight a_3 is negative because five per cent reduction in rust incidence is to result in yield gain.

Mathematical description of the function (I) is known as selection index. Thus,

$$I = b_1x_1 + b_2x_2 + .. + b_ix_i ... + b_nx_n$$

Using this function it is possible to discriminate among the superior and inferior plants. Selection index or score is calculated for all the plants and those with highest values are retained.

The expected genetic advance (Δ_i) is calculated as:

$$\frac{Z}{p} \frac{\Sigma\Sigma a_i b_i G_{ij}}{\sqrt{(\Sigma\Sigma b_i b_j p_{ij})}} \quad ... (27)$$

where Z/p is the selection intensity (i) . G_{ij} symbolises the genotypic variances and covariances of the component characters and p_{ij} represent the phenotypic variances and covariances. Genetic advance in the ith character (Δ_i) can be calculated, following Brim *et al.* (1959).

$$i = \frac{\Sigma b_i G_{ij}}{\sqrt{(\Sigma b_i G_i)}} \quad ... (28)$$

10.3.4. *Worked Example*

Twenty-eight genotypes of sorghum were raised in randomised block design with two replications. Observations were recorded on (1) Grain yield per plant (g), (2) 1000-grain weight (g), (3) Days to 50 per cent flowering and (4) Plant height (*cm*)

The X matrix, elements of which comprise of the phenotypic variances and covariances, is set up as:

$$\begin{bmatrix} \sigma_1^2 & \sigma_{12} & \sigma_{13} & \sigma_{14} \\ \sigma_{21} & \sigma_2^2 & \sigma_{23} & \sigma_{24} \\ \sigma_{31} & \sigma_{32} & \sigma_3^2 & \sigma_{34} \\ \sigma_{41} & \sigma_{42} & \sigma_{43} & \sigma_4^2 \end{bmatrix}$$

Phenotypic variance is calculated as:

$$\text{Genotypic variance} + \frac{\text{Error mean square}}{\text{No. of replications}}$$

Reader should note that what is sought here is the estimate of phenotypic and genotypic variances on plant mean basis and, therefore, error mean square is divided by number of replications. In the table of analysis of variance, value of error mean square represents the environmental variance on plot basis over *r* replications. Calculation of genotypic variance from the table of analysis of variance was described in section 4.8.2. Estimates of phenotypic covariances are obtained in like manner from the table of analysis of covariances. In the present example, the X matrix is:

$$\begin{bmatrix} 281.860 & 27.658 & 57.835 & 497.881 \\ 27.658 & 9.315 & 3.773 & 87.508 \\ 57.835 & 3.773 & 133.135 & 196.523 \\ 497.881 & 87.508 & 196.523 & 1774.695 \end{bmatrix}$$

The *G* matrix is set up as:

$$\begin{bmatrix} G_1^2 & G_{12} & G_{13} & G_{14} \\ G_{21} & G_2^2 & G_{23} & G_{24} \\ G_{31} & G_{32} & G_3^2 & G_{34} \\ G_{41} & G_{42} & G_{43} & G_4^2 \end{bmatrix}$$

Estimates of genotypic variances and covariances, for the present example, are arranged as:

$$\begin{bmatrix} 239.790 & 22.845 & -33.282 & 501.993 \\ 22.845 & 8.070 & 3.904 & 86.589 \\ -33.282 & 3.904 & 132.525 & -294.169 \\ 501.993 & 86.589 & -294.169 & 1674.005 \end{bmatrix}$$

Let us assume that the weights $a_1 = a_2 = a_3 = a_4 = 1$. Discriminant function coefficients are obtained as $G.aX^{-1}$ and hence we need an inverse of matrix X. The inverse of X matrix has been worked out in Appendix II. The X^{-1} is then

$$\begin{bmatrix} 0.0079 & -0.0044 & -0.0004 & -0.0017 \\ -0.0044 & 0.2188 & 0.0115 & -0.0104 \\ -0.0004 & 0.0115 & 0.0093 & -0.0015 \\ -0.0017 & -0.0104 & -0.0015 & 0.0017 \end{bmatrix}$$

$$X^{-1}$$

The product G. a is got as:

$$\underset{G}{\begin{bmatrix} 239.790 & 22.845 & -33.282 & 501.993 \\ 22.845 & 8.070 & 3.904 & 86.589 \\ -33.282 & 3.904 & 132.525 & -294.169 \\ 501.993 & 86.589 & -294.169 & 1674.005 \end{bmatrix}} \underset{a}{\begin{bmatrix} 1 \\ 1 \\ 1 \\ 1 \end{bmatrix}} = \underset{G.a}{\begin{bmatrix} 731.346 \\ 121.408 \\ -192.022 \\ 1968.418 \end{bmatrix}}$$

Estimate of b_1 is then obtained as:

$$b_1 = (731.346 \times 0.0079) + (121.408 \times -0.0044) + (-192.022 \times -0.0004) + (1968.418 \times -0.0017) = 1.9739$$

In like manner, other discriminant function coefficients are calculated. These are:

b_2	0.6663
b_3	–3.6347
b_4	1.1284

Selection index is then constructed as:

$$I = 1.9739x_1 + 0.6663x_2 - 3.6347x_3 + 1.128x_4$$

By substituting the mean values of x_1, x_2 x_3 and x_4 for each of the twentyeight genotypes in this selection index, scores for these genotypes are obtained. For example, the score for genotype 1 is obtained as:

$$I_1 = (42.54 \times 1.9739) + (18.30 \times 0.6663) + (65 \times -3.6347) + (191 \times 1.1284) = 75.4318$$

Scores for other genotypes are calculated in similar manner (Table 10.1).

TABLE 10.1: Calculation of selection scores for twentyeight genotypes of sorghum

Genotypes	Values of x_1	x_2	x_3	x_4	Score
1.	42.54	18.30	65	191	75.4318
2.	46.64	19.67	93	169	–42.1586
3.	25.18	16.40	69	170	1.6638
4.	17.56	13.23	57	102	–48.6042
5.	38.16	22.55	63	217	106.2257
6.	36.93	23.52	56	156	61.0547
7.	29.97	23.78	54	175	76.1985
8.	90.78	24.07	79	250	190.1871
9.	84.19	22.51	62	222	206.3344
10.	56.11	20.92	57	182	122.8854
11.	70.86	22.46	58	263	240.7922
12.	64.63	24.93	55	204	174.4691
13.	63.22	25.45	56	228	195.4792
14.	66.43	20.37	79	182	62.9262
15.	67.97	22.07	71	205	122.1295
16.	68.73	24.57	88	288	157.1627
17.	58.59	26.68	81	263	135.7861
18.	62.38	27.37	80	290	177.8285
19.	50.25	19.74	59	205	129.2159
20.	56.94	19.70	59	235	176.2466
21.	69.63	23.38	57	228	203.1180
22.	62.70	23.64	58	234	192.7478
23.	42.34	19.52	54	178	101.1625
24.	48.56	20.85	53	159	96.5214
25.	51.01	22.94	53	179	128.3180
26.	49.68	22.69	56	192	126.2912
27.	43.50	23.19	57	194	113.0478
28.	44.62	24.34	53	185	120.4080

$$\begin{bmatrix} 1.9739 \\ 0.6663 \\ -3.6347 \\ 1.1284 \end{bmatrix} =$$

It will be apparent to the reader from Table 10.1 that largest score need not be necessarily associated with highest grain yield. For example, grain yield of genotype 8 is maximum. However, the value of score for genotype 11 is largest. Selection scores of genotypes 9 and 21 are second and third, respectively, in ranking. Although grain yield is the main aim of a breeder, he is also interested in other attributes, such as plant height, days required for maturity, *etc*., which also determine the genetic worth of a plant. The scores are then arranged in descending order and the best five or ten per cent plants selected.

The expected genetic advance Δ_G, resulting from selection is calculated as:

$$i.\frac{\Sigma\Sigma a_i b_i G_{ij}}{\sqrt{(\Sigma\Sigma b_i b_j p_{ij})}}$$

For the worked example being considered, numerator is got as:

$$[1111]\begin{bmatrix} 1.9739 \\ 0.6663 \\ -3.6347 \\ 1.1284 \end{bmatrix}\begin{bmatrix} 239.70 & 22.845 & -33.282 & 501.993 \\ 22.845 & 8.070 & 3.904 & 86.589 \\ -33.282 & 3.904 & 132.525 & -294.169 \\ 501.993 & 86.589 & -294.169 & 1674.005 \end{bmatrix}$$

$$=[1111]\begin{bmatrix} 1175.7844 \\ 113.9879 \\ -745.3323 \\ 4006.7415 \end{bmatrix}$$

$$=4571.1815$$

The denominator is calculated as:

$(\Sigma\Sigma b_i b_j p_{ij})$

$$\begin{bmatrix} 281.86 & 27.658 & 57.835 & 497.881 \\ 27.658 & 9.315 & 3.773 & 87.508 \\ 57.835 & 3.773 & 133.135 & 196.523 \\ 497.881 & 87.508 & 196.523 & 1774.695 \end{bmatrix}\begin{bmatrix} 1.9739 \\ 0.6663 \\ -3.6347 \\ 1.1284 \end{bmatrix}$$

$$= [1.9739 \quad 0.6663 \quad -3.6347 \quad 1.1284] \begin{bmatrix} 926.3880 \\ 145.8310 \\ -145.4747 \\ 2329.3375 \end{bmatrix}$$

$$= 5082.9458$$

$$\therefore \quad \sqrt{\Sigma\Sigma b_i\, b_j\, p_{ij}}$$

$$= 71.2947$$

Expected genetic advance is got as:

$$i \times \frac{4571.1815}{71.294}$$

$$= i \times 64.1167$$

If five per cent superior genotypes are selected (on the basis of score values), then the expected genetic advance would be:

$$2.06 \times 64.1167$$

$$= 132.0804$$

Selection indices are usually constructed with different combinations of components, such as grain yield alone, grain yield + plant height, grain yield + plant height + days to maturity and so on. Expected genetic advances are then calculated for these selection indices, and selection index which results in maximum genetic advance is preferred for selecting plants from the segregating population.

APPENDIX II

Inversion of X matrix

Steps	Left hand side				Right hand side			
1	281.86	27.658	57.835	497.881	1	0	0	0
2		9.315	3.773	87.508	0	1	0	0
3			133.135	196.523	0	0	1	0
4				1774.695	0	0	0	1
5	281.86	27.658	57.835	497.881	1			
6.	1	0.098	0.205	1.766	0.004			
7		6.605	-1.895	38.716	-0.098	1		
8		1	-0.287	5.862	-0.015	0.151		
9			120.735	105.568	-0.233	0.287	1	
10			1	0.874	-0.002	0.002	0.608	
11				576.218	-0.988	-6.113	-0.874	1
12				1	-0.002	-0.011	-0.0015	0.0017
13.					0.0079	-0.0044	-0.0004	-0.0017
14					-0.0044	0.2188	0.0115	-0.0104
15					-0.0004	0.0115	0.0093	-0.0015
16					-0.0017	-0.0104	-0.0015	0.0017

BIBLIOGRAPHY

Allard, R.W., 1955. Biometrical approach to plant breeding. In "Brookheaven Symposium in Quantitative Biology". 9:69-88.

Allard, R.W., 1960. *Principles of plant breeding.* John Wiley & Sons. Inc. New York.

Allard, R.W. and A.D. Bradshaw, 1964. Implications of genotype-environmental interactions in applied plant breeding. *Crop Sci., 4:503-508.*

Allard, R.W. and P.E. Hansche, 1964. Some parameters of population variability and their implication in plant breeding. *Advances in Agronomy.* 16:281-324.

Anderson, V.L. and O. Kempthorne, 1954. A model for the study of quantitative inheritance. *Genetics*, 39:883-898.

Arunachalam, V., 1974. The fallacy behind the use of a modified line × tester design. *Indian J. Genet.* 34:280-287.

Arunachalam, V., 1976. Evaluation of diallel cross by graphical and combining ability methods. *Indian. J. Genet. 36:358-366.*

Askel, R. and L.V.P. Johnson, 1963. Analysis of a diallel cross: A worked example. *Advancing Front. Pl. Sci.* 2:37-54.

Becker, W.A., 1967. *Manual of procedures in quantitative genetics.* Washington State University. 2nd Ed.

Baker, R.J., 1978. Issues in diallel analysis. *Crop sci.* 18:533-536.

Brim, C.A., H.W. Johnson and C.C. Cockerham, 1959. Multiple selection criteria in soybeans. *Agron.* J. 51:42-46.

Bucio-Alanis, L., 1966. Environmental and genotype-environmental components of variability. *I. Inbred lines. Heredity, 21:3994-4005.*

Bucio-Alanis, L. and J. Hill, 1966. Environmental and genotype–environmental components of variability II. Heterozygotes. *Heredity,* 21:399-407.

Cavalli, L.L., 1952. An analysis of linkage in quantitative inheritance. In "Quantitative Inheritance". Ed. E.C.R. Reeve and C.H. Waddington, HMSO, London. pp. 135-144.

Chahal, G.S. and J.L. Jinks, 1978. A general method of detecting the additive, dominance and epistatic variation that inbred lines can generate using a single tester. *Heredity*. 40:117-125.

Chahal, G.S., T.H. Singh and D.S. Virk, 1991. Measurement and utilization of nonallelic interactions in plant breeding. Pub. *The Crop Improvement Society of India*, Ludhiana, pp. 1-63.

Cochran. W.G. and G.M. Cox, 1957. *Experimental designs*. John Wiley & Sons Inc., New York. 2nd ed.

Cockerham, C.C., 1959. Partition of hereditary variance for various genetic models. *Genetics*, 44:1141-1148.

Cockerham, C.C., 1963. Estimation of genetic variances. In "*Statistical Genetics and Plant Breeding*". NAS-NRC. pp. 53-93.

Comstock, R.E. and H.F. Robinson, 1948. The components of genetic variance in populations of biparental progenies and their use in estimating the average degree of dominance. *Biometrics*, 4:254-266.

Comstock, R.E. and H.F. Robinson, 1952. Estimation of average dominance of genes. In "*Heterosis*" Ed. G.W. Gowen. Iowa State College Press, Ames, Iowa. 494-516

Comstock, R.E. and R.H. Moll, 1963. Genotype-environment interactions. In "*Statistical Genetics and Plant Breeding*". NAS-NRC. pp. 164-196.

Coughtrey, A. and K. Mather, 1970. Interaction and gene association and dispersion in diallel crosses where gene frequencies are unequal. *Heredity*, 25:79-88.

Curnow, R.N., 1963. Sampling the diallel cross. *Biometrics*, 19:287-306.

Curnow, R.N., 1980. Selecting crosses using information from a diallel cross. *Biometrics*, 36:1-8.

Dewey, D.R. and K.H. Lu, 1959. A correlation and path coefficient analysis of components of crested wheat-grass seed production. *Agron. J.*, 51:515-518.

Dickinson, A.C. and J.L. Jinks, 1956. A generalised analysis of diallel crosses. *Genetics*, 41:65-78.

Dobzhansky. Th., 1951. *Genetics and Origin of Species*. 3rd Ed. New York. Columbia University Press.

Dobzhansky, Th., and H. Levene, 1955. Genetics of natural population XXIV. Developmental homeostasis in natural populations in *Drosophila pesudoobscura, Genetics*. 40:797-808.

Duarte, R. and M.W.Adams, 1963. Component interaction in relation to expression of a complex trait in bean cross. *Crop Sci.*, 3:185-186.

Dudley. J.W. and R.H. Moll, 1969. Interpretation and use of estimates of heritability and genetic variances in plant breeding. *Crop Sci.*, 9:257-262.

Durrant. A., 1958. Environmental conditioning of flax. *Nature*, 181:928-929.

East. E.M., 1916. Studies on size inheritance in *Nicotiana*. Genetics. 1:164-176.

Eberhart, S.A., W.A. Russell and L.H. Penny, 1964. Double cross hybrid prediction in maize when epistasis is present. *Crop Sci.*, 4:363-366 40.

Eberhart. S.A. and W.A. Russell, 1966. Stability parameters for comparing varieties. *Crop Sci.*, 6:26-40.

Eberhart. S.A. and C.O. Gardner, 1966. A general model for genetic effects. *Biometrics*, 22:864-881.

Eberhart, S.A. and W.A. Russell, 1969. Yield and stability for a 10-line diallel of single-cross and double-cross maize hybrids. *Crop Sci.*, 9:357-361.

Eisenhart, C., 1947. The assumptions underlying analysis of variance. *Biometrics*, 3:1-21.

Falconer. D.S., 1960. *Introduction to Quantitative Genetics.* Oliver and Boyd. Edinburgh. p. 362.

Feyt. H., 1976. Etude critique de *l'* analyse des croisements diallels au moyen de la simulation. *Ann. Amelior. Plantes*. 26:173-193.

Finlay. K.W., 1963. Adaptation—its measurement and significance in barley breeding. *Proc. Ist Int. Barley Genet. Symp*. Wageningen. 351-359.

Finlay, K.W. and G.N. Wilkinson, 1963. Analysis of adaptation in plant breeding programme. *Aust. J. Agric. Res.* 14:742-754.

Fisher, R.A., 1918. The correlations between relatives on the supposition of Mendelian inheritance. *Trans. Roy. Soc. Edin.*, 52:399-433.

Fisher, R.A., 1936. The use of multiple measurements in taxonomic problems. *Ann. Eugen.*, 7:179-189.

Fisher, R.A., F.R. Immer and O.Tedin, 1932. The genetical interpretation of statistics of 3rd degree in study of quantitative inheritance. *Genetics,* 17:107-124.

Ford, E.B., 1940. Polymorphism and Taxonomy. In "The New Systematics"

J. Huxley (ed.) Clarendon, Oxford, pp. 493-513.

Frey, K.J. and T. Horner, 1957. Heritability in standard units. *Agron. J.*, 49:59-62.

Frey, K.J., 1964. Adaptation reaction of oat strains selected under stress and non-stress environmental conditions. *Crop Sci.*, 4:55-58.

Gamble, E.E., 1957. Relative importance of epistatic and non-epistatic gene effects in maize. Ph.D. Thesis, Iowa State University Library, Ames, Iowa.

Gamble. E.E., 1962a. Gene effects in corn (*Zea mays*, L.) I. separation and relative importance of gene effects for yield. *Can. J. Plant Sci.*, 42:339-348.

Gamble. E.E., 1962b. Gene effects in corn (*Zea mays*, L.) II. Relative importance of gene effects for plant height and certain component attributes of yield. *Can.J. Plant Sci.* 42:349-358.

Gardner, C.O., 1961. An evaluation of effect of mass selection and seed irradiation with thermal neutrons on yield of corn crop. *Crop Sci.*, 1:241-245.

Gardner. C.O., 1963. Estimates of genetic parameters in cross-fertilising plants and their implications in plant breeding. In "*Statistical Genetics and Plant Breeding*" NAS-NRC. pp. 225-252.

Gilbert. N.E.G., 1958. Diallel cross in plant breeding. *Heredity*, 12:477-492.

Grafius, J.E., 1956. Components of yield in oats: A geometric interpretation. *Agron. J.* 48:419-423.

Grafius, J.E., 1959. Heterosis in barley. *Agron. J.* 51:551-554.

Griffing, B., 1956a. Concept of general and specific combining ability in relation to diallel crossing systems. *Aust. J. Biol. Sci.*, 9:463-493.

Griffing, B., 1956b. A generalised treatment of the use of diallel crosses in quantitative inheritance. *Heredity*, 10:31-50.

Griffing. B. and J. Langridge., 1963. Phenotypic stability of growth in self-fertilized species, *Arabidopsis thaliana.* In "*Statistical Genetics and Plant Breeding*". NAS-NRC. pp.-368-394.

Goulden, C.H., 1952. *Methods of statistical analysis*. Wiley/Tuttle.

Hardy, G.H., 1908. Mendelian proportions in mixed population. *Science*, 28:49-50.

Hayman, B.I., 1954a. The theory and analysis of diallel crosses. *Genetics*, 39:789-809.

Hayman, B.I., 1954b. The analysis of variance of diallel table. *Biometrics*, 10:235-244.

Hayman, B.I. and K. Mather, 1955. The description of genetic interactions in continuous variation. *Biometrics*, 11:69-82.

Hayman. B.I., 1957. Interaction, heterosis and diallel crosses. *Genetics*, 42:336-355.

Hayman, B.I., 1958. The separation of epistatic from additive and dominance variation in generation means. *Heredity*, 12:371-390.

Hayman, B.I., 1960. Maximum likelihood estimation of genetic components of variation. *Biometrics*, 16:369-381.

Hayman. B.I., 1963. Notes on diallel cross theory. In *''Statistical Genetics and Plant Breeding''*. NAS-NRC.

Hayward, M.D., 1979. The application of the diallel cross to out-breeding crop species. *Euphytica*, 28:729-737.

Hazel., L.N., 1943. The genetic basis for constructing selection indexes. *Genetics*, 28:476-490.

Hazel, L.N. and J.L. Lush, 1943. The efficiency of three methods of selection. *J. Hered.* 33:393-399.

Hinklemann, K., 1965. Partial triallel crosses. *Sankhya* (A) 27:173-196.

Hinklemann, K., 1968. Partial tetra-allel crosses. *Theor. Appl. Genetics*, 38:85-89.

Hinklemann, K., 1974. Two-level diallel cross experiment. *Silv. Genet.*, 23:18-22.

Hinklemann, K., 1975. Design of Genetical Experiments. In *''A survey of statistical designs and linear models''* Ed. J.N. Srivastava, North Holland.

Hinklemann, K., 1977. Diallel and multi-cross designs: What do they achieve? In *''Proceedings of International Congress on Quantitative Genetics''* Aug. 16-21, 1976. Ed. E. Pollak.,O. Kempthorne and T.B. Bailey. Iowa State University Press. Ames, Iowa.

Jayasekara, N.E.M. and J.L. Jinks, 1976. Effect of gene dispersion on estimates of components of generation means and variances. *Heredity*, 36 : 31-40.

Jinks, J.L. and B.I. Hayman. 1953. The analysis of diallel crosses. *Maize Genetics Coop. News Letter*, 27:48-54

Jinks, J.L., 1954. The analysis of continuous variation in a diallel cross of *Nicotiana rustica* varieties. *Genetics*, 39:767-788.

Jinks,. J.L., 1956. The F_2 and back cross generations from a set of diallel crosses. *Heredity*, 10:1-30.

Jinks, J.L. and R.M. Jones, 1958. Estimation of components of heterosis. *Genetics*, 43:223-234.

Jinks, J.L. and J.M. Perkins, 1970. A general method for detection of additive, dominance and epistatic components of variation. III. F_2 and back cross populations. *Heredity*, 25:419-429.

Jinks, J.L. and D.S. Virk, 1977. A modified triple test-cross analysis to test and allow for inadequate testers. *Heredity*, 39:165-170.

Johannsen. W.L., 1903. *Ueber Erblichkeit in Populationen und in reinen Leinen.* Gustav Fischer, Jena.

Johnson. L.P.V. and R. Askel, 1959. Inheritance of yielding capacity in a fifteen parent diallel cross of barely. *Can J. Genet Cytol.*, 1:208-265.

Jones, R.M., 1965. Analysis of variance on the half-diallel table. *Heredity*, 20-117-121.

Karve. A.D., 1980. Biochemical basis of stability. *Science Reporter*, April, 264-266.

Kearsey, M.J. and J.L. Jinks, 1968. A general method of detecting additive, dominance and epistatic variation for metrical traits. *Heredity*, 23:403-409.

Kempthorne, O., 1952. *The design and analysis of experiments*. John Wiley & Sons, New York.

Kempthorne, O., 1956. The theory of dillel Crosses. *Genetics*, 41:451-459.

Kempthorne, O., 1957. *An Introduction to Genetic Statistics*, John Wiley & Sons Inc., New York.

Kempthorne, O., and A.W. Nordskog, 1959. Restricted selection indices. *Biometrics*, 15:10-19.

Kempthorne, O. and R.N. Curnow, 1961. The partial diallel cross. *Biometrics*, 17:229-250.

King, J.G., J.R. Quinby. J.C. Stephens, N.W. Kramer and K.A. Lahr, 1961. An evaluation of parents of grain sorghum hybrids. Bull. Texas Agric. Exp. Stn. M.P. 510.

Langridge, J. and B. Griffing, 1959. A study of high temperature lesions in *Arabidopsis thaliana. Aust. J. Biol. Sci.*. 12:117-135.

Lewis, D., 1954. Gene-Environment interaction. A relationship between dominance, heterosis, phenotypic stability and variability. *Heredity*, 8:333-336.

Li, C.C., 1955. *Population Genetics.* The University of Chicago Press, Chicago.

Li, C.C., 1956. The concept of path coefficients and its impact on population genetics. *Biometrics,* 12:190-210.

Lush, J.L. 1943. *Animal Breeding Plans.* Iowa State College Press.

Mather, K., 1949. *Biometrical Genetics: The study of continuous variation.* Methuen & Co. Ltd., London.

Mather, K. and B.I. Harrison, 1949. The manifold effects of selection. *Heredity,* 3:1-52, 131-162.

Mather, K. and A. Vines, 1952. The inheritance of height and flowering time in a cross of *Nicotiana rustica.* Quantitative Inheritance Ed. E.C.R. Reeve and C.N. Waddington H.M.S.O. London, pp. 49-80.

Mather, K., 1967. Complementary and duplicate interactions in biometrical genetics. *Heredity,* 22:97-103.

Mather, K. and J.L. Jinks, 1971. *Biometrical Genetics: The study of continuous variation.* Chapman and Hall, London. 2nd Ed.

Mather, K. and J.L. Jinks, 1977. *Introduction to Biometrical Genetics.* Chapman and Hall, London.

Mather, K. and J.L. Jinks, 1980. *Biometrical Genetics: The study of continuous variation.* Chapman and Hall, London, 3rd. Ed.

Nelder, J.A., 1960. The estimation of variance components in certain types of experiments on quantitative genetics. In *''Biometrical Genetics''* Ed. Kempthorne, O. Pergamon Press, London.

Oakes, M.W., 1967. The analysis of diallel cross of heterozygous or multiple allelic lines. *Heredity,* 22:83-95.

Opshal, B., 1956. The discrimination of interaction and linkage in continuous variation. *Biometrics.* 12:415-432.

Panse. V.G. and Sukhatme, P.V., 1967. *Statistical methods for Agricultural workers.* Indian Council of Agricultural Research, New Delhi. 2nd Ed.

Pederson. D.G., 1971. The estimation of heritability and degree of dominance from a diallel cross. *Heredity,* 27:247-264.

Perkins, J.M. and J.L. Jinks., 1968. Environmental and genotype-environmental components of variability III. Multiple lines and crosses. *Heredity,* 23:339-356.

Perkins, J.M. and J.L. Jinks, 1970. Detection and estimation of genotype-environmental, linkage and epistatic components of variation for a metrical trait. *Heredity,* 25:157-177.

Pesek, J. and R.J. Baker, 1969. Desired improvement in relation to selection indices. *Can. J. Plant Sci.,* 49:803-804.

Pesek. J. and R.J. Baker, 1970. An application of index selection to the improvement of self-pollinated species. *Can. J. Plant Sci.,* 50:267-276.

Plaisted, R.L. and L.C. Peterson, 1959. A technique for evaluating the ability of selection to yield consistently in different locations and seasons. *Amer. Potato.* J., 36:381-385.

Pirchner, F., 1969. Population genetics in Animal Breeding. W.H. Freeman and Company, San Francisco. pp. 274.

Pooni, H.S. and J.L. Jinks, 1981. The true nature of the non-allelic interactions in *Nicotiana rustica* revealed by association crosses. *Heredity,* 47: 253-258.

Rawlings, J.E. and C.C. Cockerham, 1962a. Triallel analysis. *Crop Sci.,* 2:228-231.

Rawlings. J.E. and C.C. Cockerham, 1962b. Analysis of double cross hybrid populations. *Biometrics,* 18:229-244.

Robinson, H.F., R.E. Comstock and P.H. Harvey., 1951. Genotypic and phenotypic correlations in corn and their implications in selection. *Agron. J.,* 43:282-287.

Robinson, H.F. 1966. Quantitative genetics in relation to breeding on the centennial of Mendelism. *Indian J. Genet.* 26A: 171-177.

Sax. K., 1923. The association of size differences with seed coat pattern and pigmentation in *Phaseolus vulgaris. Genetics.* 8:552-560.

Schmidt, J., 1919. La Valeur de l' individu a titre de generateur appreciee suivant la methode du croisement diallele. Comp. Rend. Lab Carlsberg 14, No. 633.

Schwartz, D., 1960. Genetic studies on mutant enzymes in maize: Synthesis of hybrid enymes by heterozygotes. *Proc. Nat. Acad. Sci.,* 46:1210-1215.

Shank, D.B. and M.W. Adams, 1960. Environmental variability within inbred lines and single crosses of maize. *Genet.* 27:119-126.

Simmonds. N.W., 1962. Variability in crop plants, its use and conservation,. *Biol. Rev.,* 37:422-465.

Singh, D., 1973a. Diallel analysis over different environments-I. *Indian J. Genet.* 33.127-136.

Singh, D., 1973b. Diallel analysis for combining ability over several environments-II. *Indian J. Genet.* 33:469-481.

Singh, D., 1979. Diallel analysis for combining ability over environments. *Indian J. Genet.* 39:383-386.

Singh, D., 1981. Estimation of second degree genetic parameters from a set of half-diallel crosses. *Indian J. Genet.* 41:246-251.

Singh, R.K., 1972. Selection Index-Yes or No? In "Vistas Pl. Sci." II, 111-140 Ed. Verghese and Grover.

Singh, R.K. and B.D. Chaudhary, 1977., Biometrical methods in Quantitative Genetic analysis. Kalyani Publishers, New Delhi.

Smith, F., 1937. A discriminant function for plant selection. *Ann. Eugen.,* 7:240-250.

Smith, H.H. 1952. Fixing transgressive vigour in *Nicotiana rustica.* In "Heterosis," Ed. G.W. Gowen. Iowa State College Press, Ames, Iowa. pp.161-174.

Sokol, M.J. and R.J. Baker, 1977. Evaluation of the assumptions required for the genetic interpretation of diallel experiments in self-pollinating crops. *Can. J. Plant Sci.*, 57:1185-1191.

Sprague, G.F. and L.A. Tatum., 1942. General *vs.* Specific combining ability in single crosses of corn. *Jour. Amer. Soc. Agron.,* 34:923-932.

Sprague. G.F. and W.T. Federer, 1951. A Comparison of variance components in corn yield trails: II Error, year × variety, location × variety and variety components. *Agron. J.*, 43.535-541.

Stern. C., 1943. The Hardy-Weinberg Law. *Science*, 97:137-138.

Strickberger. M.W., 1968. *Genetics*. The Macmillan Company, New York.

Verma, M.M., 1975. Genotype-environment interaction, its measurement and significance in plant breeding. Punjab Agricultural University, Ludhiana.

Warner. J.N., 1952. A method for estimating heritability. *Agron. J.*, 44:427-430.

Wearden, S., 1964. Alternative analyses of the diallel cross. *Heredity,* 19:669-680.

Weinberg, W., 1909. Uber Verebungsgesetze beim Menschen. Ztschr. Abst. 4 Vererb., 1:277-280.

Whitehouse, R.H., J.B. Thompson and M.A.M. Dovalleribeiro, 1958. Studies on breeding of self-pollinating cereals. *Euphytica.* 7:147-169.

Wright, S., 1921. Correlation and causation. *J. Agric. Research*, 20:557-585.

Yates, F. and Cochran, W.G., 1938. The analysis of groups of experiments. *J. Agric. Sci., 28*:556-580.

Yates, F., 1947. Analysis of data from all possible reciprocal crosses between a set of parental lines. *Heredity,* 1:287-301.

Yule, G.V., 1906. On the theory of inheritance of quantitative compound characters on the basis of Mendel's laws—A preliminary note. Rept. Third Intern. Conf. Gen. 140-142.

INDEX